INTELLIGENT SURFACES IN BIOTECHNOLOGY

Cover image: Design concept for a diagnostic microfluidic system based on responsive polymer- and antibody-conjugated nanobeads (see Chapter 2 of this book, Figure 2.5; reproduced by permission from the Royal Society of Chemistry).

INTELLIGENT SURFACES IN BIOTECHNOLOGY

SCIENTIFIC AND ENGINEERING CONCEPTS, ENABLING TECHNOLOGIES, AND TRANSLATION TO BIO-ORIENTED APPLICATIONS

Edited by

H. Michelle Grandin
Marcus Textor

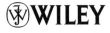WILEY

A JOHN WILEY & SONS, INC., PUBLICATION

Library of Congress Cataloging-in-Publication Data:

Intelligent surfaces in biotechnology : scientific and engineering concepts, enabling technologies, and translation to bio-oriented applications / edited by H. Michelle Grandin, Marcus Textor.
        p. cm.
   Includes bibliographical references and index.
   ISBN 978-0-470-53650-6
   1. Biomedical materials.   2. Biotechnology–Materials.   3. Smart materials.   4. Surfaces (Technology)   I. Grandin, H. Michelle.   II. Textor, Marcus.
   R857.M3I48 2012
   610.28′4–dc23

                                      2011041440

Printed in the United States of America
ISBN: 9780470536506

10 9 8 7 6 5 4 3 2 1

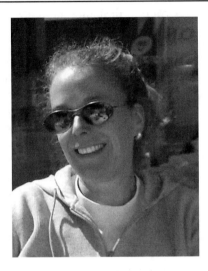

Heike Hall, PhD
December 28, 1963–July 22, 2011

The editors and contributors to this volume sadly note the passing of our colleague and friend Heike Hall, and we dedicate this volume to her. Heike was a devoted mother and wife to her family, and she was a passionate colleague and gifted scientist to us.

Heike built her scientific career at the interfaces of cells with their extracellular milieu. She carried out her PhD studies in the laboratory of Melitta Schachner at ETH Zurich, working on basic questions of how neural cells adhere to the extracellular matrix molecule laminin. In her pioneering work, she demonstrated a critical role for the carbohydrate-containing neural cell recognition molecule L1. From there, she moved to Guy's Hospital in London to work with Patrick Doherty and Frank Walsh on the role of fibroblast growth factor receptors in cell adhesion molecule-stimulated neuronal outgrowth. Following this, she moved back to Switzerland to undertake further postdoctoral studies with Jürgen Engel at the Biozentrum Basel. There she returned to her interest in L1 and expanded into the field of protein engineering, forming L1 trimers and immobilizing them on substrates to demonstrate that the trimers stimulated neuronal outgrowth much more potently than the monomeric form. With this work, she both understood more deeply L1 interactions in neurobiology, and she set the stage for the exploitation of L1 in functional nerve repair.

Following these very successful periods focused on basic biological investigations at the cell–matrix interface, Heike turned her attentions to biomedical applications of cell adhesion science, joining my laboratory at the ETH Zurich as a senior researcher, engineering cell adhesion in the context of tissue engineering and regenerative medicine. Based on her background in cellular neuroscience, Heike led our group in designing biofunctional scaffold materials for stimulating nerve repair. She continued to utilize her deep knowledge of L1 and also explored another protein, alpha dystroglycan. During this period, she also entered the field of angiogenesis and led projects developing L1-based proteins and other factors as angiogenic stimulators, inducing angiogenesis in the context of chronic wound repair.

After completing her habilitation in my laboratory, Heike joined the Department of Materials at ETH Zurich as a group leader, associated with the laboratory of Viola Vogel. There, she focused on new strategies for the development of biofunctional hydrogel matrices for integrated tissue repair, continuing to follow her passions in the repair of peripheral nerves and in the induction of angiogenesis in chronic wounds and taking on new areas of bone repair and nonviral gene delivery. These years were remarkable for their productivity and for the breadth of the science underlying Heike's work, spanning from DNA–polymer interactions in gene therapy to cell–metal interactions in orthopedics, of course with her constant work on the influence of the extracellular matrix in cellular neurobiology at the core.

In her prematurely terminated career, Heike accomplished much, in both basic science and applied. She touched many careers of students and postdoctoral fellows as a mentor. And she touched many scientists, including myself, both as a valued colleague and even more as a valued friend.

JEFFREY A. HUBBELL
October 2011
Lausanne, Switzerland

■■■■ CONTENTS

THE BORDER BETWEEN LIVING AND NONLIVING

The interface between the living and the nonliving—between cells or tissues, and materials—is, and has been for many decades, an area of science and technology where there are more questions than answers. Materials science— and particularly materials by design—is difficult; understanding "life" is even more difficult. The interface between materials and life compounds the two difficulties but adds a further, complicating twist: Biology and biochemistry at the interface with synthetic materials is—almost by definition—abnormal, and it is not even clear how much of what we know of "normal biology" can be applied in this region. Molecules normally found in interfaces *in vivo*, whatever they might be, are missing; proteins adsorb to synthetic interfaces, assume abnormal configurations, denature, and trigger the complex cascades that lead to inflammation, clotting, and bacterial attachment. It is a very important area and a very difficult one. A small area of interface with the wrong properties can trigger a large biological response.

THE PROBLEMS OF STATIC SOLUTIONS TO DYNAMIC PROBLEMS

One of the difficult problems of biointerfacial science is that most materials are static, and all of biology (over some scale of time) is dynamic. Bone and teeth remodel; cells divide, function, age, and die; skin sheds. Many synthetic materials used in biology, by contrast, are static. In some circumstances, the nonadaptive character of materials seems not to be a problem. For example, we assume—for convenience—that cells grown in plastic dishes recapitulate many of the characteristics of the same types of cells in tissue. We also know, however, that replacement of a hip joint by a construct of metal and polyethylene is good for only, perhaps, two decades and then must be replaced. We understand some of the mechanisms of failure of the synthetic joint but not others.

A concept that seems very attractive in attacking the problem of biointerfaces is that of "adaptive," or "intelligent," or "self-healing" materials. The goal is the development of materials that somehow replicate and mimic the ability of tissues and biological materials to adapt and renew. There is, however, an essential difference between "dynamic" materials and biological systems. The former are typically designed to respond to changes in environmental conditions by a change in structure and properties, and operate at, or close to, equilibrium. The latter are dissipative: Remodeling of bone involves the dissolution of existing bone by osteoclasts and redeposition of new bone by osteoblasts; both require ATP and metabolism. We do not, at the moment, know how to build dissipative biomimetic materials and structures that exist in a stable, out-of-equilibrium state, and the question is, thus, "how far can one go in building a biocompatible interface between synthetic and biological systems using the currently available tools of materials science?"

One interesting class of materials that is designed to be out of equilibrium, but is not truly dynamic in the sense of biological tissues and structures, is that intended for biodegradation and for applications such as drug delivery. These systems, rather than operating on the basis of remodeling requiring the production of ATP through metabolism, are designed to be out of equilibrium on the basis of a reactive structure. Poly(lactic acid) (PLA), for example, is thermodynamically unstable with respect to lactic acid in biological fluids, and the interface between PLA and tissue or blood is constantly renewed by hydrolysis and erosion of the polymer. In other materials and structures, the tendency of the interface to initiate unwanted biochemical processes can sometimes be accommodated by other forms of energy dissipation: For example, the tendency of a metal stent to initiate clotting in the blood passing over it is at least partially mitigated by fluid shear from this blood (which sweeps away clots) and by the slower, but also dissipative, processes that allow epithelial cells to cover the material of the stent.

WHAT IS IT THAT MAKES FOR COMPATIBILITY?

So, what makes for biological compatibility? In general, the answer is "We do not know." Although we accept cells growing in culture dishes as being useful models for studies in cell biology, we know that these cells are not fully normal; we believe (but in general cannot prove) that the compromise between the biologically abnormal environment of the culture dish, and the convenience and acceptable expense of the culture dish, justifies the use of plasticware in cell biology. In research biology, many compromises are easy to accommodate because the consequences of failure are either small or hidden. *In vivo*, and especially in humans, the stakes are much higher, and biomaterials science is still severely limited by fundamental issues in compatibility. The field still needs new ideas.

"INTELLIGENCE" IN SURFACES AND INTERFACES

Can one make "intelligent" or "adaptive" surfaces for use in biomaterials science and bioengineering? The answer is clearly "yes," but with clear caveats.

Artificial hips and knees do not fully replicate natural structures; artificial lenses allow sight but have limitations; artificial teeth work well but not perfectly; surfaces in contact with blood often remove platelets and initiate clotting. Almost all synthetic materials, over time, induce some level of inflammation and fibrosis. The successes of biomaterials science in producing acceptable solutions to the problem of biocompatibility have been remarkable, but there remains enormous opportunity for improvement. One possible direction is toward intelligent surfaces and interfaces.

"Intelligence," in this sense, is a word that is used flexibly. An "intelligent material" is one whose structure—in a particular environment—can change in a way that autonomously optimizes its performance in some application. An "intelligent child" might be one who plays Bach by the age of five. The same word "intelligent" is used in both sentences, but with very different meanings. Materials cannot have "intention," and do not sense, control, and change even as a so-called intelligent machine might. The difference between "intelligence" and "adaptability" as applied in materials science might not be important; but since the current generation of "intelligent materials" is very close to the starting point in moving from completely inert, static structures to structures optimized for performance in complex biological environments, and capable of responding to changes in them, keeping the difference between intelligence and adaptability in mind is useful in understanding how large the gap between capability and ultimate need, and how great the opportunity for new science, is in this area.

MATERIALS BY DESIGN: REDUCTIONIST SCIENCE, OR EMPIRICISM AND ENGINEERING?

In searching for solutions to difficult problems, there are always the "top-down" and "bottom-up" approaches. In one, one hopes to understand the fundamental mechanisms by which synthetic materials and biological molecules and systems interact and use that understanding in the rational design of synthetic materials having intended properties. In the second, one relies more on intuition (sometimes guided by knowledge from other areas) and empiricism to develop useful technology, even if the outcome is that the technology is not completely understood. "Biointerfaces" are still closer to empiricism than to fundamental science. Even in what appears to be the simplest cases—for example, the adsorption of proteins on the surfaces of polymers and self-assembled monolayers—and although there are quite useful empirical solutions to the design of, for example, nonabsorbing surfaces, the mechanistic basis for their activity is still not completely understood. In more complex cases—for example, the design of nonclotting surfaces for contact with blood—there is still an enormous amount to be learned even about the steps that initiate clotting.

TRADING INFORMATION ACROSS A BORDER

One of the most challenging of problems in the interfacial science of biomaterials is that of sensing or actuation. "Information" in synthetic systems is typically carried in the form of electrical current or voltage in electrically conducting wires, or as light. Information in biological systems generally takes the form of molecules interacting with receptors, or of concentration gradients in ions (or of electrochemical potentials due to these gradients) across cell membranes. It remains a challenging problem to translate between these two fundamentally different currencies. The problem is particularly difficult when the biological signal to be detected is itself problematic. "Biomarkers" for use in the diagnosis and management of disease represent a specific example of high current interest. It is unquestionably correct that biomarkers exist for some diseases: For example, the concentrations of glucose and of glycosylated hemoglobin in blood are both biomarkers relevant to the management of diabetes. For many diseases, however, the basic biology of biomarkers remains uncertain or unvalidated: The recent example of prostate-specific antigen (PSA), which has gone from "biomarker for early prostate cancer" to "clinically marginally useful, or perhaps harmful, bioanalysis" over a 20-year period, is an example. Although the field of biomarkers will certainly advance in the next years, the basic philosophy of early detection and management of disease through simple analyses (or even through a more complex recognition of patterns in multiple analyses) is still a work in progress. That uncertainty aside, however, building the technological base that allows the design and fabrication of the interfaces between electronic or photonic systems and biological systems will clearly be useful, in research and ultimately in the clinic, and remains a complex and challenging problem.

PROF. GEORGE M. WHITESIDES
Harvard University

■■■■■ PREFACE

Polymer coatings have long been studied as a versatile yet simple way to modify the characteristics of a material's surface, for example, to exhibit adhesive, insulating, or bioinert properties. More recently, the ability to impart selective, functional, and responsive properties to polymer and lipid bilayer coatings has significantly impacted a number of applications in biotechnology and medicine including biosensors, drug delivery, and tissue engineering. Such surfaces, for instance, hierarchically self-organized structures at interfaces, embody an "intelligence" mimicking natural biological systems, albethey primitive in comparison to those of even "simple" organisms or parts of them, including bacterial membranes. The nature of this research requires a multidisciplinary approach in developing the underlying scientific and engineering concepts, in enabling the technologies, and in translating these new surfaces to useful applications.

Within the pages of this book, our aim is to stimulate further research into the area of "intelligent surfaces," so eloquently described by the distinguished scientist Prof. George M. Whitesides in the "Foreword" to this book (see pp. xv), that is, the search for materials that attempt to replicate and/or mimic the ability of tissues and biological materials to adapt and/or renew, in a dynamic and ultimately dissipative manner. For the purposes of this book, our definition of intelligent surfaces will include smart materials, that is, polymers whose properties are significantly altered by external stimuli, such as temperature, pH, or electric fields, and will go beyond to include the following:

- surfaces that have one (or more) functional surface properties that can be changed in a controlled and useful fashion by external stimuli;
- surfaces that are cooperative, dynamic systems that respond or accommodate in a useful and reproducible way to environmental conditions;
- surfaces that use biological factors *in vitro* or *in vivo* to trigger a desired response, for example, controlled degradation of polymers, or the release of beneficial compounds;
- surfaces that use combinatorial and gradient surfaces as intelligent and efficient ways to test/explore the effect of multiple types or concentrations of surface cues and their combination in the interaction with the environment; and
- surfaces that provide a designed multifunctionality and/or temporospatial control in the interaction with the (bio)environment.

The authors contributing to this book are leading experts in the biomaterial and bioengineering sciences presenting valuable and inspiring views of the state of the art in this exciting, multidisciplinary field. Each chapter is designed to impart background knowledge and important design consideration for specific applications while transferring technological know-how, whenever possible, to scientists interested in the field. The first half of the book deals primarily with applications in biosensing and biodiagnostics, while the second half extends to coatings for medical devices, drug delivery, and controlled cell surface interactions.

In Chapter 1, the powerful attraction of stimulus-responsive polymers for medical sensors is presented, highlighting a need to further validate and optimize analyte specificity, detection limits, and sensor reliability/longevity. Chapter 2 presents one strategy for optimizing the use of the smart polymer, poly(N-isoproylacrylamide) (pNIPAAm), using a hybrid biosynthetic conjugate of proteins, inorganic nanoparticles, and smart polymers, for use in biosensing devices amenable to rapid near-patient point-of-care testing. Chapter 3 discusses fundamental criteria for surface-based and label-free biosensors, particularly in the nanoscale, emphasizing aspects of surface modification through self-assembly, alternative patterning strategies, and the challenges of analyte transport. A specific class of label-free biosensors, that is, the field-effect transistor-based biosensors or bio-FETs, is the topic of Chapter 4, presenting design criteria, new targets, and surface modifications strategies to facilitate signal transduction and amplification. Chapter 5 presents another approach to intelligent surface coatings inspired by nature, namely, supported lipid bilayers incorporating transmembrane proteins, with a focus on their application as sensors for ion channel activity.

Modification of biomaterial and medical device surfaces with intelligent surfaces that prevent infection, such as antibacterial and anti-inflammatory coatings, including grafting of bioactive molecules and coatings that release antibacterial agents, is discussed in Chapter 6. Chapter 7 presents layer-by-layer (LBL) sequential polymer deposition as a means to generate intelligent mulitlayered polymer films, incorporating cargo, for controlled release with a focus on applications in the important area of drug delivery. To further understand the interactions of cells on surfaces, micro- and nanopatterning of active biomolecules provides a useful tool as outlined in Chapter 8. And finally, Chapter 9 further discusses the use of responsive polymers for drug delivery, along with two other important uses of these intelligent coatings, namely, chromatography and the emerging field of cell sheet engineering for regenerative medicine.

Together, the chapters of this book provide an impressive insight into the exciting field of intelligent surfaces in biotechnology and should inspire scientists in the fields of biomaterials, polymer chemistry, bioengineering, and medical devices and technology to make further contributions to this important area of multidisciplinary science. The comparatively simple level of intelligence embodied in today's surfaces, with respect to natural systems, is an indicator that the major proponent of the work required to develop surface solutions approaching the intelligence found in nature, for example, in the context of time- and space-dependent organization of macromolecular entities or release of multiple soluble cues, remains a task for the future.

The editors wish to express a heartfelt thank you to all chapter authors for their outstanding contributions and for their effort and patience in bringing this book to life. A special thank you is extended to Prof. George Whitesides for providing an erudite "Foreword" and to Prof. Jeffrey Hubbell for providing a special "Dedication" as described below. Furthermore, the editors wish to thank Ms. Josephine Baer for her dedication to the completion of this work.

Regrettably, our friend and colleague Dr. Heike Hall (coauthor of Chapter 6, "Antimicrobial and Anti-Inflammatory Intelligent Surfaces") passed away during the writing of this volume. Despite her illness, she continued to be actively involved in the writing and revising of her chapter, thereby demonstrating her commitment to the science that captivated her attention. We wholeheartedly dedicate this work to her and are thankful to Prof. Jeffrey Hubbell for providing a special "Dedication" detailing the scientific achievements of Dr. Heike Hall (see pp. v).

H. Michelle Grandin
Marcus Textor

Yoshikatsu Akiyama, Institute of Advanced Biomedical Engineering and Science, Tokyo Women's Medical University, Tokyo, Japan

Daniel Aydin, Department of New Materials and Biosystems, Max Planck Institute for Intelligent Systems, Stuttgart, Germany, and Department of Biophysical Chemistry, University of Heidelberg, Heidelberg, Germany

Ashutosh Chilkoti, Department of Biomedical Engineering, Duke University, Durham, North Carolina

Laurent Feuz, Biological Physics, Department of Applied Physics, Chalmers University of Technology, Göteborg, Sweden

Allison L. Golden, Department of Bioengineering, University of Washington, Seattle, Washington

Hans J. Griesser, Ian Wark Research Institute, University of South Australia, Mawson Lakes, Australia

Stefani S. Griesser, Ian Wark Research Institute, University of South Australia, Mawson Lakes, Australia

Heike Hall, Cells and BioMaterials, Department of Materials, ETH Zurich, Zurich, Switzerland

Vera C. Hirschfeld-Warneken, Department of New Materials and Biosystems, Max Planck Institute for Intelligent Systems, Stuttgart, Germany, and Department of Biophysical Chemistry, University of Heidelberg, Heidelberg, Germany

John M. Hoffman, Department of Bioengineering, University of Washington, Seattle, Washington

Fredrik Höök, Biological Physics, Department of Applied Physics, Chalmers University of Technology, Göteborg, Sweden

Andreas Janshoff, Institute of Physical Chemistry, University of Göttingen, Göttingen, Germany

Toby A. Jenkins, Department of Chemistry, University of Bath, Bath, United Kingdom

Kazunori Kataoka, Department of Materials Engineering, Graduate School of Engineering, The University of Tokyo, Tokyo, Japan, and Division of Clinical Biology, Center for Disease Biology and Integrative Medicine, Graduate School of Medicine, The University of Tokyo, Tokyo, Japan

James J. Lai, Department of Bioengineering, University of Washington, Seattle, Washington

Ilia Louban, Department of New Materials and Biosystems, Max Planck Institute for Intelligent Systems, Stuttgart, Germany, and Department of Biophysical Chemistry, University of Heidelberg, Heidelberg, Germany

Alexandra P. Marques, 3B's Research Group—Biomaterials, Biodegradables and Biomimetics, University of Minho, Headquarters of the European Institute of Excellence on Tissue Engineering and Regenerative Medicine, Guimarães, Portugal; and 3 ICVS/3B's Laboratório Associado, PT Government Associate Laboratory, Guimarães, Portugal

Akira Matsumoto, Institute of Biomaterials and Bioengineering, Tokyo Medical and Dental University, Tokyo, Japan

Yuji Miyahara, Institute of Biomaterials and Bioengineering, Tokyo Medical and Dental University, Tokyo, Japan

Kenichi Nagase, Institute of Advanced Biomedical Engineering and Science, Tokyo Women's Medical University, Tokyo, Japan

Masamichi Nakayama, Institute of Advanced Biomedical Engineering and Science, Tokyo Women's Medical University, Tokyo, Japan

Michael A. Nash, Department of Bioengineering, University of Washington, Seattle, Washington

Teruo Okano, Institute of Advanced Biomedical Engineering and Science, Tokyo Women's Medical University, Tokyo, Japan

Rogério P. Pirraco, Institute of Advanced Biomedical Engineering and Science, Tokyo Women's Medical University, Tokyo, Japan; 3B's Research Group—Biomaterials, Biodegradables and Biomimetics, University of Minho, Headquarters of the European Institute of Excellence on Tissue Engineering and Regenerative Medicine, Guimarães, Portugal; and ICVS/3B's Laboratório Associado, PT Government Associate Laboratory, Guimarães, Portugal

Erik Reimhult, Laboratory for Biologically Inspired Materials, Department of NanoBiotechnology, University of Natural Resources and Life Sciences, Vienna, Austria

Rui L. Reis, 3B's Research Group—Biomaterials, Biodegradables and Biomimetics, University of Minho, Headquarters of the European Institute of Excellence on Tissue Engineering and Regenerative Medicine, Guimarães,

Portugal; and ICVS/3B's Laboratório Associado, PT Government Associate Laboratory, Guimarães, Portugal

Joachim P. Spatz, Department of New Materials and Biosystems, Max Planck Institute for Intelligent Systems, Stuttgart, Germany, and Department of Biophysical Chemistry, University of Heidelberg, Heidelberg, Germany

Brigitte Städler, Interdisciplinary Nanoscience Centre (iNano), Aarhus University, Aarhus, Denmark

Patrick S. Stayton, Department of Bioengineering, University of Washington, Seattle, Washington

Claudia Steinem, Institute of Organic and Biomolecular Chemistry, University of Göttingen, Göttingen, Germany

Vinalia Tjong, Department of Biomedical Engineering, Duke University, Durham, North Carolina

Krasimir Vasilev, Mawson Institute, University of South Australia, Mawson Lakes, Australia

Masayuki Yamato, Institute of Advanced Biomedical Engineering and Science, Tokyo Women's Medical University, Tokyo, Japan

Stefan Zauscher, Department of Mechanical Engineering and Materials Science, Duke University, Durham, North Carolina

Alexander N. Zelikin, Department of Chemistry, Aarhus University, Aarhus, Denmark

Jianming Zhang, Department of Mechanical Engineering and Materials Science, Duke University, Durham, North Carolina

Stimulus-Responsive Polymers as Intelligent Coatings for Biosensors: Architectures, Response Mechanisms, and Applications

VINALIA TJONG, JIANMING ZHANG, ASHUTOSH CHILKOTI, and STEFAN ZAUSCHER

1.1 INTRODUCTION

Stimulus-responsive polymers (SRPs) are used in biomedical applications that range from drug delivery,[1,2] regenerative medicine,[3,4] tissue engineering,[5,6] to biosensing.[7–9] The function of SRPs in these applications is predicated on their ability to change conformation, surface energy, or charge state in response to a stimulus. Common stimuli include changes in temperature, light, pH, ionic strength, redox potential, mechanical force, the strength of electric and magnetic fields, and changes in the biomolecular and chemical composition of the environment.[10,11] When SRPs are coated onto surfaces, they often retain their stimulus-responsive behavior, which can be harnessed for sensing applications. The use of SRP coatings in biosensor applications is schematically illustrated in Figure 1.1, where the coatings function as both the reaction matrix and the responsive layer, which produces a measurable output signal.[10,11]

In this chapter, we discuss the use of SRPs as responsive coatings for biosensor applications. We specifically focus on the different SRP architectures, the various transduction mechanisms that underpin the use of SRPs as sensor platforms, and highlight selected applications of SRPs in a biomedically relevant context. Finally, we discuss the limitations and challenges in the application of SRPs as coatings for biosensors.

Intelligent Surfaces in Biotechnology: Scientific and Engineering Concepts, Enabling Technologies, and Translation to Bio-Oriented Applications, First Edition.
Edited by H. Michelle Grandin and Marcus Textor.

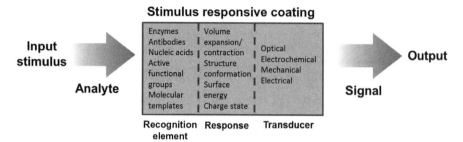

Figure 1.1 Schematic showing the role of stimulus-responsive polymer coatings in the biosensor transduction paradigm. In this paradigm, the SRP coating serves as both a matrix for analyte interaction and as a responsive coating that transduces an input stimulus into a measurable signal.

1.2 SRP ARCHITECTURES FOR BIOSENSOR APPLICATIONS

To be useful for sensing applications,[12–14] the architectures of SRP coatings for biosensors are designed to undergo large, and often reversible, structural changes in response to small changes in the local solvent environment or in response to specific binding events.[15–17] Four types of SRP architectures are commonly used for biosensor applications: (i) cross-linked polymer networks (hydrogels), (ii) end-grafted polymer chains (polymer brushes), (iii) self-assembled multilayered polymer films (layer-by-layer [LBL] thin films), and (iv) molecularly imprinted polymer (MIP) coatings, as illustrated in Figure 1.2. To achieve better signal amplification, hybrid coatings are being developed that combine an analyte-specific matrix with transduction-enhancing materials (e.g., electrochemically or optically sensitive materials).

1.2.1 Cross-Linked Polymer Networks (Hydrogels)

In cross-linked polymer networks (Fig. 1.2a), individual polymer chains are cross-linked to yield a 3-D mesh of interconnected polymer chains. Due to this interconnectivity, polymer networks can be used as freestanding materials or as thin films on a support. The cross-links maintain network integrity and impart flexibility so that the network can swell and shrink upon exposure to a particular stimulus such as a change in the solvent conditions,[18,19] temperature,[20,21] pH,[22] ionic strength,[23] metabolite concentration,[24,25] or other environmental changes.[26,27] Acrylamide-based polymers such as poly(N-isopropylacrylamide) (pNIPAM), acrylic acid-based polymers such as poly(hydroxyethyl methacrylic)acid (pHEMA), and copolymers such as poly(vinyl alcohol)–poly(acrylic acid) (pVA–pAA) are common SRP coatings (see also Table 1.1).

Two major synthetic approaches are used to prepare hydrogel coatings for sensors. In one approach, the reaction mixture, containing monomers, a cross-linking agent, and an initiator, is coated onto the substrate (e.g., by spin

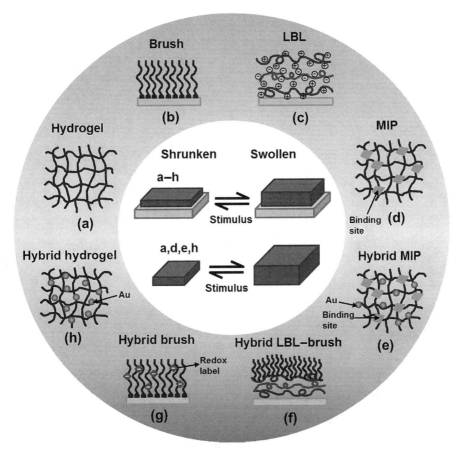

Figure 1.2 The four main architectures of stimulus-responsive polymers are (a) hydrogels, (b) polymer brushes, (c) layer-by-layer (LBL) multilayers, and (d) molecularly imprinted polymers (MIPs). Furthermore, biosensor platforms with hybrid structures that embed inorganic (AuNPs) or organic reporter molecules (redox label ferrocene) in the polymer matrix are shown (e, g, and h), and the combination of the two main structures (LBL and polymer brush) are illustrated in (f). Adapted with permission from references [8], [13], and [132]. (See color insert.)

coating) and reacted *in situ* to form a cross-linked polymer network. These polymer networks are most often synthesized by free radical polymerization techniques, such as UV-initiated polymerization,[28,29] redox-initiated polymerization,[30] and plasma polymerization.[31-34] In the other synthesis approach, polymer chains contain photoreactive (e.g., benzophenone or 4-cinnamoylphenyl methacrylate)[35-37] or chemically reactive (e.g., 1,4-diiodobutane or carboxylic acids)[38-42] pendant groups or monomers that upon UV irradiation, high temperature, or cross-linking agents, form cross-linked networks. Alternatively, high-energy irradiation (e.g., electron beam, γ-rays, UV light) that causes

TABLE 1.1 Transduction Mechanism

Architecture	Mechanical		Polymerized Colloidal Crystal	Optical			Electrochemical
	QCM	Microcantilever		Hologram	Fiber Optics	SPR	Voltammetry
Hydrogel Gelatin, Dextran Cellulose pHEMA pHEMA-MAA pMAA pNIPAM pVA-pAA	Moisture[34] Temperature[34] Glucose[72] pH[39] Protein[105, 133] Protease[108] Ionic strength[134]	pH[116, 117]	pH[40, 78] Metal ion[28, 77-81, 86] Glucose[75, 77, 82, 84, 88, 89, 135] Creatinine[83] Ammonia[85] Ethanol[87]	Water content[18] Alcohol[19] Ionic strength[23] Metabolite[65] Glucose[24, 65, 90, 93, 136] Lactate[25] pH[62, 76, 94] Metal ion[23, 29, 64, 65, 76, 94] Trypsin[92]	pH[76, 97] Glucose[97, 98] DNA[67]	pH[59, 99, 100] Glucose[72]	Temperature[37] Glucose[72] pH[70] Cholesterol[103]
Polymer Brush p4VP, p2VP pAA pDMA pMEM pMMA pNIPAM pNIPAM-VI pNIPAM-A		Glucose[119, 122] pH[116, 117, 120] Solvents[118, 137] Ionic strength[138] Fragrance[137]				pH[17, 54, 57]	pH[63, 68]
Layer-by-Layer pAA pAH pEI pMAA pSS pVP	Nucleotide[123]	Glucose[122] Organophosphor[121]				pH[55, 139]	Ion[49, 50] pH[61] Ascorbic acid[104]
Molecular Imprint Polymer p2VP Hydrogel polymer	Nucleotide[107, 123] Herbicide[106] Monosaccharide[107]			Dopamine[26] Atrazine[27] Adrenaline[58] Cholesterol[60]			

p2VP, poly(2-vinylpyridine); p4VP, poly(4-vinylpyridine); pAA, poly(acrylic acid); pAH, poly(allylamine hydrochloride); pEI, polytheyleneimine; pHEMA, poly(2-hydroxyethyl methacrylate); pHEMA-MAA, poly(2-hydroxyethyl methacrylate-co-methacrylic acid); pMAA, poly(methacrylic acid); pMEM, poly(2-dimethylamino ethyl methacrylate); pNIPAM, poly(N-isopropylacrylamide); pNIPAM-VI, poly(N-isopropylacrylamide-co-N-vinylimidazole); pNIPAM-A, poly(N-isopropylacrylamide-co-

random chain scission can be used to cross-link polymeric thin films. Comprehensive reviews on hydrogel synthesis can be found in the literature.[41,43,44]

1.2.2 End-Grafted Polymer Chains (Polymer Brushes)

Stimulus-responsive, end-grafted polymer chains (SRP brushes) (Fig. 1.2b,g) are another important architecture that has been extensively used for biosensor applications. Polymer brushes are an ensemble of densely packed polymer chains, immobilized on a surface by physisorption or by covalent attachment of one chain end. The dense lateral packing of polymer chains in the brush leads to steric repulsive interactions between the packed chains and causes them to extend away from the substrate surface.[13] Chain attachment is achieved through either a "grafting-to" or a "grafting-from" approach. In the grafting-to approach, suitably end-functionalized polymer chains are chemically reacted with the substrate surface. Although this approach is straightforward, the polymer brush layer typically has a low grafting density because steric hindrance from previously deposited polymer chains prevents incoming chains to interact with the substrate surface. In contrast, the grafting-from approach, in which monomers are polymerized from immobilized initiators on the surface (surface initiated polymerization), yields a high grafting density. For an extensive discussion on the synthesis of polymer brushes, the reader is referred to a number of recent review articles.[45–47]

Similar to other SRP systems, the application of external stimuli can cause a conformational reorganization in the polymer brush through stretching or contraction of polymer chains, which results in large, and possibly reversible, changes in the overall brush thickness, adhesion, wettability, or affinity to a particular analyte. Examples of polymer brushes used as sensor coatings are listed in Table 1.1.

1.2.3 Self-Assembled Polyelectrolyte (PEL) Multilayers (LBL Thin Films)

In the LBL assembly, schematically shown in Figure 1.2c, an organized, multilayer thin film is assembled on a solid support by harnessing attractive interactions between the polymer layers.[48] LBL polymer films are most often prepared by the multiple, sequential deposition of positively and negatively charged PEL chains. For example, when a net negatively charged substrate (e.g., silica) is immersed in a solution of positively charged PEL, such as poly(diallyldimethylammonium chloride) (PDDA), poly(allylamine hydrochloride) (pAH), or polyethyleneimine (PEI), and subsequently rinsed with pure water to remove loosely adsorbed chains, the substrate becomes positively charged because of the adsorption and charge overcompensation by the cationic PEL. Subsequent immersion in a negatively charged PEL solution, such as poly(styrene sulfonate) (pSS), poly(vinyl sulfonate) (pVS), or poly(acrylic acid) (pAA), results in the reversal of the net charge on the substrate. Using sequential deposition of oppositely charged PELs, multilayers with a desired structure, chemical composition, and thickness can be assembled on the substrate. To improve the stability of the multilayer, the films are often chemically attached to the substrate and are internally cross-linked by functionalizing the PEL with photoreactive groups.[49,50]

Due to the short- and long-range interactions between the layers in the polymer film assembly, stimuli that perturb the equilibrium of these interactions will cause volumetric expansion or contraction of the layers. Similar to other responsive polymer coatings, the change in the layer conformation upon exposure to an analyte or stimulus can be exploited to transduce a binding event or change in the solvent environment.

1.2.4 Molecularly Imprinted Polymers

Molecularly Imprinted Polymers (MIPs) coatings consist of cross-linked polymer chains that form a 3-D network (Fig. 1.2d,e), similar to that of hydrogel networks described earlier. In molecular imprinting, cross-linking monomers that bear, for example, vinyl or acrylic groups are copolymerized in the presence of the target analyte to yield weakly cross-linked polymer networks with a highly porous structure. Removal of the "imprinted" analyte through solvent extraction or chemical cleavage creates a molecular template that is subsequently available for analyte binding with high specificity. For a detailed discussion of MIP, readers are referred to several reviews.[51,52]

1.2.5 Hybrid Coatings

Hybrid coatings that couple a polymer's stimulus responsiveness to embedded, stimuli-responsive reporter materials provide a useful strategy to further exploit the properties of SRP coatings. For example, to enhance the response of the polymer coating, reporter molecules, such as optically or electrochemically sensitive materials, have been embedded in hydrogels, polymer brushes, LBL films, and MIPs (Fig. 1.2e,g,h) to increase the sensing sensitivity of the polymer coating.[17,26,27,53–60] Hybrid coatings that are composed of two different SRP types allow the hybrid coating to respond to two stimuli; for example, a pNIPAM brush grafted onto a pAH/pAA multilayer (Fig. 1.2f) can respond to changes in temperature and pH.[61]

1.3 MECHANISMS OF RESPONSE

1.3.1 Sensing Selectivity

A broad range of analytes including pH,[62,63] ionic groups,[28,29,64] metabolites,[65] small molecules[26,27] and biomolecules[66,67] have been detected or evaluated using SRP sensing platforms. These analytes typically interact with the SRP coating in one of two ways: (i) by altering the solvent environment in which the sensing platform is operated, for example, by changing pH or ionic strength, or (ii) by reacting with specific molecular recognition elements present in the polymer chains or the polymer matrix, for example, by DNA hybridization, antibody–antigen interactions, molecular template recognition, or receptor–ligand interactions.[17,26,27,58,60,62–64,66–69]

Typically two strategies are used to impart sensing selectivity to SRP coatings. The first strategy employs polymer chains that intrinsically respond to the stimulus; for example, PELs respond conformationally to changes in the solvent pH.[17,62,68] The second strategy achieves selectivity through incorporating functional elements into the polymer chains, for example, by copolymerization with functionalized monomers,[64,69] through incorporating specific molecular recognition elements (e.g., antibodies) into the polymer matrix by copolymerization,[24] molecular interactions,[28] chemical conjugation,[65] physical entrapment,[70] or through molecular imprinting a template for the recognition element of interest.[58,60]

1.3.2 Conformational Reorganization of SRP Coatings

The interactions of analytes with SRPs or specific recognition moieties often cause significant conformational responses of SRP coatings. These conformational changes typically arise from changes in the osmotic swelling pressure or the charge density of the polymer, and for hydrogels, from changes in the cross-link density, and can be measured by various transduction strategies discussed later in this chapter.

1.3.2.1 Changes in Osmotic Swelling Pressure   The conformational response of SRP coatings often occurs due to changes in their osmotic swelling state,[71] which can be triggered by changes in solvent composition, solvent temperature, pH, or soluble ion concentration. The osmotic pressure equilibrium of the polymer matrix with its surrounding environment typically depends on three additive contributions: (i) a contribution that arises from the free energy of mixing between polymer chains and solvent (π_{mix}), (ii) a contribution that arises from the elastic restoring force associated with stretching of the polymer chains (π_{el}), and (iii) a contribution that arises from the difference in mobile ion concentration inside and outside of the polymer matrix (π_{ion}).[7] Any stimulus that leads to a change in one or more of the pressure terms will shift the osmotic equilibrium in the matrix and cause the polymer to swell or shrink. For example, PELs are useful for pH sensing applications as a pH change is transduced into macroscopic swelling of the PEL.[17,62,68] Similarly, binding of soluble metal ions, such as Na^+, K^+, Ca^{2+}, Mg^{2+}, Zn^{2+} or Pb^{2+} to recognition elements (e.g., crown ethers that function as chelators of metal ions) that are incorporated into the polymer chains through copolymerization also changes the osmotic swelling pressure in the polymer matrix measurably through the change in mobile ion concentration (π_{ion}).[28, 29, 64]

Some illustrative examples that harness osmotic swelling pressure changes for the detection of analytes other than pH or ionic strength are briefly highlighted next. For example, direct detection of glucose is possible with coatings that contain boronic acid functionalities that function as synthetic glucose receptors. This approach was employed by Gabai et al.,[72] who utilized the swelling response of an m-acrylamidophenylboronic acid-acrylamide hydrogel coating upon glucose binding for glucose detection. The ensuing swelling response was transduced into an electrical signal by resultant changes in the electron-transfer ability, mediated by the presence of a redox probe, and measured by faradaic impedance spectroscopy. Molecular templates, imprinted into the SRP matrix during fabrication, have been used for the detection of dopamine,[26] atrazine,[27] adrenaline,[58] and cholesterol.[60] Direct binding of these analytes into the molecular recognition cavities in the polymer matrix caused swelling of the SRP matrix, which was measured by the shift in the plasmon absorbance peak or the change in the minimum angle of reflectance.

Alternatively, the swelling response of the SRP coating has been triggered indirectly by harnessing the catalytic action of enzymes on their respective substrates, which often results in the generation of acidic or basic products that alter the local solvent pH. For example, the catalytic oxidation of glucose by glucose oxidase (GOx) yields anionic species that arise from the further reduction of the oxidation product and cause swelling of the polymer matrix.[28] Another interesting example in that regard is the SRP-based sensor developed by Marshall et al. to detect urea and penicillin.[65] In that work, the concentration of the metabolites is monitored through pH changes associated with the specific catalytic reaction of urease and penicillinase. While urease catalyzes the hydrolysis of urea to ammonium bicarbonate and causes an increase in the local pH, penicillinase's catalytic reaction leads to the formation of penicilloic acid, which decreases the local pH. This local pH change ionizes the pendent functional groups of the polymer chains and causes the overall polymer matrix to swell as a result of electrostatic and osmotic forces.

1.3.2.2 Changes in Apparent Cross-Link Density

A response mechanism relevant to SRP hydrogels is the change in the apparent cross-link density or the change in the equilibrium length of elastically active network chains upon exposure to the stimulus, and reveals itself as a shrinking or swelling of the polymer gel. This response mechanism has been applied to detect DNA hybridization, antibody–antigen interaction, and glucose binding. For example, Murakami and Maeda[73] used gel shrinkage due to the shortening of cross-links to detect binding of a complementary target DNA strand to single-stranded DNA probes embedded in the polymer matrix. Yuan et al.[74] used an analogous strategy to detect binding of ATP to the enzyme adenylate kinase 3 (AK) that was immobilized in the polymer network. Furthermore, an increase in the cross-link density due to glucose binding to two pendant boronate groups in the polymer network was exploited for glucose detection at high ionic strengths.[75] Finally, Miyata et al.[66] used the free antigen-induced decrease in antigen–antibody mediated cross-link density to detect free antigen.

1.4 SENSING AND TRANSDUCTION MECHANISMS

For SRP coatings to be useful in sensing applications, the SRPs' response to a stimulus has to be transduced into a measurable output. The response of an SRP often results in volumetric changes that are measurable as changes in the physical properties such as optical density, refractive index, electron-transfer ability (voltage and current), mass, and mechanical stress. Here we limit our review to optical, electrochemical, and mechanical sensors that are commonly used to transduce the response of SRPs. In Table 1.1, we provide an overview of transduction mechanisms and SRP types and architectures that are used for the detection of a broad range of biologically relevant analytes.

1.4.1 Optical Transduction

Incorporation of micro- and nanostructures into the SRP coating enables the transduction of the volumetric swelling/shrinking response through measurable changes of the optical properties of the polymer coating. For example, hydrogel thin films that shrink significantly often appear opaque, with a low optical transmission coefficient; however, upon swelling, the hydrogel returns to a clear and more transparent state.[76] Furthermore, light diffraction from a crystalline colloidal array, polymerized within a stimulus-responsive hydrogel film, can translate the swelling/shrinking of the polymer gel into a measurable change of the diffraction peak.[77] Alternatively, gold nanoparticles (AuNPs) incorporated into SRP polymer brushes allow for the sensitive detection of changes in the solvent pH by measuring concomitant changes in the optical absorbance peak.[17]

Three optical measurement modes, (i) diffraction, (ii) reflection, and (iii) transmission, have been employed to transduce the response of SRP coatings (Fig. 1.3).

For *diffraction mode* transduction, a diffraction grid on or within the SRP coating is obtained (i) by polymerizing a crystalline colloidal array of polymer spheres within the SRP hydrogel film,[28,75,77–88] (ii) by harnessing the periodically ordered, dielectric structure of interconnected porosity in the hydrogel film,[89–91] or (iii) by the formation of silver gratings on the polymer coating surface.[18,19,23–25,29,62,64,65,90,92–94] Upon exposure to a stimulus, the responsive polymer coating will swell or shrink and, consequently, the lattice spacing between the elements of diffraction grating will change. These changes can be detected and measured by monitoring changes in the diffraction wavelengths as light passes through the SRP coating.

In *reflection mode* transduction, the swelling/shrinking and the change in the overall refractive index of the SRP coating is translated into measurable

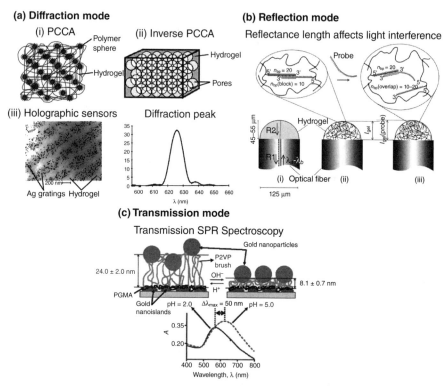

Figure 1.3 Various optical measurement modes that are exploited to transduce the response of stimulus-responsive polymer coatings. (a) In the diffraction mode, the swelling/shrinking of the polymer matrix shifts the diffraction peaks generated by (i) ordered polymer spheres, (ii) ordered porosity, or (iii) metal gratings in a hydrogel matrix. (b) In the reflection mode, the swelling and shrinking of hydrogels coated on the tip of fiber optics change the reflectivity of the coating. The volumetric response in the gel arises from the disruption in oligonucleotide junctions and changes the optical path length (top panel): (i) Hemispherical hydrogel coating at the end of the optical fiber, (ii) sensing (blue) and blocking (red) oligonucleotides in their hybridized state, and (iii) destabilization of the hybridization junctions due to the addition of probe nucleotides (green) cause the gel to swell. (c) In the transmission mode, the extension and contraction of a polymer brush due to the change in pH are coupled to the plasmon response of Au nanoislands (anchored by cross-linked thin layer of polyglycidyl methacrylate [PGMA]) and nanoparticles, which generates a shift in the absorbance peak. Adapted with permission from references [17], [29], [67], [88], and [91]. (See color insert.)

signals such as changes in the optical path length, changes in light reflection within the polymer matrix,[95] or changes in the minimum angle of reflectance of the polymer coating on a Au-coated glass slide.[26] To enhance the sensitivity, hybrid polymer coatings with AuNPs embedded in the polymer matrix are often used.[26,27,55] In addition to the change in the refractive index of the coating, the swelling/shrinking of the polymer changes the interparticle plasmon coupling of the AuNP in the polymer matrix, which is then translated into the shift in the minimum angle of reflectance.

In *transmission mode* transduction, the change in the optical density (i.e., index of refraction) of the polymer coating is used to transduce the response to a stimulus. For example, hydrogels in the shrunken state often appear opaque, with low optical transmission coefficients, while in the swollen state, they are significantly more transparent.[76] In addition, for hybrid SRP coatings, in which optically sensitive materials are incorporated into the polymer matrix, the swelling or shrinking of the polymer matrix changes the interparticle distance of the embedded materials, which in turn changes their optical coupling within the polymer matrix.[59,96]

1.4.1.1 Examples of SRP Sensors That Use Optical Transduction Principles

Next, we discuss four major classes of SRP sensors, shown in Figure 1.3, that use optical transduction principles: (i) polymerized crystalline colloidal arrays[28,75,77–88]; (ii) holographic-based biosensors,[18,19,23–25,29,62,64,65,90,92–94] which employ diffraction mode transduction; (iii) fiber optic sensors[67,95,97,98]; and (iv) plasmonic sensors,[17,26,27,53–60,99,100] which employ transmission and reflection mode transduction, respectively.

Asher et al. have developed a range of versatile colorimetric hydrogel-based sensors that respond to metal ions,[28,77–80,86] glucose,[28,75,77,82,84,88] temperature,[78] creatinine,[78,83] ammonia,[85] pH,[78,87] and ethanol[87] by changes in the diffraction behavior of the hydrogel. The sensor consists of a mesoscopic, periodic crystalline colloidal array (PCCA) of polymer spheres (~100 nm) polymerized within a stimulus-responsive hydrogel film (Fig. 1.3a). The hydrogel film swells or shrinks in response to external stimuli, which induces a change in the spacing of the colloidal array and hence shifts the diffraction peak as light passes through the hydrogel. Furthermore, the volumetric change of the hydrogel can be tailored specifically to the type of analyte of interest by incorporating analyte-specific groups into the polymer matrix. This design flexibility allows this sensing platform to be useful for a broad range of applications. Early work on the PCCA platform was focused on the detection of lead $Pb,^{2+}$ $Ba,^{2+}$ K^+, and glucose.[28,77,79] Specificity for cations was obtained by incorporating 18-crown-6 ether as a cation binding element into an acrylamide-based hydrogel, while glucose sensitivity was achieved by conjugation of GOx or β-galactosidase to the embedded polystyrene (PS) colloids, using biotin–avidin linkers. For high-ionic-strength glucose sensing in biological fluid, the crystalline colloidal array was embedded within a polyacrylamide–poly(ethylene glycol) (PEG) hydrogel with pendant phenylboronic acid groups.[75] Further development of this glucose sensor has resulted in colorimetric PCCA-based sensors that exhibit a fast response to glucose concentration in tear fluid with a ~1-μM detection limit.[82,84]

Inverse opal responsive hydrogels (inverse PCCA, Fig. 1.3a) provide an alternate sensing platform that also uses a diffraction-based transduction strategy. Here, instead of having a crystalline colloidal array of polymeric spheres embedded in the hydrogel matrix, an inverse opal structure with periodically ordered interconnecting porosity is created in the hydrogel matrix by first embedding a close-packed colloidal silica structure into the hydrogel mixture during polymerization, followed by selective etching of the silica by hydrofluoric acid. The interaction of light with the ordered pores results in distinct diffraction spectra that correspond to the lattice spacing of the pores. The pore spacing is modulated by swelling or shrinking of the hydrogel matrix in response to external stimuli and causes measurable shifts in the diffraction spectra. Kataoka group[91] and Braun group[135] have used this sensing strategy for glucose detection, while Asher group[87] used it for ethanol detection and pH sensing. An extension of this detection strategy for glucose sensing applications was developed by Takeoka group,[89] who polymerized a phenylboronic acid functionalized, acrylamide-based hydrogel in the pores and thus confined the swelling of the hydrogel to within the inverse opal structured, porous polymer matrix.

In holographic sensors, the change in SRP conformation is transduced by changes in the spacing between the fringes of a diffraction grating (typically colloidal silver) developed on the surface of an SRP coating as shown in Figure 1.3a. Similar to PCCA-based sensors, the specificity in holographic sensors is obtained through a rational design of the polymer matrix; for example, a pH sensor was fabricated by incorporating ionizable monomers into the hydrogel matrix[62]; an ionic strength sensor was made from charged sulfonate and quaternary ammonium monomers that were incorporated into polymeric hydrogel films[23]; and a sensor made of acrylamide hydrogel film bearing the glucose binding ligand,[24,25,93] 3-acrylamidophenylboronic acid (3-APB), and 2-acrylamido-5-fluorophenylboronic acid (5-F-2-MAPB) was used to detect glucose or lactate.

Lowe group pioneered the use of hydrogel-based holographic sensors, containing poly(2-hydroxyethyl methacrylate) (pHEMA) copolymerized or modified with analyte-sensitive groups, for measuring proteases,[92] pH,[62] metal ions,[29,64] ionic strength,[23] lactate,[25] glucose,[24,90,93] and metabolites[65] of enzymatic reactions, as well as spores,[94] ethanol,[19] and humidity.[18]

The low cost, robustness, and calibration stability of fiber optics have motivated their use as transducers to detect optical changes in hydrogels upon swelling and shrinking. Early work by Seitz group[76] demonstrated the utility of fiber optic detection for pH sensing by measuring the changes in the reflected intensity transmitted through an optical fiber that was coated at its end with a pH-sensitive hydrogel. Later, Stokke group[95] used the interference of light guided by the optical fiber and light reflected from a hydrogel coating at the end of the fiber to measure gel swelling and shrinking with ~2-nm precision. This interference configuration has also been used to measure glucose concentration[97,98] and DNA hybridization (Fig. 1.3b).[67]

A surface plasmon is described as an oscillation of free electron density against the fixed, positive metal ions. Since surface plasmons are electromagnetic waves that propagate parallel to the metal/dielectric interface, any changes that alter the dielectric properties at this interface, such as the adsorption of molecules, will affect the oscillations/resonance of the electromagnetic waves. There are two primary modes of surface plasmon resonance (SPR) sensing: (i) conventional or planar SPR, exhibited by planar films of gold or silver, and (ii) localized surface plasmon resonance (LSPR), which is exhibited by AuNP or silver nanoparticle (NP). In addition, there are hybrid detection modalities in which noble metal NPs are combined with planar SPR to amplify the response of one or both of these transduction modalities.[17,53,56,57,59]

For planar SPR sensing, the signal is typically transduced in reflectivity mode using the Kretschmann configuration,[101] where the change in the angle of minimum reflected intensity is tracked as a function of dielectric changes on the sensing surface. In LSPR, the signal is transduced in transmission mode by measuring the plasmon resonance of, for example, AuNPs in terms of light absorption and scattering.[102] The principle of detection enhancement through LSPR coupling was shown, among others, by Gupta et al.[53,54] In their approach, they first grafted solvent-responsive PS brushes and pH-responsive poly(2-vinylpyridine) (p2VP) brushes onto silicon/glass surfaces and subsequently adsorbed AuNPs to the PS brush. The AuNPs then nucleated the growth of silver NPs on the p2VP brush. They then showed that brush swelling increased the interparticle distances and caused a distinct blue shift of the absorbance peak. The effect of changes in the interparticle distance on LSPR coupling has been demonstrated for other coating structures as well. For example, Lee and Perez-Luna[56] linked AuNPs to linear carboxylated dextran chains that were attached to a silane-functionalized glass surface. Upon exposure to a nonpolar solvent, the dextran gel shrank, causing the AuNPs to aggregate, which induced a red shift in the absorption spectrum and broadened the plasmon absorption peaks. Lupitsky et al.[57] used LSPR sensing to detect changes in pH. They first grew pH-responsive p2VP brushes on 200-nm silica core particles and then decorated the brushes with 15-nm AuNPs. Cyclic pH changes in the range between pH 2.5 and 6.0 caused a volumetric swelling/shrinking response of the polymer brush that affected the distance between AuNPs. This change in interparticle spacing was accompanied by a significant wavelength shift in the absorption peak, which translated into a color change from purple to blue as the pH changed from 2.5 to 6.0.

Planar SPR and LSPR can readily be coupled by simply mixing the metal NPs into the polymer matrix,[59] by physical adsorption,[17,53] or by covalent attachment of these NPs to the end chain of the polymer brush,[56,57] thereby creating a hybrid responsive coating. For example, Tokareva et al.[17] demonstrated the enhancement of LSPR sensing by grafting pH-responsive polymer brushes onto gold islands and then adsorbing AuNPs (~13 nm in diameter) to the brush surface (Fig. 1.3c). Upon changing the pH from 5 to 2, the distance change between the AuNPs and the gold islands also changed the extent of interparticle coupling in LSPR, which resulted in a wavelength shift of the absorption peak maximum of 50 nm, as compared with only 6 nm in the absence of the NPs. Another example of enhanced LSPR sensing was reported by Jiang et al.,[55] who modulated the packing of AuNP in a multilayer film of pAH and pSS prepared by LBL deposition on gold by changes in pH. Using the planar SPR mode, they showed that pH-induced changes in the packing of the AuNPs strongly affected the SPR response. The enhanced SPR shifts in response to pH were explained by electromagnetic coupling between the LSPR of the AuNPs and the SPR of the gold film. A similar SPR signal enhancement strategy was applied to detect cholesterol,[60] adrenaline,[58] dopamine,[26] and atrazine.[27] For these sensing applications, however, the hydrogel coatings were molecularly imprinted with a recognition template specific to the analyte of interest.

Periodically arrayed, nanostructured metallic patterns provide another platform to exploit the SPR phenomenon. The plasmonic response in this platform can be excited with incident light and exhibits a complex, multipeak transmission spectrum in the visible and near-infrared region. By coating the metallic nanopattern with a stimulus-responsive hydrogel, this sensor can measure analytically relevant parameters. For example, Mack and coworkers[99] coated a 500-nm-thick pH-responsive pHEMA hydrogel film onto gold-coated nanowell arrays. They found that summing the absolute magnitudes of the difference spectra over all wavelengths yielded an integrated plasmonic response that directly correlated with pH-dependent changes in the hydrogel coating. Based on the same principle, Sabarinathan and coworkers[100] fabricated a hydrogel-based pH sensor by coating the surface of a gold nanocrescent array pattern with pHEMA.

1.4.2 Electrochemical Transduction

Electrical signals are among the simplest sensor outputs to measure, and efforts have thus been made to translate volume changes in the SRP coating to changes in current (resistance) or voltage (conductance). This detection strategy is generally exploited with SRPs that are used as electrode coatings for electrochemical devices.[63,68,70,72,103,104] Here, the ability of the matrix to swell or shrink is used to control the accessibility of a redox label to the electrode interface and thus to increase or decrease the electron-transfer resistance, respectively.[72,105–108]

For electrochemical transduction, signals are typically measured by one of three methods: (i) by *potentiometry*, which measures electrostatic potential or charge accumulation at zero current; (ii) by *voltammetry*, which measures ionic strength in terms of conductance and impedance; and (iii) by *amperometry*, which measures the current at a fixed voltage. Of these measurement methods, amperometry is the most popular, largely due to its simplicity, sensitivity, and low cost.

To impart specificity to the sensing surface of electrochemical sensing devices, the electrodes are typically coated with a polymer matrix that contains receptors for an analyte of interest. In addition to providing an analyte-specific binding substrate, the polymer matrix can also increase the loading capacity of the sensor surface by transforming a 2-D substrate into a 3-D matrix that can contain additional signal amplifying components.

1.4.2.1 Examples of SRP Sensors That Use Electrochemical Transduction Principles

The use of SRP coatings for electrochemical sensing is largely confined to the supporting polymer matrix, which immobilizes the recognition elements and embeds redox-active molecules such as ferrocene and methylene blue. Various types of SRPs have been utilized as coatings on the electrode surfaces of electrochemical sensors, including pH[63,68,109] and glucose-sensitive[110] polymer brushes, pH-sensitive LBL films,[104] glucose-sensitive hydrogels,[70,72] and hydrogel coatings to detect cholesterol.[103] SRPs imbue polymer coatings with an electrochemical switching functionality in which a redox reaction on the electrode surface occurs or is blocked when the SRPs are in the swollen "on" state or in the collapsed "off" state, respectively.

For example, Zhou et al.[68] used electrochemical polymerization to coat Au electrodes with pAA brushes. They then showed the pH-sensitive switching of the pAA brushes through cyclic voltammetry (CV) and electrical impedance spectroscopy (EIS) in the presence of anionic ferricyanide ions $[Fe(CN)_6]^{3-/4-}$. Here, a switch from acidic to basic pH resulted in a measurable increase of electron-transfer resistance due to repulsion of $[Fe(CN)_6]^{3-/4-}$ from the electrode surface and hence could be exploited as a pH sensor. Furthermore, Zhou et al. used pAA brushes as a matrix to demonstrate the pH-driven, reversible immobilization of cytochrome c (Cyt c) on Au electrode surfaces using CV and EIS. Cyt c below pH 10 is a basic redox metalloprotein that bears several positive charges, while pAA above pH 7 is a negatively charged PEL, as illustrated in Figure 1.4a. Thus, attractive electrostatic interactions that occur in weakly basic conditions cause the pAA brush to take up Cyt c, and repulsive interactions that occur in acidic conditions cause the pAA brush to release Cyt c. Using a similar approach, Tam et al.[63] demonstrated pH sensing with Indium tin oxide (ITO) electrodes that were functionalized with poly(4-vinylpyridine) (p4VP) brushes. At pH 4.5, the p4VP brush has a positively charged pyridine group that causes the hydrophilic brush to swell, which increases the permeability of the polymer matrix and allows anionic species, such as $[Fe(CN)6]^{4-}$, to permeate through the polymer brush and to undergo an electrochemical redox reaction at the electrode surface (Fig. 1.4b). At pH 9.1, the polymer brush is deprotonated and hence collapses onto the surface, which prevents $[Fe(CN)_6]^{4-}$ to permeate through the coating, thus inhibiting any redox processes at the electrode surface.

An LBL PEL thin film containing $[Fe(CN)_6]^{3-}$ was used for the electrocatalytic detection of ascorbic acid in the concentration range from 1 to 50 mM. This film, composed of pAH and carboxymethyl cellulose (CMC), was coated onto the surface of a Au disk electrode.[104] Upon exposure to weakly acidic or neutral solutions, $[Fe(CN)_6]^{3-}$ ions are confined to the film, while in basic solution, $[Fe(CN)_6]^{3-}$ ions are repelled from the film. The ability of pAH/CMC LBL

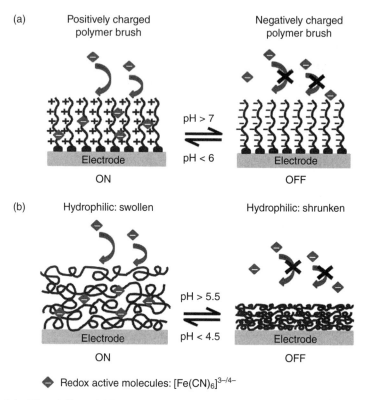

Figure 1.4   The ability of SRP to respond to changes in pH is exploited to enhance electrochemical signal transduction. (a) A pAA brush undergoes a pH-induced switch from a positively charged (on) to a negatively charged (off) state, which in turn attracts and repels redox-active species. (b) An acrylamide-based hydrogel coating undergoes a pH-induced conformational change from the swollen (hydrophilic) "on" state to the collapsed (hydrophobic) "off" state in which redox-active species are excluded from the coating. Adapted with permission from reference [63].

films to produce clear redox peaks, mediated by the acid concentration-driven confinement or release of $[Fe(CN)_6]^{3-}$ ions, can thus be exploited for sensing.

Gabai and coworkers[72] used an m-acrylamidophenylboronic acid-functionalized acrylamide hydrogel coated on Au electrodes for the electrochemical detection of glucose. In the presence of the redox probe $[Fe(CN)_6]^{3-}:[Fe(CN)_6]^{4-}$ (1:1), an increase in glucose concentration caused swelling of the polymer matrix, which in turn decreased the electron-transfer resistance as measured by faradaic impedance spectroscopy. Other examples of glucose sensing have utilized a hydrogel matrix to immobilize soluble enzyme such as GOx.[70] In one study, a ferrocene-containing hydrogel was mixed with the enzyme to obtain glucose-oxidizing electrodes. In the presence of glucose, but in the absence of GOx, only the redox response from ferrocene moieties was detected. In the presence of GOx, however, the anodic current increased strongly. This indicates the effective wiring of redox-active polymers with the active center of the reduced GOx, which, in the presence of glucose, amplifies the electrochemical signal generated by the glucose–GOx reaction.

1.4.3 Mechanical Transduction

Volumetric transformations in SRPs involve stretching and contraction of polymer chains to accommodate the change in the system's osmotic pressure. For sensing applications, SRPs are typically immobilized on a solid support, and this surface confinement restricts the ability of the polymer coating to expand or to contract freely as compared to the bulk polymer, and leads to the generation of large interfacial stresses. These stresses are harnessed for sensing applications using, for example, SRP-coated microcantilevers, where the stress-induced cantilever bending can be amplified and recorded (Fig. 1.5a).[13,111,112] *Optical* (optical lever and interferometry) and *electrical* (piezoresistive and piezoelectric) detection schemes are commonly used to monitor

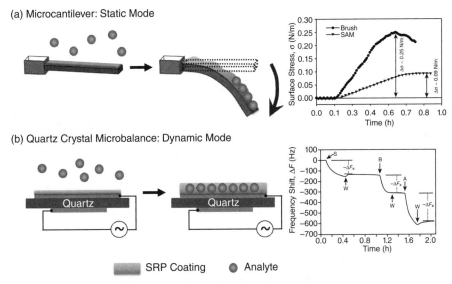

Figure 1.5 Two examples of mechanical signal transduction: (a) static microcantilever deflection where an SRP coating on the topside of the cantilever causes an increase in surface stress upon analyte binding. Right graph: surface stress plotted as a function of time for two glucose-sensitive coatings. The SRP coating provides a faster and more sensitive response upon glucose binding (10 mM) compared with self-assembled monolayers (SAMs). (b) Dynamic transduction mode using a QCM sensor. The SRP coating on the quartz crystal provides a scaffold for the analyte to bind, which causes a decrease in the resonance frequency. Right graph: frequency plotted as a function of time, showing the frequency response when a streptavidin-coated crystal (S) is exposed to biotinylated BSA (B). After a wash step (W) and exposure to anti-BSA (A), a further drop in resonance frequency is observed. Adapted with permission from references [105] and [119]. (See color insert.)

microcantilever deflection. For example, in optical lever deflection detection, laser light is reflected from the back of the microcantilever onto a position-sensitive photodetector, and small cantilever deflections are thus translated into easily measurable detector voltages. For piezoresistive deflection detection, the change in resistance of a piezoresistive material embedded in the microcantilever is measured. This approach allows the measurement of large cantilever deflections and obviates the need for a complex alignment procedure, which is often a serious problem in optical-based detection methods.

Another mechanical transduction approach is provided by quartz crystal resonators that translate changes in mass on the crystal surface into measurable frequency changes (Fig. 1.5b). For these sensing approaches, the SRP coating serves as a matrix for direct analyte binding, which increases the coupled mass,[72,105–107] or as a matrix that swells due to interaction with the surrounding solvents, which increases the water retention and thus the overall mass.[113]

The transduction approach for quartz crystal microbalance (QCM) relies on the shift of resonance frequency of an oscillating quartz crystal and the change of mass on the QCM crystal surface.[114] The sensitivity of QCM thus relies on the accurate measurement of changes in the crystal's resonance frequency.

1.4.3.1 *Examples of SRP Sensors That Use Mechanical Transduction Principles*   For mechanical transduction schemes, a reactive and analyte-specific SRP coating in contact with the transducer surface is needed to detect chemical or biological molecules.[111,115] For microcantilever sensing, several types of SRP coatings, including hydrogels,[116,117] polymer brushes,[118–120] and LBL films,[121,122] have been employed. For example, Hilt et al.[116] coated microcantilevers with cross-linked pAA-PEG copolymer hydrogels to detect pH changes. The Zauscher group[118,119] demonstrated the use of pNIPAM copolymer brushes, grown on one side of a microcantilever, to detect changes in pH, ionic strength, and glucose concentration (Fig. 1.5a). Similarly, Yan et al.[122] used cantilevers modified with GOx/PEI multilayers to detect glucose. Glucose concentration was also measured by QCM using a glucose-sensitive hydrogel copolymer (*m*-acrylamidophenylboronic acid-co-acrylamide) electropolymerized on QCM electrodes.[72] Biotin-functionalized hydrogel coatings for QCM sensors were developed for protein immobilization and antibody assays, and, for example, the specificity of the coating for bovine serum albumin (BSA) antibody was measured in real time using QCM sensors (Fig. 1.5b).[105] In addition, MIP coatings that are specific to nucleotides,[107,123] monosaccharides,[107] and herbicides[106] were developed, and the specificity of the imprinted molecular template to the target was verified using QCM. QCM also provides a convenient technique to study the conformational change in SRP coatings in real time.[39,113,124] For example, Richter et al.[39] used pVA-co-pAA hydrogels, spin coated on the quartz crystal, to map the hydrogel's swelling hysteresis in response to changes in pH.

1.5 LIMITATIONS AND CHALLENGES

SRPs have an extraordinarily large potential for biosensing applications as a result of the broad range of SRP architectures, the rich palette of analyte-specific modifications, and the large number of possible transduction approaches. Nevertheless, to date, many studies have only focused on "proof of concept" demonstration of SRPs as sensor platforms, and not yet on improving sensor performance. Several figures of merit are important in the evaluation of sensor performance, including the limit of detection (LOD), sensitivity, selectivity, working range, response time, reliability, and long-term stability. Next, we will briefly discuss the strengths and limitations of SRPs as sensor coatings in the light of these figures of merit and discuss some challenges that need to be overcome to improve the performance of SRP-based sensors.

1.5.1 LOD and Sensitivity

Two important measures of sensor performance are the LOD and the ability to produce a large response as a function of analyte concentration, generally referred to as the sensor's sensitivity. When SRPs are used as sensor coatings, the LOD and sensitivity are largely limited by the ability of the SRP matrix to respond to the lowest concentration of the analyte. Two important factors for the responsiveness of SRP coatings are their capacity to interact with the target analyte and the accessibility of recognition elements embedded in the coating. Typically, SRP coatings increase the sensing volume per unit area of sensor surface, which in turn can increase the LOD and sensitivity. However, an increase in sensing volume must be weighed against an ensuing barrier for analyte diffusion, which may impede the analyte's access to recognition sites throughout the coating.[125]

A factor to consider with SRP gel coatings is their cross-link density. Cross-link density affects both the volumetric swelling response of the gel upon exposure to a stimulus and its mechanical integrity. The lower the cross-linking density, the larger is the relative volume change upon exposure to a stimulus and consequently, the larger is the sensitivity of the gel. However, gel coatings with low cross-link density have little mechanical integrity, which could compromise the stability and robustness of the coating during use.

Although the use of SRP coatings in biosensors allows the label-free detection of analytes, the LOD of SRP sensors is generally inferior compared to sensing approaches that use a label. For example, the LOD of SRP-based sensors for biologically relevant samples including electrolytes, glucose, or metabolites is in the micro- to millimolar concentration range. While this LOD is sufficient for detecting common metabolites, many applications require detection of biomolecules (biomarkers) or toxic chemicals in the pico- to nanomolar range.[11] In many cases, such small analyte concentrations may be insufficient to cause changes in the SRP coatings directly. Thus, SRP coatings with amplification potential, for example, through reaction cascades, need to be developed to further improve the performance of SRP coatings.

1.5.2   Selectivity

SRP coatings can be engineered to selectively detect a wide range of analytes. This selectivity is typically obtained by incorporating analyte-specific recognition elements into the SRP coating. However, despite a range of available strategies to impart selectivity, nonspecific interactions with SRPs can limit signal-to-noise ratios. An important issue for SRP coating design is thus to develop strategies that minimize nonspecific interactions while simultaneously maximizing the desired interactions of the SRP coating with the analyte.[29]

1.5.3   Working Range

For SRP-based biosensors, the working range of the sensor, determined by the range of conditions in which the polymer matrix is responsive to the presence of stimuli, must be considered carefully. For example, for a sensor that has to operate under physiological conditions, an appropriate polymer type and subsequent modification for the recognition of a specific analyte has to be selected to work at the physiological pH of 7.4.[62,90] This constraint challenges the biological relevance of some proof of concept SRP biosensor studies where the operating conditions are often far outside the physiological range.

Another issue that can compromise the sensor working range is that surface-attached SRP thin films can differ in their physicochemical properties compared to those of the same polymer in bulk. For example, the apparent pKa of a pAA hydrogel in bulk is ~4.7; however, when this gel is coated as a thin film on a QCM sensor surface, the apparent pKa drops to ~2.2.[39] For pVA-co-pAA thin films, this phenomenon was observed for a coating thickness of less than 400 nm.

Thus, to further extend the utility of SRP coatings for biosensing applications, careful consideration of the appropriate working range needs to be given in the design and choice of the SRP coating.

1.5.4   Response Time

The response time of SRP-based coatings is determined by the kinetics of their response. In general, the response kinetics depends on the polymer chain dynamics, the diffusivity of the analyte, and the kinetics of the chemical reactions within the polymer matrix.[126] As the primary response in most SRP-based transduction approaches is in the form of volumetric changes of the film, the response kinetics can often be determined from the swelling kinetics. The thickness of the SRP coating has a strong influence on the swelling kinetics. For example, for an SRP gel, the swelling rate depends inversely proportional on the square of the gel thickness and on the diffusion coefficient of the polymer network.[127] It was found that when the thickness of the polymer coating is in the nanometer range, a sensor responds within a few hundred milliseconds, whereas a film thickness on the order of 100 μm results in a response time of several minutes.[9]

Other factors such as chain dynamics and inter- and intramolecular interactions may play an important role in the response kinetics of SRP sensors. For example, a strong swelling–shrinking hysteresis observed in multilayer films was attributed to the low mobility of polymer segments in hydrophobic domains of the PEL backbone.[11] The kinetics of ionization is another important factor that affects the response time of ionic SRP coatings.[9]

Finally, the response time can be strongly affected by other forces that constrain the swelling process of the polymer coating. For example, microcantilever sensors that use the mechanical work of SRP coatings for transduction have a slower response time in addition to significant swelling hysteresis[128] compared with the response of the free swelling SRP.[39]

1.5.5 Reliability and Long-Term Stability

Reliability is another important figure of merit of SRP-based sensors and is defined as the ability of the sensor to produce a consistent and accurate signal from repeated exposures to a relevant stimulus for an extended period of time. SRP coatings often display a significant swelling hysteresis, which is caused by changes in the microscopic structure of the polymer chains in the network and the tendency for polymer chains to attain an equilibrium conformation.[39] For sensing, this requires a number of conditioning cycles before a consistent response signal is attained and measurement accuracy can be achieved.[9]

Delamination of the polymer layer from the sensor platform/substrate is another problem that can affect the reliability of SRP coatings. For example, SRP gel coatings are typically anchored to a solid substrate, where the strong osmotic swelling pressure in the lateral dimension can put a swollen film under biaxial compressive stress.[41] This mechanical stress can be large enough to overcome the adhesion forces and can cause wrinkling of the free surface of the film and lead to its delamination from the substrate.[129,130] Several strategies, such as using an adhesion promoter,[36] enclosing the hydrogel element in a microelectromechanical device,[131] and using a very thin SRP layer,[39] can help to avoid delamination.

SRP-based sensors are designed to provide selectivity by incorporating a recognition element in the coating and to exploit the ability of the SRP coating to respond to a specific stimulus. For biologically relevant applications, the recognition elements are often biomolecules such as enzymes or antibodies, which are prone to denaturation. Despite the practical importance of this issue, there are no studies to date that rigorously validate the long-term viability of the biomolecular recognition elements in SRP-based biosensor coatings.

1.6 CONCLUSION AND OUTLOOK

The recent developments in SRP coatings for biosensor applications have significantly expanded the toolset available to detect a broad range of analytes, including metal ions, metabolites, biomolecules, and biomolecular binding events. These developments are mainly driven by the availability and design of a wide range of functional polymer coatings, the ability to impart sensing selectivity, and a broad choice of signal transduction mechanisms. In this chapter, we discussed and summarized recent research trends in the field of SRP-based biosensors, with focus on the architecture of the polymer coatings, the mechanism of SRP response to analytes, and the transduction of the SRP response into a measurable signal. To date, the research carried out in the field has focused on the "proof-of-principle" demonstration of the detection principles and the development of creative signal transduction mechanisms. Although SRP-based biosensors possess many attractive attributes, their broad implementation requires further research in the validation and optimization of their properties, such as analyte specificity, detection limits, working range, reliability, and the long-term performance of the sensor.

ACKNOWLEDGEMENTS

Stefan Zauscher and Ashutosh Chilkoti thank the National Science Foundation for support through grants NSF NIRT CBET-0609265 and NSF CBET-1033621.

REFERENCES

1. Alexander, C. & Shakesheff, K.M. Responsive polymers at the biology/materials science interface. *Advanced Materials* **18**, 3321–3328 (2006).
2. Schmaljohann, D. Thermo- and pH-responsive polymers in drug delivery. *Advanced Drug Delivery Reviews* **58**, 1655–1670 (2006).
3. Yamato, M. et al. Temperature-responsive cell culture surfaces for regenerative medicine with cell sheet engineering. *Progress in Polymer Science* **32**, 1123–1133 (2007).
4. Elloumi-Hannachi, I., Yamato, M., & Okano, T. Cell sheet engineering: a unique nanotechnology for scaffold-free tissue reconstruction with clinical applications in regenerative medicine. *Journal of Internal Medicine* **267**, 54–70 (2010).
5. Lee, K.Y. & Mooney, D.J. Hydrogels for tissue engineering. *Chemical Reviews* **101**, 1869–1879 (2001).
6. Ulijn, R.V. et al. Bioresponsive hydrogels. *Materials Today* **10**, 40–48 (2007).
7. Gawel, K., Barriet, D., Sletmoen, M., & Stokke, B.T. Responsive hydrogels for label-free signal transduction within. *Biosensors Sensors* **10**, 4381–4409 (2010).
8. Hu, J.M. & Liu, S.Y. Responsive polymers for detection and sensing applications: current status and future developments. *Macromolecules* **43**, 8315–8330 (2010).

9. Richter, A. et al. Review on hydrogel-based pH sensors and microsensors. *Sensors* **8**, 561–581 (2008).

10. Roy, D., Cambre, J.N., & Sumerlin, B.S. Future perspectives and recent advances in stimuli-responsive materials. *Progress in Polymer Science* **35**, 278–301 (2010).

11. Tokarev, I., Motornov, M., & Minko, S. Molecular-engineered stimuli-responsive thin polymer film: a platform for the development of integrated multifunctional intelligent materials. *Journal of Materials Chemistry* **19**, 6932–6948 (2009).

12. Ratner, B.D. surface modification of polymers—chemical, biological and surface analytical challenges. *Biosensors & Bioelectronics* **10**, 797–804 (1995).

13. Stuart, M.A.C. et al. Emerging applications of stimuli-responsive polymer materials. *Nature Materials* **9**, 101–113 (2010).

14. Uhlmann, P., Merlitz, H., Sommer, J.-U., & Stamm, M. Polymer brushes for surface tuning. *Macromolecular Rapid Communications* **30**, 732–740 (2009).

15. Alarcon, C.D.H., Pennadam, S., & Alexander, C. Stimuli responsive polymers for biomedical applications. *Chemical Society Reviews* **34**, 276–285 (2005).

16. Gil, E.S. & Hudson, S.M. Stimuli-responsive polymers and their bioconjugates. *Progress in Polymer Science* **29**, 1173–1222 (2004).

17. Tokareva, I., Minko, S., Fendler, J.H., & Hutter, E. Nanosensors based on responsive polymer brushes and gold nanoparticle enhanced transmission surface plasmon resonance spectroscopy. *Journal of the American Chemical Society* **126**, 15950–15951 (2004).

18. Blyth, J., Millington, R.B., Mayes, A.G., Frears, E.R., & Lowe, C.R. Holographic sensor for water in solvents. *Analytical Chemistry* **68**, 1089–1094 (1996).

19. Mayes, A.G., Blyth, J., Kyrolainen-Reay, M., Millington, R.B., & Lowe, C.R. A holographic alcohol sensor. *Analytical Chemistry* **71**, 3390–3396 (1999).

20. Miyata, T., Onakamae, K., Hoffman, A.S., & Kanzaki, Y. Stimuli-sensitivities of hydrogels containing phosphate groups. *Macromolecular Chemistry and Physics* **195**, 1111–1120 (1994).

21. Lee, W.F. & Yuan, W.Y. Thermoreversible hydrogels XIII: synthesis and swelling behaviors of [N-isopropylacrylamide-co-sodium 2-acrylamido-2-methylpropyl sulfonate-co-N,N-dimethyl(acrylamido propyl) ammonium propane sulfonate] copolymeric hydrogels. *Journal of Polymer* **7**, 29–40 (2000).

22. Brannonpeppas, L. & Peppas, N. A. Time-dependent response of ionic polymer networks to ph and ionic-strength changes. *International Journal of Pharmaceutics* **70**, 53–57 (1991).

23. Marshall, A.J. et al. Holographic sensors for the determination of ionic strength. *Analytica Chimica Acta* **527**, 13–20 (2004).

24. Kabilan, S. et al. Holographic glucose sensors. *Biosensors & Bioelectronics* **20**, 1602–1610 (2005).

25. Sartain, F.K., Yang, X.P., & Lowe, C.R. Holographic lactate sensor. *Analytical Chemistry* **78**, 5664–5670 (2006).

26. Matsui, J. et al. SPR sensor chip for detection of small molecules using molecularly imprinted polymer with embedded gold nanoparticles. *Analytical Chemistry* **77**, 4282–4285 (2005).

27. Matsui, J. et al. Molecularly imprinted nanocomposites for highly sensitive SPR detection of a non-aqueous atrazine sample. *Analyst* **134**, 80–86 (2009).

28. Holtz, J.H., Holtz, J.S.W., Munro, C.H., & Asher, S.A. Intelligent polymerized crystalline colloidal arrays: novel chemical sensor materials. *Analytical Chemistry* **70**, 780–791 (1998).

29. Mayes, A.G., Blyth, J., Millington, R.B., & Lowe, C.R. Metal ion-sensitive holographic sensors. *Analytical Chemistry* **74**, 3649–3657 (2002).

30. Reuber, J., Reinhardt, H., & Johannsmann, D. Formation of surface-attached responsive gel layers via electrochemically induced free-radical polymerization. *Langmuir* **22**, 3362–3367 (2006).

31. Bullett, N.A., Talib, R.A., Short, R.D., McArthur, S.L., & Shard, A.G. Chemical and thermo-responsive characterisation of surfaces formed by plasma polymerisation of N-isopropyl acrylamide. *Surface and Interface Analysis* **38**, 1109–1116 (2006).

32. Forch, R. et al. Recent and expected roles of plasma-polymerized films for biomedical applications. *Chemical Vapor Deposition* **13**, 280–294 (2007).

33. Pan, Y.V., Wesley, R.A., Luginbuhl, R., Denton, D.D., & Ratner, B.D. Plasma polymerized N-isopropylacrylamide: synthesis and characterization of a smart thermally responsive coating. *Biomacromolecules* **2**, 32–36 (2001).

34. Tamirisa, P.A. & Hess, D.W. Water and moisture uptake by plasma polymerized thermoresponsive hydrogel films. *Macromolecules* **39**, 7092–7097 (2006).

35. Guenther, M. et al. Chemical sensors based on multiresponsive block copolymer hydrogels. *Sensors and Actuators. B, Chemical* **126**, 97–106 (2007).

36. Kuckling, D., Harmon, M.E., & Frank, C.W. Photo-cross-linkable PNIPAAm copolymers. 1. Synthesis and characterization of constrained temperature-responsive hydrogel layers. *Macromolecules* **35**, 6377–6383 (2002).

37. Matsukuma, D., Yamamoto, K., & Aoyagi, T. Stimuli-responsive properties of N-isopropylacrylamide-based ultrathin hydrogel films prepared by photo-cross-linking. *Langmuir* **22**, 5911–5915 (2006).

38. Hayward, R.C., Chmelka, B.F., & Kramer, E.J. Crosslinked poly(styrene)-block-poly(2-vinylpyridine) thin films as swellable templates for mesostructured silica and titania. *Advanced Materials* **17**, 2591–2595 (2005).

39. Richter, A., Bund, A., Keller, M., & Arndt, K.F. Characterization of a microgravimetric sensor based on pH sensitive hydrogels. *Sensors and Actuators. B, Chemical* **99**, 579–585 (2004).

40. Sorber, J. et al. Hydrogel-based piezoresistive pH sensors: investigations using FT-IR attenuated total reflection spectroscopic Imaging. *Analytical Chemistry* **80**, 2957–2962 (2008).

41. Tokarev, I. & Minko, S. Stimuli-responsive hydrogel thin films. *Soft Matter* **5**, 511–524 (2009).

42. Tokarev, I., Orlov, M., & Minko, S. Responsive polyelectrolyte gel membranes. *Advanced Materials* **18**, 2458–2460 (2006).

43. Kopecek, J. & Yang, J.Y. Review—hydrogels as smart biomaterials. *Polymer International* **56**, 1078–1098 (2007).

44. Mathur, A.M., Moorjani, S.K., & Scranton, A.B. Methods for synthesis of hydrogel networks: a review. *Journal of Macromolecular Science—Reviews in Macromolecular Chemistry and Physics* **C36**, 405–430 (1996).

45. Advincula, R.C., Brittain, W.J., Caster, K.C., & Ruhe, J. *Polymer Brushes: Synthesis, Characterization, Applications*. Weinheim, Germany: Wiley (2004).

46. Edmondson, S., Osborne, V.L., & Huck, W.T.S. Polymer brushes via surface-initiated polymerizations. *Chemical Society Reviews* **33**, 14–22 (2004).

47. Minko, S. Responsive polymer brushes. *Polymer Reviews* **46**, 397–420 (2006).

48. Tang, Z.Y., Wang, Y., Podsiadlo, P., & Kotov, N.A. Biomedical applications of layer-by-layer assembly: from biomimetics to tissue engineering (vol. 18, p. 3203, 2006). *Advanced Materials* **19**, 906–906 (2007).

49. Park, M.K., Deng, S.X., & Advincula, R.C. pH-sensitive bipolar ion-permselective ultrathin films. *Journal of the American Chemical Society* **126**, 13723–13731 (2004).

50. Kang, E.H., Liu, X.K., Sun, J.Q., & Shen, J.C. Robust ion-permselective multilayer films prepared by photolysis of polyelectrolyte multilayers containing photo-cross-linkable and photolabile groups. *Langmuir* **22**, 7894–7901 (2006).

51. Haupt, K. & Mosbach, K. Molecularly imprinted polymers and their use in bio-mimetic sensors. *Chemical Reviews* **100**, 2495–2504 (2000).

52. Haupt, K. Molecularly imprinted polymers in analytical chemistry. *Analyst* **126**, 747–756 (2001).

53. Gupta, S. et al. Gold nanoparticles immobilized on stimuli responsive polymer brushes as nanosensors. *Macromolecules* **41**, 8152–8158 (2008).

54. Gupta, S. et al. Immobilization of silver nanoparticles on responsive polymer brushes. *Macromolecules* **41**, 2874–2879 (2008).

55. Jiang, G. et al. Signal enhancement and tuning of surface plasmon resonance in Au nanoparticle/polyelectrolyte ultrathin films. *Journal of Physical Chemistry* **C111**, 18687–18694 (2007).

56. Lee, S. & Perez-Luna, V.H. Surface-grafted hybrid material consisting of gold nanoparticles and dextran exhibits mobility and reversible aggregation on a surface. *Langmuir* **23**, 5097–5099 (2007).

57. Lupitsky, R., Motornov, M., & Minko, S. Single nanoparticle plasmonic devices by the "grafting to" method. *Langmuir* **24**, 8976–8980 (2008).

58. Matsui, J. et al. Composite of Au nanoparticles and molecularly imprinted polymer as a sensing material. *Analytical Chemistry* **76**, 1310–1315 (2004).

59. Tokarev, I., Tokareva, I., & Minko, S. Gold-nanoparticle-enhanced plasmonic effects in a responsive polymer gel. *Advanced Materials* **20**, 2730–2734 (2008).

60. Tokareva, I., Tokarev, I., Minko, S., Hutter, E., & Fendler, J.H. Ultrathin molecularly imprinted polymer sensors employing enhanced transmission surface plasmon resonance spectroscopy. *Chemical Communications* **31**, 3343–3345 (2006).

61. Fulghum, T.M., Estillore, N.C., Vo, C.D., Armes, S.P., & Advincula, R.C. Stimuli-responsive polymer ultrathin films with a binary architecture: combined layer-by-layer polyelectrolyte and surface-initiated polymerization approach. *Macromolecules* **41**, 429–435 (2008).

62. Marshall, A.J., Blyth, J., Davidson, C.A.B., & Lowe, C.R.P. H-sensitive holographic sensors. *Analytical Chemistry* **75**, 4423–4431 (2003).

63. Tam, T.K. et al. Reversible "closing" of an electrode interface functionalized with a polymer brush by an electrochemical signal. *Langmuir* **26**, 4506–4513 (2010).

64. Gonzalez, B.M., Christie, G., Davidson, C.A.B., Blyth, J., & Lowe, C.R. Divalent metal ion-sensitive holographic sensors. *Analytica Chimica Acta* **528**, 219–228 (2005).

65. Marshall, A.J., Young, D.S., Blyth, J., Kabilan, S., & Lowe, C.R. Metabolite-sensitive holographic biosensors. *Analytical Chemistry* **76**, 1518–1523 (2004).

66. Miyata, T., Asami, N., & Uragami, T. A reversibly antigen-responsive hydrogel. *Nature* **399**, 766–769 (1999).

67. Tierney, S. & Stokke, B.T. Development of an oligonucleotide functionalized hydrogel integrated on a high resolution interferometric readout platform as a label-free macromolecule sensing device. *Biomacromolecules* **10**, 1619–1626 (2009).

68. Zhou, J., Lu, X., Hu, J., & Li, J. Reversible immobilization and direct electron transfer of cytochrome c on a pH-Sensitive Polymer Interface. *Chemistry—a European Journal* **13**, 2847–2853 (2007).

69. Miyata, T., Asami, N., & Uragami, T. Preparation of an antigen-sensitive hydrogel using antigen-antibody bindings. *Macromolecules* **32**, 2082–2084 (1999).

70. Bunte, C., Prucker, O., Konig, T., & Ruhe, J. Enzyme containing redox polymer networks for biosensors or biofuel cells: a photochemical approach. *Langmuir* **26**, 6019–6027 (2010).

71. Shibayama, M. & Tanaka, T. Volume phase-transition and related phenomena of polymer gels. *Advances in Polymer Science* **109**, 1–62 (1993).

72. Gabai, R. et al. Characterization of the swelling of acrylamidophenylboronic acid-acrylamide hydrogels upon interaction with glucose by faradaic impedance spectroscopy, chronopotentiometry, quartz-crystal microbalance (QCM), and surface plasmon resonance (SPR) experiments. *Journal of Physical Chemistry B* **105**, 8196–8202 (2001).

73. Murakami, Y. & Maeda, M. DNA-responsive hydrogels that can shrink or swell. *Biomacromolecules* **6**, 2927–2929 (2005).

74. Yuan, W.W., Yang, J.Y., Kopeckova, P., & Kopecek, J. Smart hydrogels containing adenylate kinase: translating substrate recognition into macroscopic motion. *Journal of the American Chemical Society* **130**, 15760–15761 (2008).

75. Alexeev, V.L. et al. High ionic strength glucose-sensing photonic crystal. *Analytical Chemistry* **75**, 2316–2323 (2003).

76. Shakhsher, Z., Seitz, W.R., & Legg, K.D. Single fiberoptic pH sensor-based on changes in reflection accompanying polymer swelling. *Analytical Chemistry* **66**, 1731–1735 (1994).

77. Holtz, J.H. & Asher, S.A. Polymerized colloidal crystal hydrogel films as intelligent chemical sensing materials. *Nature* **389**, 829–832 (1997).

78. Reese, C.E., Baltusavich, M.E., Keim, J.P., & Asher, S.A. Development of an intelligent polymerized crystalline colloidal array colorimetric reagent. *Analytical Chemistry* **73**, 5038–5042 (2001).

79. Asher, S.A., Peteu, S.F., Reese, C.E., Lin, M.X., & Finegold, D. Polymerized crystalline colloidal array chemical-sensing materials for detection of lead in body fluids. *Analytical and Bioanalytical Chemistry* **373**, 632–638 (2002).

80. Asher, S.A., Sharma, A.C., Goponenko, A.V., & Ward, M.M. Photonic crystal aqueous metal cation sensing materials. *Analytical Chemistry* **75**, 1676–1683 (2003).

81. Reese, C.E. & Asher, S.A. Photonic crystal optrode sensor for detection of Pb^{2+} in high ionic strength environments. *Analytical Chemistry* **75**, 3915–3918 (2003).

82. Alexeev, V.L., Das, S., Finegold, D.N., & Asher, S.A. Photonic crystal glucose-sensing material for noninvasive monitoring of glucose in tear fluid. *Clinical Chemistry* **50**, 2353–2360 (2004).

83. Sharma, A.C. et al. A general photonic crystal sensing motif: creatinine in bodily fluids. *Journal of the American Chemical Society* **126**, 2971–2977 (2004).

84. Ben-Moshe, M., Alexeev, V.L., & Asher, S.A. Fast responsive crystalline colloidal array photonic crystal glucose sensors. *Analytical Chemistry* **78**, 5149–5157 (2006).

85. Kimble, K.W., Walker, J.P., Finegold, D.N., & Asher, S.A. Progress toward the development of a point-of-care photonic crystal ammonia sensor. *Analytical and Bioanalytical Chemistry* **385**, 678–685 (2006).

86. Baca, J.T., Finegold, D.N., & Asher, S.A. Progress in developing polymerized crystalline colloidal array sensors for point-of-care detection of myocardial ischemia. *Analyst* **133**, 385–390 (2008).

87. Xu, M., Goponenko, A.V., & Asher, S.A. Polymerized polyHEMA photonic crystals: pH and ethanol sensor materials. *Journal of the American Chemical Society* **130**, 3113–3119 (2008).

88. Muscatello, M.M.W., Stunja, L.E., & Asher, S.A. Polymerized crystalline colloidal array sensing of high glucose concentrations. *Analytical Chemistry* **81**, 4978–4986 (2009).

89. Honda, M., Kataoka, K., Seki, T., & Takeoka, Y. Confined stimuli-responsive polymer gel in inverse opal polymer membrane for colorimetric glucose sensor. *Langmuir* **25**, 8349–8356 (2009).

90. Lee, M.C. et al. Glucose-sensitive holographic sensors for monitoring bacterial growth. *Analytical Chemistry* **76**, 5748–5755 (2004).

91. Nakayama, D., Takeoka, Y., Watanabe, M., & Kataoka, K. Simple and precise preparation of a porous gel for a colorimetric glucose sensor by a templating technique. *Angewandte Chemie (International ed. in English)* **42**, 4197–4200 (2003).

92. Millington, R.B., Mayes, A.G., Blyth, J., & Lowe, C.R. A holographic sensor for proteases. *Analytical Chemistry* **67**, 4229–4233 (1995).

93. Kabilan, S. et al. Glucose-sensitive holographic sensors. *Journal of Molecular Recognition* **17**, 162–166 (2004).

94. Bhatta, D., Christie, G., Madrigal-Gonzalez, B., Blyth, J., & Lowe, C.R. Holographic sensors for the detection of bacterial spores. *Biosensors & Bioelectronics* **23**, 520–527 (2007).

95. Tierney, S., Hjelme, D.R., & Stokke, B.T. Determination of swelling of responsive gels with nanometer resolution. Fiber-optic based platform for hydrogels as signal transducers. *Analytical Chemistry* **80**, 5086–5093 (2008).

96. Shakhsher, Z.M., Odeh, I., Jabr, S., & Seitz, W.R. An optical chemical sensor based on swellable dicarboxylate functionalized polymer microspheres for pH copper and calcium determination. *Microchimica Acta* **144**, 147–153 (2004).

97. Tierney, S., Falch, B.M.H., Hjelme, D.R., & Stokke, B.T. Determination of glucose levels using a functionalized hydrogel-optical fiber biosensor: toward continuous monitoring of blood glucose in vivo. *Analytical Chemistry* **81**, 3630–3636 (2009).

98. Tierney, S., Volden, S., & Stokke, B.T. Glucose sensors based on a responsive gel incorporated as a Fabry-Perot cavity on a fiber-optic readout platform. *Biosensors & Bioelectronics* **24**, 2034–2039 (2009).

99. Mack, N.H. et al. Optical transduction of chemical forces. *Nano Letters* **7**, 733–737 (2007).

100. Jiang, H., Markowski, J., & Sabarinathan, J. Near-infrared optical response of thin film pH-sensitive hydrogel coated on a gold nanocrescent array. *Optics Express* **17**, 21802–21807 (2009).

101. Homola, J. Surface plasmon resonance sensors for detection of chemical and biological species. *Chemical Reviews* **108**, 462–493 (2008).

102. Anker, J.N. et al. Biosensing with plasmonic nanosensors. *Nature Materials* **7**, 442–453 (2008).

103. Tokarev, I., Orlov, M., Katz, E., & Minko, S. An electrochemical gate based on a stimuli-responsive membrane associated with an electrode surface. *Journal of Physical Chemistry B* **111**, 12141–12145 (2007).

104. Wang, B., Noguchi, T., & Anzai, J.-I. Layer-by-layer thin film-coated electrodes for electrocatalytic determination of ascorbic acid. *Talanta* **72**, 415–418 (2007).

105. Chen, H.M., Huang, T.H., & Tsai, R.M. A biotin-hydrogel-coated quartz crystal microbalance biosensor and applications in immunoassay and peptide-displaying cell detection. *Analytical Biochemistry* **392**, 1–7 (2009).

106. Pogorelova, S.P., Bourenko, T., Kharitonov, A.B., & Willner, I. Selective sensing of triazine herbicides in imprinted membranes using ion-sensitive field-effect transistors and microgravimetric quartz crystal microbalance measurements. *Analyst* **127**, 1484–1491 (2002).

107. Sallacan, N., Zayats, M., Bourenko, T., Kharitonov, A.B., & Willner, I. Imprinting of nucleotide and monosaccharide recognition sites in acrylamidephenylboronic acid-acrylamide copolymer membranes associated with electronic transducers. *Analytical Chemistry* **74**, 702–712 (2002).

108. Stair, J.L., Watkinson, M., & Krause, S. Sensor materials for the detection of proteases. *Biosensors & Bioelectronics* **24**, 2113–2118 (2009).

109. Amir, L. et al. Biofuel cell controlled by enzyme logic systems. *Journal of the American Chemical Society* **131**, 826–832 (2009).

110. Nagel, B., Warsinke, A., & Katterle, M. Enzyme activity control by responsive redoxpolymers. *Langmuir* **23**, 6807–6811 (2007).

111. Singamaneni, S. et al. Bimaterial microcantilevers as a hybrid sensing platform. *Advanced Materials* **20**, 653–680 (2008).

112. Chen, G.Y., Thundat, T., Wachter, E.A., & Warmack, R.J. Adsorption-induced surface stress and its effects on resonance frequency of microcantilevers. *Journal of Applied Physics* **77**, 3618–3622 (1995).

113. Harnish, B., Robinson, J.T., Pei, Z.C., Ramstrom, O., & Yan, M.D. UV-cross-linked poly(vinylpyridine) thin films as reversibly responsive surfaces. *Chemistry of Materials* **17**, 4092–4096 (2005).

114. Sauerbrey, G. Verwendung Von Schwingquarzen Zur Wagung Dunner Schichten Und Zur Mikrowagung. *Zeitschrift Fur Physik* **155**, 206–222 (1959).

115. Alvarez, M. & Lechuga, L.M. Microcantilever-based platforms as biosensing tools. *Analyst* **135**, 827–836 (2010).

116. Hilt, J.Z., Gupta, A.K., Bashir, R., & Peppas, N.A. Ultrasensitive biomems sensors based on microcantilevers patterned with environmentally responsive hydrogels. *Biomedical Microdevices* **5**, 177–184 (2003).

117. Zhang, Y.F., Ji, H.F., Snow, D., Sterling, R., & Brown, G.M. A pH sensor based on a microcantilever coated with intelligent hydrogel. *Instrumentation Science & Technology* **32**, 361–369 (2004).

118. Abu-Lail, N.I., Kaholek, M., LaMattina, B., Clark, R.L., & Zauscher, S. Micro-cantilevers with end-grafted stimulus-responsive polymer brushes for actuation and sensing. *Sensors and Actuators. B, Chemical* **114**, 371–378 (2006).

119. Chen, T. et al. Glucose-responsive polymer brushes for microcantilever sensing. *Journal of Materials Chemistry* **20**, 3391–3395 (2010).

120. Zhou, F., Shu, W.M., Welland, M.E., & Huck, W.T.S. Highly reversible and multi-stage cantilever actuation driven by polyelectrolyte brushes. *Journal of the American Chemical Society* **128**, 5326–5327 (2006).

121. Karnati, C. et al. Organophosphorus hydrolase multilayer modified microcantilevers for organophosphorus detection. *Biosensors & Bioelectronics* **22**, 2636–2642 (2007).

122. Yan, X., Ji, H.-F., & Lvov, Y. Modification of microcantilevers using layer-by-layer nanoassembly film for glucose measurement. *Chemical Physics Letters* **396**, 34–37 (2004).

123. Kanekiyo, Y. et al. "Molecular-imprinting" of AMP utilising the polyion complex formation process as detected by a QCM system. *Journal of the Chemical Society, Perkin Transactions 2*, 2719–2722 (1999).

124. Ruan, C., Zeng, K., & Grimes, C.A. A mass-sensitive pH sensor based on a stimuli-responsive polymer. *Analytica Chimica Acta* **497**, 123–131 (2003).

125. Jain, P., Baker, G.L., & Bruening, M.L. Applications of polymer brushes in protein analysis and purification. *Annual Review of Analytical Chemistry* **2**, 387–408 (2009).

126. Hinsberg, W., Houle, F.A., Lee, S.W., Ito, H., & Kanazawa, K. Characterization of reactive dissolution and swelling of polymer films using a quartz crystal microbalance and visible and infrared reflectance spectroscopy. *Macromolecules* **38**, 1882–1898 (2005).

127. Tanaka, T. & Fillmore, D.J. Kinetics of swelling of gels. *Journal of Chemical Physics* **70**, 1214–1218 (1979).

128. Trinh, Q.T., Gerlach, G., Sorber, J., & Arndt, K.F. Hydrogel-based piezoresistive pH sensors: design, simulation and output characteristics. *Sensors and Actuators. B, Chemical* **117**, 17–26 (2006).

129. Tanaka, T. et al. Mechanical instability of gels at the phase-transition. *Nature* **325**, 796–798 (1987).

130. Orlov, M., Tokarev, I., Scholl, A., Doran, A., & Minko, S. pH-Responsive thin film membranes from poly(2-vinylpyridine): water vapor-induced formation of a microporous structure. *Macromolecules* **40**, 2086–2091 (2007).

131. Gerlach, G. et al. Application of sensitive hydrogels in chemical and pH sensors. *Macromolecular Symposia* **210**, 403–410 (2004).

132. Tokarev, I. & Minko, S. Multiresponsive, hierarchically structured membranes: new, challenging, biomimetic materials for biosensors, controlled release, biochemical gates, and nanoreactors. *Advanced Materials* **21**, 241–247 (2009).

133. Carrigan, S.D., Scott, G., & Tabrizian, M. Real-time QCM-D immunoassay through oriented antibody immobilization using cross-linked hydrogel biointerfaces. *Langmuir* **21**, 5966–5973 (2005).

134. Sannino, A., Pappad, S., Giotta, L., Valli, L., & Maffezzoli, A. Spin coating cellulose derivatives on quartz crystal microbalance plates to obtain hydrogel-based fast sensors and actuators. *Journal of Applied Polymer Science* **106**, 3040–3050 (2007).

135. Lee, Y.J., Pruzinsky, S.A., & Braun, P.V. Glucose-sensitive inverse opal hydrogels: analysis of optical diffraction response. *Langmuir* **20**, 3096–3106 (2004).

136. Kabilan, S. et al. Selective holographic glucose sensors. Proceedings of the IEEE Sensors 2004, **1–3**, 1003–1006 (2004).

137. Lang, H.P. et al. An artificial nose based on microcantilever array sensors. *Journal of Physics: Conference Series* **61**, 663–667 (2007).

138. Valiaev, A., Abu-Lail, N.I., Lim, D.W., Chilkoti, A., & Zauscher, S. Microcantilever sensing and actuation with end-grafted stimulus-responsive elastin-like polypeptides. *Langmuir* **23**, 339–344 (2007).

139. Kozlovskaya, V. et al. Ultrathin layer-by-layer hydrogels with incorporated gold nanorods as pH-sensitive optical materials. *Chemistry of Materials* **20**, 7474–7485 (2008).

CHAPTER 2

Smart Surfaces for Point-of-Care Diagnostics

MICHAEL A. NASH, ALLISON L. GOLDEN, JOHN M. HOFFMAN, JAMES J. LAI, and PATRICK S. STAYTON

2.1 INTRODUCTION

Sensitive biomarker testing can potentially help in the identification and epidemiological tracking of many diseases, as well as in monitoring patients' response to treatment.[1] The results of routine biomarker tests performed in centralized laboratories usually take several hours, sometimes days, to reach the patient from the time of sample collection.[2] Point-of-care (POC) diagnostic devices have received much attention in recent years due to the potential of these devices to address many of the current challenges in the biodiagnostics and healthcare fields.[3] With rising healthcare costs plaguing an aging medical infrastructure, POC tests are thought to be an alternative to centralized laboratory testing and a potential contributor to shortened patient stays and a general movement from inpatient to outpatient settings.

POC or "near-patient" tests are typically performed outside the central laboratory environment with very short therapeutic turnaround times. In addition to the well-utilized glucose tests, POC tests are also applicable for a wide range of clinically relevant biomarkers such as human chorionic gonadotrophin for pregnancy, cardiac markers for myocardial infarction, various infectious disease markers, and cholesterol.[4-10] Over the years, the introduction of transportable, handheld instruments has allowed POC testing to be available in a range of medical environments including the workplace, home, disaster sites, and convenience clinics.

The global market for POC tests has shown consistent growth of approximately 6% annually, a trend that is projected to continue through 2013. The POC testing market is estimated to grow from $12.8 billion in 2008 to $16.4

Intelligent Surfaces in Biotechnology: Scientific and Engineering Concepts, Enabling Technologies, and Translation to Bio-Oriented Applications, First Edition.
Edited by H. Michelle Grandin and Marcus Textor.
© 2012 John Wiley & Sons, Inc. Published 2012 by John Wiley & Sons, Inc.

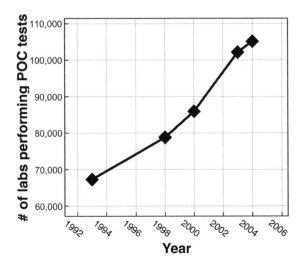

Figure 2.1   Increase in the number of laboratories with a CLIA waiver for point-of-care analytes and test systems, 1993–2004.[152] The number of labs performing near-patient rapid point-of-care tests is rapidly growing.

billion by 2013.[11] This trend is reflected in the growth in the number of labs possessing certificates of waiver from the Clinical Laboratory Improvement Amendments (CLIA) Act, shown in Figure 2.1. Such CLIA waivers are obtained by labs performing simple rapid near-patient POC tests and are indicative of the rise in POC testing in general.

2.1.1   POC Testing Challenges

Achieving clinically relevant immunoassay limits of detection for biomarkers has typically required more time-consuming methods and specialized equipment found in centralized and higher-resource laboratory facilities. In settings outside the hospital, most POC tests do not meet the quality standards offered by lab-based tests. As an example, POC tests for malaria are suitable for detecting higher levels of antigen released by parasitized red blood cells but are not adequate for the detection of low-level parasitemia common in patients from nonendemic regions with clinical disease,[12–14] or in cases of subpatient parasitemia levels that can serve as transmission reservoirs.[15,16]

A major challenge in low-cost diagnostic test development is to lower the limit of detection (LOD) of the assays toward the range of those used in hospital laboratories.[17] Specimen quality and quantity are intrinsically associated with assay performance. For example, the biomarker concentration and the specimen volume define the absolute mass quantity available for detection. The rarity of infectious disease antigens or nucleic acids in a broad sample background can lead to crippling signal-to-noise problems due to nonspecific interactions between contaminating biomolecules and device surfaces. Additionally, the rare antigens and nucleic acids themselves can be lost at various places when they are adsorbed nonspecifically to the device surfaces. Therefore, chromatography has been employed for purifying and concentrating biomarkers prior to diagnostic testing.[18,19] However, current chromatographic approaches exhibit disadvantages such as a requirement for complicated multistep protocols, costly reagents and resins, the need for refrigeration and well-equipped laboratories, and experienced lab technicians. There is a major need for a simple yet highly efficient biological sample handling platform[20] that is integrated into a simple yet highly sensitive detection module.

Additionally, POC devices are limited in use for infectious species discrimination, which can be important for correct treatment choice and monitoring.[21,22] By improving detection limits and developing multiplex assays, rapid diagnostic technologies can move to the forefront of providing accurate diagnosis across the spectrum of medical needs rather than simply providing faster results for conventional methods.

2.2 STANDARD METHODS FOR BIOMARKER PURIFICATION, ENRICHMENT, AND DETECTION

Affinity chromatography has been a mainstay in the biotechnology industry for several decades.[23] This suite of techniques employs matrix-immobilized capture molecules (e.g., protein A and antibodies) for the specific purification, enrichment, and subsequent recovery of target molecules from a biological sample. The sample solution is run through a column containing a packed solid phase with a high surface area-to-volume ratio. Alternatively, the sample solution can be contacted with the solid phase media in batch mode followed by centrifugation, washing, and recovery of the product. A variety of solid phase materials have been used, including activated gels and agarose beads, and many commercial products are available. These micro- and nanoporous affinity chromatography supports have enjoyed widespread application and success in a variety of formats despite their associated limitations. Typical affinity chromatography columns with tightly packed beads, for example, exhibit large fluidic resistance due to the tortuous fluid path through the packed media. A large fluidic resistance is associated with a high back pressure upstream of the column and therefore necessitates the use of high-pressure pumps that are not easily adapted for use in low-resource settings, such as for POC biomarker purification and enrichment.

For biomarker detection, the enzyme-linked immunosorbent assay (ELISA) has been, since its invention in the 1960s, a valuable tool in both fundamental research and clinical diagnostics.[24-26] Similar to immunoaffinity chromatography, this broad class of heterogeneous immunoassays takes advantage of the specific binding between antibodies immobilized at surfaces and antigens in the sample. Prior to the invention of ELISA, immunoassays were typically quantified using radioisotope labels that were difficult to produce and handle (e.g., iodine-131 emitting β- and γ-radiation). These radioactive immunoassay labels required specialized facilities and were associated with health risks to laboratory personnel and generation of radioactive medical waste. The arrival of ELISA with secondary antibody–enzyme conjugates as a readout reagent was welcomed because it circumvented the use of radioisotopes and could be quantified using simple spectrophotometry or fluorescence instead of a specialized radioisotope counting equipment.

Receptor–ligand binding during an ELISA must occur at a solid–liquid interface, resulting in mass transport barriers that can limit the efficiency of bioselective binding processes. ELISAs therefore suffer from slow reaction kinetics due to the presence of an unstirred surface layer that limits the flux of biomolecules to the surface. These slow reaction kinetics result in long incubation times that are unsuitable for POC applications where a fast therapeutic turnaround time is necessary. Additionally, the presence of a large solid–liquid interface in conventional ELISA means there is a large area where nonspecific binding can occur, increasing the assay noise and hurting the LOD.

These challenges faced by conventional affinity chromatography and ELISA have created a need for a simple yet robust biomarker processing, enrichment, labeling, and detection system. The need is particularly evident in the context of recent global health initiatives where simple self-powered POC assay devices and readout methods are required.[9,10] The need for integrated enrichment and detection strategies that are compatible with use in low-resource settings away from centralized laboratories is now greater than ever before.

2.3   SMART REAGENTS FOR BIOMARKER PURIFICATION AND PROCESSING

As an alternative to affinity chromatography and ELISA, over the past two and a half decades, a multitude of affinity thermoprecipitation reagents for biomarker processing and detection have been developed by our group and several others.[27–69] Synthetic polymers have been used in bioprocessing and bioseparation systems to achieve liquid-phase affinity separation of target molecules. These homogeneous separation and enrichment systems overcome the mass transport limitations associated with heterogeneous ELISA because the binding of target molecules to capture ligands occurs in solution where molecular diffusion facilitates rapid mass transport equilibration. As such, incubation times can be decreased from hours to minutes in many cases without compromising sensitivity. Since a large bulk solid phase is not present during the immunospecific capture step, nonspecific binding is minimized.

In a classical phase separation immunoassay, depicted in Figure 2.2, a stimuli-responsive polymer that is sensitive to the local environment is

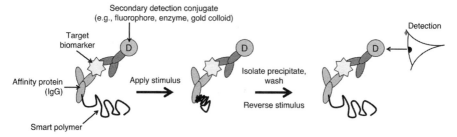

Figure 2.2 Schematic of affinity thermoprecipitation immunoassay. The smart capture reagent (e.g., IgG–pNIPAAm conjugate) and the secondary detection conjugate bind to the target biomarker, forming a sandwich immunocomplex. The stimulus (e.g., temperature and pH) is applied, causing the smart polymer to collapse and the sandwich immunocomplex to precipitate from the solution. The precipitate is isolated by centrifugation or membrane filtration, and the amount of the optical label is measured and correlated with the amount of the target biomarker.

conjugated to a targeting ligand (e.g., antibody). These single- or multi-ligand-bearing polymers are mixed with a biological sample containing the target biomarker, and a secondary detection conjugate (e.g., enzyme–antibody conjugate). After the association of the targeting ligand with the target molecule, the environmental stimulus (e.g., heat) is applied, causing the polymer to change conformation from an extended hydrated coil to a collapsed hydrophobic globule. The collapsed hydrophobic polymer chains further self-associate and undergo a time-dependent aggregation and precipitation process. A separation step (e.g., membrane filtration and centrifugation) can then be used to isolate the precipitated immunocomplex containing the target from the remaining aqueous supernatant. The amount of the secondary detection conjugate is then measured and quantitatively correlated with the amount of target biomarker in the original sample. This basic framework for smart polymer-based affinity precipitation has been utilized to separate and detect a wide range of analytes, including clinically relevant biomarkers[27,49,66,70] with analytical sensitivity comparable to conventional ELISA.

One of the most commonly used thermally responsive polymers is poly(*N*-isopropylacrylamide) (pNIPAAm). Other thermally responsive polymers include similarly structured poly(N-substituted acrylamides) (e.g., poly(N, N'-diethylacrylamide)). These thermally responsive polymers in general all contain both hydrophobic and hydrophilic characters within each monomer unit, such that the polymer is at the edge of solubility. Aqueous solutions of pNIPAAm exhibit a lower critical solution temperature (LCST) below which the pNIPAAm chains are solvated by surrounding water molecules. The driving force behind the solubility of pNIPAAm below the LCST is an exothermic enthalpy change due to hydrogen bonding of water molecules to the amide groups of the N-isopropylacrylamide (NIPAAm) monomer units. The competing force favoring polymer collapse is the caged or clathrate-like water surrounding the hydrophobic isopropyl groups, which are unable to form hydrogen bonds with the polymer. These sequestered water molecules result in decreased system entropy. The LCST is reached when the unfavorable confined entropy of water around the isopropyl groups overcomes the favorable enthalpy of hydrogen bonding to the amide groups. The LCST signals the polymer's transition from soluble to collapsed, which proceeds rapidly as an endothermic process driven by the balance between hydrogen bonding and entropy gain due to the release of caged water molecules.[71]

Experimentally, the LCST is measured by observing a rapid increase in turbidity over a few degrees Celsius due to scattering of light by the large polymer aggregates. Some of the earliest reports on pNIPAAm solution properties used such "cloud-point" measurements to determine the LCST[31], and this method remains today the easiest method for determining a polymer's LCST. The LCST is not strongly dependent on the concentration of the polymer provided it is not too dilute.[71] The molecular weight of the polymer also has little effect on LCST; however, smaller polymer molecular weights may correspond with broader cloud-point curves. Figure 2.3 shows a typical cloud-point curve, where percent response is measured by spectrophotometric optical density (i.e., solution turbidity). After smart polymer collapse, the stimulus can be reversed, causing rehydration of the collapsed polymers; however, the rate of smart polymer rehydration is often much slower than the rate of aggregation because water molecules must permeate into the entangled polymer aggregates, which requires time.

Several environmental stimuli in addition to heat have been used to trigger smart polymer phase transitioning, including pH[28,55,70,72–77] and light.[52] NIPAAm

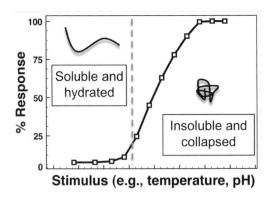

Figure 2.3   Diagram of smart polymer phase transition. A smart polymer undergoes a conformational change from a hydrophilic random coil to a hydrophobic globule upon a small change in an environmental stimulus. Poly(N-isopropylacrylamide) is a thermally responsive polymer with a lower critical solution temperature (LCST) of ~32°C. Smart polymers can be conjugated to proteins and nanoparticles to confer their phase transition behavior to the biohybrid macromolecules.

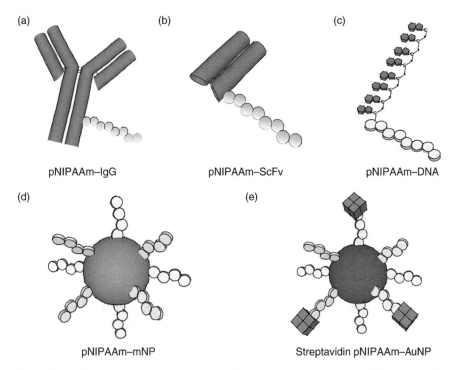

(a)   (b)   (c)

pNIPAAm–IgG   pNIPAAm–ScFv   pNIPAAm–DNA

(d)   (e)

pNIPAAm–mNP   Streptavidin pNIPAAm–AuNP

Figure 2.4 Examples of smart reagents for biomarker detection. The thermally responsive polymer chains are depicted as repeating yellow disks in each schematic of the biohybrid reagent. (a) pNIPAAm-conjugated mono- or polyclonal immunoglobulin G (IgG). (b) pNIPAAm-conjugated single-chain antibody variable segment (ScFv). (c) pNIPAAm-conjugated nucleic acid (e.g., DNA and RNA). (d) pNIPAAm-conjugated magnetic nanoparticle (mNP) and (e) streptavidin–pNIPAAm-conjugated gold nanoparticle (AuNP). (See color insert.)

monomers can be copolymerized with monomers that contain titratable groups (e.g., amine and carboxyl), and the ionization state and hydrophilicity of the comonomers will modulate the LCST properties of NIPAAm copolymers. This approach has been used to produce polymers that are both pH and temperature responsive.[68,78]

For applications in biomarker processing and detection, hybrid bioconjugates of thermally responsive polymers and targeting ligands (e.g., antibodies and nucleotides) are typically prepared. Figure 2.4 shows schematic diagrams of some commonly used smart conjugates for applications in biodetection. Protein–polymer conjugates can be prepared such that there are multiple proteins per polymer, or multiple polymers per protein, depending on the polymerization and bioconjugation techniques used. Smart polymers can be synthesized with a variety of polymerization techniques (e.g., reversible addition–fragmentation chain transfer [RAFT] and atom transfer radical polymerization [ATRP]) to produce polymers with telechelic or semitelechelic functional groups, or alternatively pendant amine-reactive or sulfhydral-reactive groups along the backbone of the polymer. These functional groups can be randomly or site-specifically conjugated to functional groups on proteins using conventional bioconjugation techniques such as carbodiimide coupling or maleimide chemistry.

2.3.1   IgG Antibody–pNIPAAm Conjugates

In one of the earliest demonstrations of a simple enzyme-based phase separation immunoassay, Auditore-Hargreaves et al.[27] prepared an IgG–pNIPAAm conjugate that was used in conjunction with a peroxidase-conjugated secondary antibody to detect hepatitis B surface antigen (HB-Ag) in human serum samples. The authors first prepared an N-hydroxysuccinimide (NHS) ester of 4-vinylbenzoic acid, which was randomly conjugated to amine groups on the IgG antibody. NIPAAm monomers were then copolymerized with the vinyl benzoate-conjugated antibodies resulting in antibody-conjugated pNIPAAm. After the sandwich immunocomplex was formed in solution, the temperature was increased above the polymer LCST, causing precipitation of the polymer and coprecipitation of the associated antigen and enzyme-labeled secondary antibody. After centrifugation and removal of the unbound enzyme-conjugated secondary antibody, the immunoassay result was quantified by colorimetric or fluorescent substrate development and measurement by an absorbance/fluorescence reader. These results demonstrated sensitive detection limits for the HB-Ag around 0.5–1.0 ng/mL, depending on the type of substrate used.

Another early example of a phase separation immunoassay was reported by Chen and Hoffman[30] The authors prepared a conjugate of protein A and pNIPAAm and used it to deplete fluorescently labeled human IgG from solution. The authors began by preparing a ca. 24-kDa random copolymer of N-acryloxy succinimide and NIPAAm and found that the polymer had ~5.5 active ester groups per polymer. The copolymer was then randomly conjugated to lysine amine groups on protein A, which complexed with human IgG in solution due to the affinity between protein A and the Fc region of the IgG antibody. The sample was then heated and centrifuged to separate the complexed IgG molecules. In the study by Chen et al.,[30] nonconjugated free pNIPAAm polymer was included in the reaction mixture as a precipitation aid. Free polymer additives result in larger aggregates as compared with aggregated solutions without free polymer. Such additives are important in smart separations that depend on aggregate size (e.g., centrifugation and magnetic separation).

In other early studies using antibody–pNIPAAm conjugates, Monji et al. expanded the format of the standard phase separation immunoassay by demonstrating how the centrifugation step could be circumvented using membrane filtration of the aggregates.[48,66] The authors performed a conventional phase separation immunoassay except that, after applying the thermal stimulus, the sample solution was flowed through a microporous membrane using vacuum suction. When heated, the smart polymer conjugates above the LCST formed large aggregates that did not pass through the porous filters with appropriately chosen pore sizes. After flow through the membrane, the fluorescence of the membrane surface was measured to quantify the amount of antigen in the starting sample. In the absence of the antigen, the labeled secondary antibodies with fluorescein or R-phycoerythrin dyes flowed through the membrane and were not strongly accumulated, which provided a low background. The authors demonstrated an assay for human IgM that was linear across an analyte range from 0 to 50 ng/mL using an R-phycoerythrin fluorescently labeled secondary antibody.

2.3.2 Single-Chain Antibody–pNIPAAm Conjugates

Single-chain antibody Fv fragments (ScFvs) are small fusion proteins of IgG heavy (V_H) and light (V_L) chains that exhibit similar bioactivity and specific binding to antigens as the parent IgG molecule. Whole IgG antibody production in eukaryotic organisms (e.g., yeast) is oftentimes difficult, requiring expensive and complicated handling, culture, analysis, and storage. ScFv fragments are easily genetically modified and expressed in *Echerichia coli* and in many cases can be expressed in the folded state.

There have been several reports on the use of ScFv antibodies in pNIPAAm-based affinity thermoprecipitation. Fong et al.[37] reported the expression and conjugation of an ScFv fragment targeting hen egg white lysozymes. After polyhistidine tag purification of the ScFv fragment in *E. coli*, the authors randomly conjugated an 8.5 kDa pNIPAAm with a semitelechelic N-hydroxysuccinimidyl ester group to the N-terminus and lysine amine groups on the ScFv. The authors demonstrated 80% depletion of 10 nM fluorescently labeled hen egg white lysozyme spiked in samples of 10% bovine serum.

In a related work, Kumar et al.[61] demonstrated purification of polyhistidine-tagged ScFv antibodies from *E. coli* cell culture supernatants using metal chelate affinity thermoprecipitation. They produced a 161 kDa copolymer containing ~15% 1-vinylimidazole and ~85% NIPAAm. The copolymer was then loaded with Cu(II) or Ni(II) ions in aqueous solution. After purifying the metal ion-loaded polymers by threefold thermal precipitation, they used the metal chelates to bind extracellularly expressed His_6-ScFv antibody fragments. The precipitation of the His_6-ScFv fragments was found to be strongly pH dependent, with optimum precipitation in the range of pH 6.0–7.0 for the Cu(II)-loaded copolymers and pH 7.0–8.0 for the Ni(II)-loaded copolymers. At these optimum pH values, the authors reported 80–90% precipitation of the target ScFv fragments, which were present in the *E. coli* culture supernatants at ~24 µg/mL. After thermoprecipitation, the captured protein was recovered by elution with 50 mM EDTA buffer at pH 8.0.

2.3.3 Nucleotide–pNIPAAm Conjugates

Covalent conjugates of pNIPAAm and DNA have been reported and used by several groups for affinity thermoprecipitation and purification of nucleotides. For example, Costioli et al.[79] demonstrated how a pNIPAAm-DNA reagent could be used for the purification of plasmid DNA via triple-helix affinity thermoprecipitation. After the capture of the plasmid and the redissolution of the complex below the LCST, the target plasmid DNA was released by increasing the pH. The authors reported capture efficiencies between 70% and 90%, while nonspecific capture was below 7%. Safak et al.[80] demonstrated how a similar reagent comprising a block copolymer of DNA and pNIPAAm could be used for the purification of polymerase chain reaction (PCR) products. The authors prepared a 6-kDa synthetic pNIPAAm segment blocked with a 1147-base pair nucleic acid segment. In a related work, Mori and Maeda[81] prepared a graft copolymer of NIPAAm and DNA and showed how the pNIPAAm-g-DNA reagent formed stable colloidal particles above the LCST. They further showed how the graft copolymer could be used to discriminate between target DNA and single base pair point mutant DNA by observing the change in pNIPAAm particle light scattering upon hybridization to the target sequence.

Fong et al.[38] used complementary DNA base pairing for the noncovalent attachment of pNIPAAm to streptavidin. They prepared a linear 8.5 kDa pNIPAAm with a semitelechelic NHS ester group that was used for conjugation to an amine-terminated 20 mer of DNA. The complementary DNA sequence was site-specifically conjugated to a streptavidin E116C mutant. The complementary DNA sequences on the polymer and streptavidin molecules underwent sequence-specific hybridization and allowed the affinity thermoprecipitation of biotinylated alkaline phosphatase and tritiated biotin.

2.3.4 Magnetic Nanoparticle (mNP)–pNIPAAm Conjugates

mNPs are commonly used in bioseparation, enrichment, and detection,[82–84] and more recently have also been applied to POC diagnostics.[85,86] Small magnetizable particles (e.g., iron oxide) act as single-domain net magnetic dipoles and experience an applied magnetic force in the presence of a magnetic field gradient. The separability of a particular mNP species is a function of many physical parameters, including the magnetic dipole moment, diffusion coefficient, hydrodynamic drag coefficient, and the field gradient. These particles are superparamagnetic and, as such, retain no residual magnetization after the magnetic field has been removed. This property is advantageous because after magnetic capture/enrichment has taken place, the particles do not remain magnetically agglomerated but can disaggregate into a carrier fluid and remain soluble.

During the magnetic separation step, the target protein is removed from a complex sample matrix containing proteins and lipids that may cause interference in conventional POC immunoassay. For example, in lateral-flow immunochromatography, a high-dose "hook" effect can occur when excess sample antigen occupies the binding sites on the solid phase, preventing the gold-labeled antigen from binding.[87] This effect can confound the results of conventional assays because it results in lower signal strength at high antigen concentrations. Magnetic separation eliminates the high-dose hook effect because only bound antigen molecules are separated and applied to the flow strip. Magnetic separation/enrichment of the sample can therefore not only increase the sensitivity of immunoassays but can also eliminate sample matrix-derived interferences.

Typically, mNPs may be used in concentration/enrichment style immunoassays, wherein specific targeting ligands (e.g., antibodies) are bound to the magnetic carrier and act as a primary capture antibody. These primary antibody–mNP conjugates bind the target biomarker in the sample and may also nonspecifically bind other target proteins in the sample. A secondary detection conjugate comprising an antibody that has been labeled using an enzyme, fluorophore, nanoparticle, or other optical label is bound to a secondary epitope on the target biomarker, and the sandwich immunocomplex is separated using a magnetic field. The amount of separated label can then be quantitatively correlated with the amount of target biomarker in the original sample. In this style of immunoassay, micron-scale particles consisting of polymeric microbeads impregnated with iron oxide nanoparticles are often used.[88,89] Biological media are not susceptible to the magnetic field and therefore are not separated, although some residual nonspecific binding of proteins to the mNPs and walls of the carrying vessel will occur. Due to these unique physical properties and associated advantages, separation/enrichment of mNPs and surface-bound ligands has developed into a major bioprocessing technology.

Recently, several groups have reported the synthesis, characterization, and/or use of pNIPAAm-coated mNP in biodiagnostics and bioseparation applications.[43,44,50,51,90–97] A unique feature of pNIPAAm-coated mNPs that distinguishes them from conventional magnetic microparticle technologies is their thermally triggered magnetophoretic behavior. Above the LCST, polymer-induced flocculation of pNIPAAm-coated mNPs increases the effective particle size "seen" by the magnetic field, resulting in rapid magnetophoresis of the aggregates. This property allows for the use of very small pNIPAAm-coated magnetic particles for affinity separations while still preserving their ability to be magnetically separated.

Particle size considerations are important in designing magnetic particle capture systems for biodiagnostics. Small particles (<100 nm) are desirable in affinity separations because their small size enables rapid diffusive mixing and binding to the target analyte. Additionally, smaller particles have higher specific surface area per gram. However, small particles are typically difficult to separate using modest magnetic fields because thermal diffusion dominates over the miniscule magnetic forces applied to the small magnetic dipoles of the individual solvated particles. Grafting or stabilizing the mNPs with pNIPAAm overcomes this size limitation on the separability because after binding to the target, polymer-induced aggregation of the particles can be used to increase the effective magnetophoretic mobility and to overcome thermal diffusion. The thermally triggered magnetophoresis[43,44,51,90–93,98] of pNIPAAm-functionalized mNPs has been reported by several groups, and such particles are also sold commercially.

Several groups have used pNIPAAm mNPs for affinity separations of cells and proteins. For example, Furukawa et al.[90] prepared a thermally responsive copolymer of pNIPAAm and a biotin-containing monomer. The magnetic particles were used in conjugation with avidin and biotinylated IgG antibodies for the targeted separation of yeast cells. Narain et al.[50] prepared oleic acid-functionalized mNPs (10 nm in diameter) and performed a ligand exchange reaction with a 22 kDa pNIPAAm that had been functionalized with a semitelechelic biotin group using maleimide chemistry. The resulting particles were found to bind streptavidin with high affinity when the streptavidin was free in solution or bound to the surface of a Biacore SPR chip.

Lai et al.[43] developed a straightforward method for preparing small (<10 nm) pNIPAAm-modified mNPs in a single step. The authors prepared an amphiphilic pNIPAAm copolymer (5 or 15 kDa) that contained a semitelechelic dodecyl hydrocarbon group that directed the polymers to form micelles in aqueous buffers and polar solvents. The authors loaded the micelle cores with iron pentacarbonyl, which thermally decomposed when the temperature was raised to 190°C, resulting in the formation of pNIPAAm-modified iron oxide nanoparticles. X-ray diffraction and Mössbauer spectroscopy on the particles demonstrated that they were made from γ-Fe$_2$O$_3$ (maghemite). These particles were ~5 nm in diameter and exhibited a thermally triggered magnetophoretic behavior, as reported for pNIPAAm-modified mNPs prepared through other synthetic routes.

2.3.5   Gold Nanoparticle (AuNP)–pNIPAAm Conjugates

AuNPs have become a major contributing technology in the biodiagnostics field due to their unique nanoscopic physical and chemical properties. Although bulk gold is nominally an "expensive" precious metal, only minute amounts of metal are typically used at low concentrations in diagnostics assays, making colloidal gold conjugates very affordable for use in biosensing. AuNPs can be prepared in bulk quantities with very narrow size distributions (<10% standard deviation [SD]) and are readily functionalized with affinity ligands through a variety of conjugation schemes, including thiol chemisorption and nonspecific protein adsorption. Additionally, AuNPs are stable for long periods of time and can be stored in a dry format and later rehydrated with good preservation of specific binding activity.

The intense red color of AuNPs is attributable to the interaction of free conduction band electrons in the metal with an oscillating electrical field provided by the incoming incident light. The collective oscillation of the electrons, known as localized surface plasmon resonance (LSPR), results in the particles acting as antennas for incoming light, which is absorbed or scattered by the particles with extremely high efficiency. The electromagnetic field at the surface of AuNPs is enhanced by a factor of 10^6 or more.[99] This enhanced near-field is the basis for many surface-enhanced spectroscopic techniques, including surface-enhanced Raman spectroscopy,[100,101] and surface-enhanced fluorescence,[102,103] both of which have been adapted to sensitive biological sensing applications.[104,105]

The particle extinction coefficient depends on the size and shape of the AuNPs, as well as the dielectric constant of the solvent. A typical extinction coefficient for 20 nM AuNPs is ~10^9 M/cm, while that of 80 nm AuNPs is ~10^{10} M/cm. With such high extinction coefficients, which are four to five orders of magnitude larger than typical organic dyes,[106] high-sensitivity detection can be achieved using AuNP reagents without the need for advanced optical instrumentation. This remarkable optical extinction property is a major driver of the use of AuNPs in POC biodetection applications.

The peak wavelength of the LSPR is extremely sensitive to the interparticle distance. When AuNPs come within 1.0–1.5 particle diameters of each other, the electric dipoles induced by the incident electromagnetic field experience plasmonic coupling, resulting in a shift of the LSPR to lower energies (longer wavelengths). This plasmonic red shift has been exploited in biodetection assays[107,108] in which the presence of a target molecule (e.g., nucleotide and protein) causes agglutination of AuNPs that have been functionalized with a biospecific recognition molecule, resulting in a color change from red to purple.

pNIPAAm-functionalized AuNPs have received increased attention in recent years for use in tunable plasmonic devices and for biodetection. Several groups have reported that the red shift of the LSPR can be controlled via smart polymer-induced aggregation. For example, Zhu et al.[109] prepared a 4.6 kDa pNIPAAm with a semitelechelic thiol group and used the polymer to functionalize 13-nm AuNPs. They reported that upon application of a thermal stimulus, the LSPR was red shifted from 527 to 566 nm. In addition to a red shift in the optical resonance, polymer-induced aggregation also resulted in an increase in solution turbidity and Rayleigh scattering from the aggregates. Yusa et al.[110] prepared a similar smart pNIPAAm–AuNP conjugate by end modifying a semitelechelic trithiocarbonate polymer end group to produce pNIPAAm with a terminal thiol. This polymer was adsorbed onto citrate-capped AuNPs, and the plasmonic red shift was measured as the solution temperature was raised above the polymer LCST. The authors reported a plasmon shift from 523 to 580 nm and also showed how increasing NaCl could be used to decrease the critical plasmonic red shift temperature.

In addition to thiol functionalized polymers, polymers incorporating amine groups can also be used to stabilize pre-extant AuNPs or alternatively can be used to catalytically self-assemble polymer-functionalized AuNPs *in situ* by utilizing the ability of tertiary amine groups to reduce Au^{3+} to Au^0 at basic pH. Using this approach, Li et al.[111] synthesized a diblock copolymer containing NIPAAm and 2-(dimethylamino)ethyl methacrylate and mixed the polymer with NaAuCl$_4$ at 50°C. They found that such a reaction resulted in *in situ* reduction of the gold ions by the polymer and in self-assembly of gold-decorated vesicles that exhibited similar stimuli responsiveness of the dual pH/temperature-responsive diblock copolymers. These authors reported that the thiol group functionality was not necessary for successful modification of AuNPs when amine-containing polymers were used.

Further pursuing amine-containing polymers as dual reductants and colloidal stabilizing agents, Nash et al.[51] prepared a diblock copolymer of NIPAAm and 2-(dimethylamino) ethyl acrylamide. This diblock copolymer was used to stabilize iron oxide nanoparticles through a thermal decomposition of iron pentacarbonyl precursors. After purification of the mNP reagent, it was found that the ability of the amine-containing polymer to reduce gold cations was retained and conferred to the mNPs. This allowed for *in situ* reduction of gold anions onto the mNP cores, forming core–shell nanoparticles that exhibited both the magnetic properties of the iron oxide, and the optical extinction of the gold. However, the obtained particle mixtures were found to be heterogeneous in size and Au/Fe ratio, which limited applications in diagnostic assays.

Very few reports are found in the current literature describing the use of pNIPAAm-functionalized AuNPs in a biodetection assay. Although Uehara et al.[112] reported a homogeneous colorimetric assay for glutathione based on the color change of a pNIPAAm-functionalized AuNP reagent, their assay did not rely on the thermal phase transition of the pNIPAAm itself. They prepared a water-soluble pNIPAAm-co-acryloyldiethyletriamine random copolymer and used it to functionalize citrate-stabilized AuNPs. The sol was not colloidally stable and therefore a red-shited LSPR was observed. Upon addition of glutathione, the polymers were liberated from the particles resulting in a blue shift of the LSPR back to ~520 nm. The thermal phase transition of the pNIPAAm chains was therefore not an important aspect of the reported assay.

2.4 SAMPLE-PROCESSING MODULES FOR SMART CONJUGATE BIOASSAYS

A variety of sample-processing modules have been utilized in conjunction with the aforementioned smart conjugate reagents in bioassays to isolate, purify, and detect clinically relevant biomarkers and/or model protein analytes (e.g., streptavidin). Bulk centrifugation and removal of the sample supernatant is a common and straightforward method to enrich and purify target biomarkers bound to thermally precipitated conjugates of smart polymers and affinity proteins (e.g., pNIPAAm–IgG conjugates).[27,77] This method, however, is not readily adapted for use in low-resource POC testing because it requires an experienced technician and the use of a high-speed centrifuge. Centrifugation is not easily incorporated into microfludic devices, although recent progress in this area[113,114] may offer new microfluidic-based centrifugal sample-processing modules for smart conjugate bioassays in the future.

In addition to bulk centrifugation, microfluidic sample-processing modules have been utilized in conjunction with microfabricated heating elements to achieve localized heating and capture of smart reagents in predefined regions of microchannels. Malmstadt et al.,[45,47] for example, showed that latex nanobeads comodified with pNIPAAm and biotinylated poly(ethylene glycol) (PEG) could be reversibly immobilized in heated regions of poly(laminate) microfluidic devices. Biotinylated monoclonal antidigoxin antibodies were attached to the latex nanobeads via streptavidin linkage. The antibody-functionalized beads were then reversibly immobilized in a heated region of the microchannel through nonspecific hydrophobic polymer adhesion to the poly(ethylene terephthalate) (PET) microfluidic channel walls. This format allowed for capture reagent immobilization in a specified region of the device immediately prior to the analytical measurement. The approach was developed into a competitive fluorescent immunoassay for digoxin with micromolar sensitivity.

In this early work on microfluidic-based smart nanobead capture, the microdevice surfaces were not modified with a smart polymer. The surface hydrophobicity was sufficient to accommodate polymer adhesion and nanobead immobilization above the LCST. More recent studies[35,115–117] have focused on smart conjugate bioassays in which the device surfaces themselves, in addition to the capture reagents, have been modified with smart polymers, as depicted in Figure 2.5. Approaches relying on modified device surfaces have an advantage in that rehydration of the surface-grafted polymers upon cooling the device below the LCST can facilitate conjugate release from the capture surface.

2.4.1   Grafting of pNIPAAm from Microchannel Surfaces

Microfluidic platforms have a demonstrated potential for applications in clinical diagnostics and in POC settings.[10,118] Unfortunately, the potential of this technology has not been fully realized and several challenges remain. One important outstanding need is the purification and enrichment of dilute biomarkers from complex biological fluids.[119] The use of smart polymer–protein conjugates together with smart polymer-grafted microchannel surfaces has emerged as a viable approach to address these deficiencies in the microfluidics field.

Numerous materials have been used to construct microfluidic devices, including glass, PET, and poly(dimethylsiloxane) (PDMS). PDMS is commonly used in microfluidics research due to the ease with which PDMS devices can be rapidly prototyped on a laboratory scale. The utility of PDMS is compromised by its hydrophobicity and chemical inertness; channels are difficult to wet with aqueous solutions and proteins nonspecifically bind to the surface. Organic solvents, meanwhile, partition and diffuse into bulk PDMS[120]. In general, this property is considered a limitation of PDMS and makes it unsuitable in applications that require the use of organic solvents in microfluidic

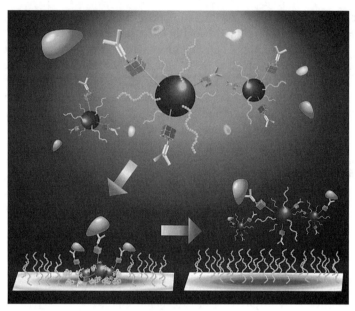

Figure 2.5 Design concept for a microfluidic system that utilizes smart nanobeads having both smart polymers and antibodies on the surface. The microchannel walls are also modified with the smart polymers to allow the trapping of smart nanobeads above the LCST. First, suspended smart beads are loaded into the microfluidic channel together with the sample to allow for capture of the target biomarker (top). Next, the stimulus (e.g., heat) is applied to collapse the smart polymers at selected locations in the channel and to capture selectively the smart nanobeads to achieve fractionation, purification, and enrichment of the target molecules (lower left). Finally, the surface is cooled below the LCST to release the captured beads into the flow stream for downstream analysis (lower right). Reproduced from Ebara et al.[35] by permission from the Royal Society of Chemistry. (See color insert.)

devices. However, the bulk partitioning of solvents into PDMS has in some cases been exploited for applications in two-phase fluidic systems, for example, where one phase can be selectively extracted into the channel walls.[121] The hydrophobic partitioning of small organic molecules into PDMS can also be exploited to functionalize specific regions of PDMS microchannels with free radical initiators that can initiate polymerization from the surface.

In the work by Malmstadt et al.,[45,47] the aggregated smart nanobeads showed relatively uneven distributions on the channel walls. Additionally, the release of the captured beads upon cooling below the LCST was found to be incomplete because some beads were not able to detach from the channel sidewalls. These effects led to heterogeneous adsorption and desorption kinetics that compromised analytical performance. These limitations led to the development of complementary surface traps that could be applied to PDMS and other polymeric microdevice surfaces.[35,115,116] The surface traps were constructed by grafting pNIPAAm to the PDMS channel walls, which then provided a switchable surface that worked in concert with the smart conjugate reagents (e.g., pNIPAAm nanobeads or IgG–pNIPAAm conjugates) to produce more uniform adsorption/desorption profiles, resulting in higher capture and release efficiencies and more reproducible analytical measurements.

To modify PDMS device surfaces, Ebara et al.[115] used ultraviolet (UV)-mediated grafting of pNIPAAm from PDMS. The protocol for this method is described in Methods Box 2.1. A UV-activated hydrogen-abstracting initiator (benzophenone) was reacted with pendant methyl groups at the PDMS channel surface, resulting in the formation of free radicals that initiated the polymerization of monomers in solution. This polymerization technique was shown to be versatile and allowed for surface grafting of a wide range of vinyl-containing monomers, including temperature-responsive NIPAAm monomers, pH-responsive acrylic acid monomers, and nonfouling PEG monomers to prevent nonspecific adsorption to the PDMS. This work also showed that surface grafting of PEG from microchannel surfaces reduces pNIPAAm conjugate surface capture.

In general, UV graft polymerization is a highly attractive method for surface modification of microfluidic devices, particularly when the surfaces have no chemically reactive groups. UV irradiation generates free radicals at the channel surface, despite the absence of organic functional groups available for conjugation of initiators. Also, UV graft polymerization can be spatially patterned through lithographic masking, permitting control of functionalization within specific regions of the microdevice. Ebara et al.[35,115] showed that the polymer graft density could be controlled by irradiation time and that the

---

METHODS BOX 2.1   MODIFYING PDMS WITH SMART POLYMERS

Benzophenone is dissolved in acetone (20%) and flowed through a PDMS microfluidic channel for approximately 1 minute, allowing sufficient time for the acetone/benzophenone mixture to diffuse into the channel walls. The channel is then washed with water. An aqueous solution containing the vinylated monomer (e.g., NIPAAm, 10%), NalO$_4$ (0.5 mM), and benzyl alcohol (0.5 wt %) is loaded into the channel and irradiated with a broad spectrum UV lamp (2.95 mW/cm^2 at 365 nm) for 15 minutes under stopped flow. The channel is then washed extensively with water, resulting in a pNIPAAm-grafted microchannel surface. PEG and poly(acrylic acid)-grafted surfaces can be prepared using the same protocol by substituting PEG–acrylate or acrylic acid for NIPAAm in the monomer solution.

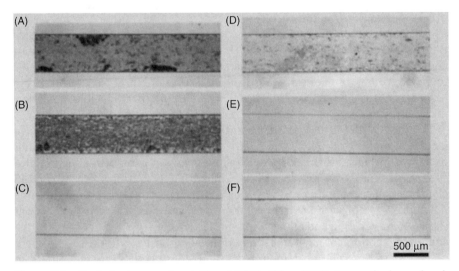

Figure 2.6   Optical micrographs at 40 and 20°C of the pNIPAAm-grafted nanobeads on the channel surfaces of ungrafted (A,D), pNIPAAm-grafted (B,E), and PEG-grafted (C,F) PDMS microfluidic channels. The beads were flowed through the channel for 5 minutes at 40°C and then were rinsed for 5 minutes at 20°C (D–F). The pNIPAAm-grafted microchannels show the most uniform capture and sharp/complete release. Reproduced from Ebara et al.[35] by permission from the Royal Society of Chemistry.

molecular weight of the polymer surface grafts was influenced by the concentration of the photosensitizer benzophenone.

UV-initiated polymer grafting from PDMS surfaces was demonstrated as a means to modulate interactions between the channel walls and the smart nanobeads. When the channel temperature was raised above the LCST of pNIPAAm, the beads flowing through the channel aggregated and adhered to the walls of the pNIPAAm-modified channel, while the PEG-grafted PDMS did not show a trapping effect. The smart nanobeads adhered more uniformly to pNIPAAm-grafted PDMS than to bare PDMS. When the temperature was reversed back below the LCST, the pNIPAAm beads detached quickly and eluted from the pNIPAAm-grafted channel walls completely, as shown in Figure 2.6. When the same experiment was performed with unmodified PDMS or unmodified PET devices, some beads were not eluted, even under high shear conditions. These results demonstrated that the pNIPAAm surface traps achieve more uniform adsorption and desorption profiles as compared with bare PDMS, which is crucial for performing reproducible analytical bioassays.

2.4.2   Grafting of pNIPAAm from Porous Membranes

Flow-through micro- and nanoporous membranes have a long history in biomolecule capture, separation, and detection. Lateral-flow immunochromatography devices made from nonwoven materials such as nitrocellulose, for example, are widely manufactured and sold to consumers. Such membranes have large surface area-to-volume ratios allowing efficient capture of biomolecules that are transported through the membrane via convective fluid flow.

Porous membranes incorporating surface-grafted smart polymers have also been used in the bioseparations field to perform separations on the basis of porosity, hydrophobicity, or surface accessibility (Methods Box 2.2).[122–131] Smart grafted membranes are particularly appealing when used jointly with smart conjugate reagents such as IgG–pNIPAAm conjugates. The synergistic switching of responsive membrane surfaces in concert with the switching of smart conjugate reagents in solution can be used to direct separation and enrichment of target biomarkers bound to the smart capture reagents at the membrane surface. For example, porous temperature-responsive pNIPAAm-grafted membrane surfaces can serve as microchannel-compatible concentrators of pNIPAAm-conjugated antibodies and their biomarker targets when heated. After capture and/or detection at the membrane surface, the smart polymers can be switched off by lowering the temperature below the LCST to facilitate release of the bound biomarkers for further downstream processing.

Golden et al.[117] developed a system of smart antibody conjugates and porous grafted membranes for the purpose of separating and concentrating immunocomplexes within a microfluidic channel. The concentrator system consisted of two stimuli-responsive modules: (i) a porous membrane and (ii) smart antibody conjugates. Above the LCST, hydrophobic polymer–polymer interaction directed the capture of antibody conjugates with bound ligands at the membrane. Upon lowering the temperature, the transition to a hydrophilic state rapidly ejected the bound polymer conjugates into the flow stream, resulting in a sharp immunoconjugate release profile.

To prepare the responsive porous membranes, Golden et al.[117] modified hydroxyl groups on nylon membranes with a trithiocarbonate-containing chain transfer agent (CTA) via Steglich esterification. pNIPAAm chains were then grafted from the CTA-conjugated membranes using RAFT polymerization, as shown in Figure 2.7. The molar ratio of CTA to initiator during the polymerization was kept at 5:1. The solution polymer was retained and its polydispersity was compared to that of the membrane-grafted polymer.

One advantage of the conjugation scheme used by Golden et al.[117] was that the polymers were conjugated to the nylon membranes by a relatively labile ester bond. These ester bonds could be cleaved by base hydrolysis, enabling direct purification and characterization of the surface-grafted polymers. After base hydrolysis for 1 hour using 1N sodium hydroxide at 70°C, recovered and purified product obtained from approximately 3 cm^2 of membrane yielded milligram quantities of a soluble polymer product. The polymer chains cleaved from the membranes were dissolved in dimethylformamide and characterized using gel permeation chromatography (GPC) to determine their number average molecular weight (Mn). In comparison to the polymers obtained from the solution-based polymerization, the polydispersity index (PDI) of the surface-grafted polymers was found to be slightly larger. PDIs of 1.2–1.4 were

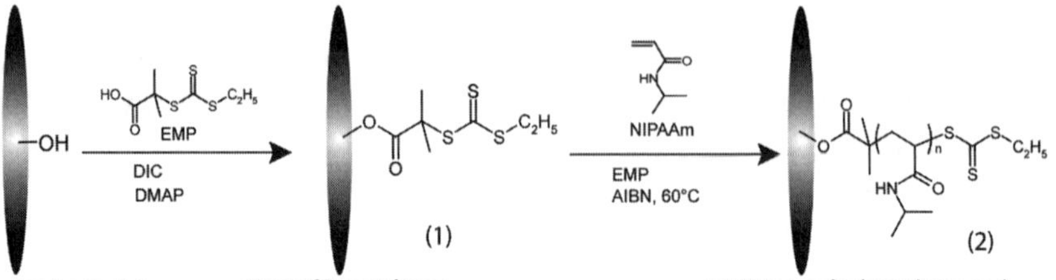

(1)   (2)

Hydroxylated nylon 6,6   Macro-CTA membrane   pNIPAAm-grafted membrane and
(LoProdyne, Pall)   solution pNIPAAm

Figure 2.7 Synthesis of pNIPAAm-polymerized membranes. Membranes were prepared by first coupling the RAFT chain transfer agent (CTA) via esterification to produce a macro-CTA membrane (1). Next, the membrane was immersed in a RAFT-mediated polymerization of NIPAAm with additional CTA and free radical initiator to yield a solution-phase homopolymer and a covalently linked surface polymer. Reproduced from Golden et al.[117] by permission from the American Chemical Society.

METHODS BOX 2.2   MODIFYING POROUS MEMBRANES WITH SMART POLYMERS

Membranes with grafted pNIPAAm are prepared by combining the RAFT CTA 2-ethylsulfanylthiocarbonylsulfanyl-2-methyl propionic acid (EMP, 100 mM), diisopropylcarbodiimide (DIC, 100 mM), and dimethylamino-pyridine (DMAP, 10 mM) in 10 mL anhydrous dimethylformamide (DMF) and the mixture to a vacuum-dried LoProdyne nylon membrane. The reaction is stirred for 48 hours at room temperature. Membranes are then washed in acetone and ethanol, dried by vacuum at room temperature, and stored under ambient conditions. The membrane with bound CTA is then immersed in a solution-phase RAFT polymerization reaction containing the EMP CTA (13.2 or 40 mmol), N-isopropylacrylamide monomer (0.2 g/mL), and azobisisobutyronitrile initiator (2.7 or 8 mmol) in DMF. Following purging the vessel with N_2, polymerization proceeds at 60°C for 18–24 hours. Membranes are then removed and washed extensively with acetone and ethanol, and dialyzed for 48 hours at 4°C with several changes of deionized water to remove noncovalently adsorbed or entangled polymer.

---

obtained for the polymer surface grafts, while PDIs of the solution-based polymers were ~1.2.

The temperature-sensitive surface was designed to provide a thin, flow-through platform to capture antibodies and targets and to release them rapidly upon change of stimulus, as shown in Figure 2.8. The RAFT-mediated pNIPAAm modification of the porous membrane surface resulted in a surface capable of high percentage capture and release of antigens and the ability to concentrate the antigen from dilute solutions. These specific results are further outlined in Section 6.2.

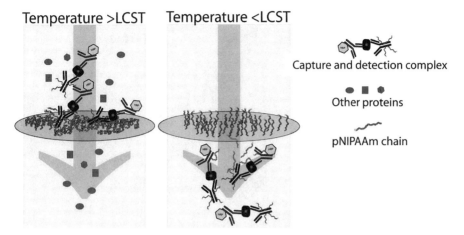

Figure 2.8   Schematic system design for immunocomplex capture and concentration under conditions of capture (>LCST) and release (<LCST). Covalently modified pNIPAAm-antibody, bound antigen, and detection antibody are captured at the membrane during polymer aggregation above the LCST, while unconjugated plasma components flow through. When the membrane region of the device is cooled, the polymer becomes hydrophilic and molecular conjugates are released back into the flow stream, carrying their cargo of antigen and detection antibody with them. Reproduced from Golden et al.[117] by permission from the American Chemical Society.

2.4.3   Magnetic Processing Modules

Batch mode magnetic separation is the simplest and most easily implemented magnetic processing module. In batch mode magnetic separation, magnetic particles are conjugated to a targeting ligand (e.g., antibody) that binds to a specific biomarker target in the sample. The application of an external magnetic field then causes the magnetically labeled biomolecules to be captured along the sidewall of the carrying vessel while the remainder of the reaction mixture is removed. This type of separation can be used to achieve biomarker enrichment by redissolving the captured precipitate into a manyfold smaller volume of carrier fluid. Commercial immunoassay systems utilizing batch separation of magnetic beads have been developed and sold worldwide. For example, the Elecsys® immunoassay system by Roche utilizes batch mode separation of magnetic microbeads conjugated to antibodies and currently has ~100 approved biomarker tests worldwide.

In addition to batch mode magnetic separation, continuous-flow magnetic separation systems have been used to achieve continuous separation of cells and proteins in microfludic channels. Lai et al.[44] demonstrated how continuous-flow magnetic separation could be used in conjunction with dual pH/temperature-responsive smart mNPs to achieve continuous separation of fluorescently labeled proteins, as shown in Figure 2.9. The authors combined an H-filter microfluidic device with a smart pH-responsive mNP reagent that

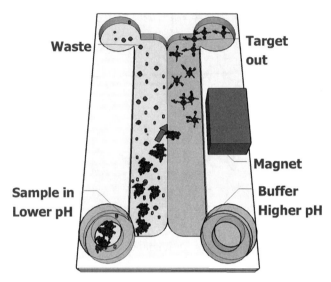

Figure 2.9 Target analyte separation in a microfluidic channel facilitated by pH-responsive magnetic nanoparticles (mNPs) under isothermal conditions. The channel contains two flow streams. The left stream (green) is the sample that has been preincubated with mNPs. mNP aggregation is triggered by the lower pH buffer in this sample flow stream. The pH of the right stream (pink) is chosen to reverse mNP aggregation. A magnet provides a sufficient field to pull the aggregates laterally into the higher pH flow stream. The conjugate aggregates move out of the sample flow stream and in to the higher pH stream, where they return to a dispersed state, carrying the bound target analyte with them. Movement of other molecules across this interface is limited by diffusion due to the laminar flow conditions. Reproduced from Lai et al.[44] by permission from the Royal Society of Chemistry. (See color insert.)

could be reversibly aggregated by lowering the solution pH. The system was designed to pull aggregated mNPs and their bound biomarker targets from one laminar flow stream across the laminar fluid interface into an adjacent flow stream. The adjacent flow stream with an alkaline pH caused the mNPs to disaggregate. Instead of being caught at the surface of the magnet, the disaggregated mNPs with low magnetophoretic mobility flowed freely by the magnet via the second laminar flow stream to the second fork of the H-filter device, enabling further downstream processing.

The pH-responsive polymer used by Lai et al.[44] was composed by random copolymerization of *tert*-butyl methacrylate (tBMA) and NIPAAm. The tBMA was deprotected during the high-temperature mNP synthesis procedure and resulted in a pH-responsive carboxyl group displayed on the surface ofthe mNPs. Using this deprotection scheme, approximately 40% of the *tert*-butyl groups were converted to methacrylic acid groups, as determined by proton nuclear magnetic resonance spectroscopy.

The general strategy for achieving continuous-flow separation of fluorescently labeled streptavidin used by Lai et al.[44] was to introduce the pH-responsive mNP conjugates containing biotinylated polymer as dispersed nanoparticles to the sample to facilitate binding to the target. The sample solution pH was lowered to induce mNP aggregation outside of the microchannel. The solution was then introduced into the microfluidic channel into a laminar flow stream at low pH where the mNPs remained aggregated. As the aggregates flowed through a magnetic field, they were magnetophoresed laterally across the laminar fluid interface and into the adjacent higher pH buffer stream, carrying the fluorescently labeled streptavidin with them. Because the polymer coating was sharply pH responsive, the aggregates redissolved rapidly and continued to flow as individual particles with low magnetophoretic mobility in the receiving stream rather than being captured at the channel surface near the magnet. Movement of other molecules into the second flow stream, meanwhile, was limited by diffusion due to the low Reynolds number (laminar) fluid flow thereby achieving continuous purification of the target in the device.

In another smart magnet nanoparticle processing module, Lai et al.[43] showed how biotinylated pNIPAAm magnetic particles could bind to streptavidin and be reversibly immobilized in a locally heated region of a PEGylated PDMS microfluidic device adjacent to a magnet. The PDMS microfluidic channel was modified with PEG using the photoinitiator method developed by Ebara et al.[35,115] The magnetic field was introduced by embedding a magnet at the lower side of the channel. The mNPs below the LCST were soluble and freely flowed into the heated region. Upon entering the heated region, the mNPs aggregated but did not stick to the nonfouling PEGylated channel walls in the absence of an applied magnetic field. The mNPs were captured onto the PEGylated channel walls only when the temperature was raised above the LCST and the magnetic field was applied. The reversal of the temperature and applied magnetic field resulted in the redissolution of the aggregated mNPs and their diffusive reentry into the flow stream.

Recently, Nash et al.[132] demonstrated a novel mechanism for achieving batch magnetic separation of AuNPs. The bioseparation/enrichment system consisted of a mixture of magnetic and AuNPs, each with a smart polymer corona. AuNPs (~25-nm diameter) were modified with a biotinylated amine-containing diblock copolymer, and mNPs (~10-nm diameter) were synthesized directly with a homo-pNIPAAm polymer surface coating. When mixtures of these two particle types were heated above the polymer LCST, the particles coaggregated as a result of hydrophobic interactions between the collapsed polymers. Eight-kilodalton homo-pNIPAAm (2 mg/mL) was added to the particle mixture to facilitate mNP and AuNP cross-aggregation. The aggregates contained both magnetic (iron oxide) and gold aggregates with a strongly enhanced magnetophoretic mobility that allowed them to be rapidly coseparated in a modest applied magnetic field gradient. By resuspending the magnetically captured particle aggregates into a smaller volume of fluid, the

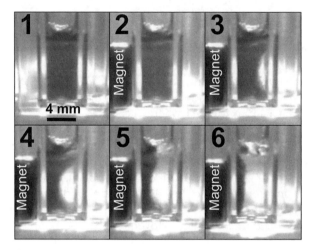

Figure 2.10 Video stills of dual AuNP/mNP coaggregation and magnetic separation. For the purposes of the video, the sample comprised 250 μL of an AuNP/mNP/homo-pNIPAAm mixture in phosphate buffered saline. Two hundred fifty microliters of 5 M NaCl was used to trigger the pNIPAAm phase transition seconds before image 1 was acquired. The magnet was then applied for a total of 20 minutes. A comparable magnetic separation behavior was observed for mixtures that were coaggregated using a thermal stimulus. Reproduced from Nash et al.[132] by permission from the American Chemical Society. (See color insert.)

gold-labeled model target biomarker streptavidin could be concentrated manyfold. The enriched gold-labeled half immunosandwich could then be directly analyzed and visualized with an antistreptavidin immunochromatographic flow strip. Time-lapse images of the magnetic separation of AuNPs via coaggregation with pNIPAAm mNPs are shown in Figure 2.10.

2.5 DEVICES FOR USE IN SMART CONJUGATE BIOASSAYS

A variety of device formats have been used in conjunction with the aforementioned smart separation modules for detecting target biomarkers using smart protein and smart nanoparticle conjugate reagents. In designing devices for smart conjugate bioassays, it is important to consider the end user of the technology. In general, simpler devices that require no electricity or controlled pressure sources (e.g., syringe pumps and vacuum control) will, in the long term, be more amenable for use in POC settings where the resource/technology level may be low. For this reason, membrane-based fluid flow systems such as those found in immunochromatographic flow strips are a highly attractive method for controlling timing and delivery of smart reagents and target biomarkers to detection and/or filtration zones within the devices. Recently, there has been resurgence in interest in paper-based diagnostic systems,[133–137] and this trend is expected to continue and to carry smart polymer-based diagnostic technologies forward.

2.5.1 Lateral-Flow Immunochromatography Devices

Lateral-flow immunoassays (LFIAs), also referred to as "immunochromatographic tests" or "dipstick assays," represent a current major dominant technology in POC testing. An aqueous sample containing biomolecules is applied to an absorbent pad and flows via capillary wicking through the chromatographic strip. The flow strips can be made from a variety of nonwoven materials, most commonly nitrocellulose, but also including other materials such as nylon, poly(ethersulfone), and poly(ethylene). Capillary wicking drives movement and eventual absorption of the liquid by an absorbent pad located at the distal end of the flow strip. The fluid flow conveys biomolecules in the sample through the capture zones of the membrane where predeposited reagents (e.g., antibodies) exert specific biomolecular affinity for target biomarkers in the sample. The fluid flux through the capture zone results in concentration of the analyte at the test line, which can be visualized using a variety of optical labels.

Many tests rely on dissolution of colloidal gold–antibody conjugates from a "conjugate pad" located just downstream of the sample application port. The liquid in the sample dissolves the colloidal gold–antibody conjugates, which are stored in dried form and are stable under ambient conditions for long periods of time. Following dissolution, the gold conjugate binds to the target in the sample and flows through the nitrocellulose to the test line. The colloidal gold–antigen complex then binds to the complementary antibody at the test line and is detected visually by the eye. A second line of capture reagents with specific affinity for the antibodies on the gold colloid serves as an internal procedural control, ensuring the test runs correctly.

A variety of optical labels have been used in LFIA including colloidal gold,[138–142] colored latex,[143] or quantum dots.[144] Silver enhancement of colloidal gold labels through reduction catalysis at the gold particle surface has also been shown to increase the sensitivity of LFIAs.[145–147] Colloidal gold is easily detected by the naked eye below nanomolar concentrations and is the most widely used type of optical label in POC LFIAs.[140] Studies comparing the effects of colloidal gold size on LFIA performance have shown that sensitivity of the tests increased with increasing nanoparticle size.[148–150] However, larger particles are less colloidally stable and are prone to agglomeration. Practically speaking, most assays are run with particles that are 40 nm in diameter, a size that represents a balance between colloidal stability and signal generation.

Researchers have demonstrated approaches to making LFIAs more quantitative by incorporation of illumination sources and optical detectors into "readers" that accept disposable lab cards or LFIA test strips. The readers measure the intensity of the label at the test line. Better accuracy is oftentimes achieved by normalizing the signal at the test line to that at the control line. Thanks to advances in miniaturization and manufacturing technology, the costs of readers have decreased dramatically over the past 15 years. The use of readers greatly diminishes subjective user interpretation, enables electronic data storage and integration with centralized laboratory information systems, and is more sensitive than detection by the eye.

Smart nanoparticle conjugates have been adapted by Nash et al.[132] for use in lateral-flow immunochromatography devices to detect model proteins and clinically relevant malaria biomarkers. They described a system for achieving magnetic separation and enrichment of AuNP biomarker "half immunosandwiches" that was advantageous because it enabled direct enrichment of the active gold biomarker detection reagent, analogous to what is formed after the dissolution of the conjugate pad in a typical immunochromatographic biosensor. Magnetic enrichment of AuNPs was achieved via polymer-induced coaggregation and separation with pNIPAAm-coated mNPs. After enrichment, the enriched particle mixture was directly applied to the lateral-flow membranes, and the target biomarker was visualized by the eye at the test line of the immunochromatographic flow strip.

2.5.2   Wicking Membrane Flow-Through Devices

An alternative immunoassay format utilizing membrane-based capillary flow has been demonstrated by Golden et al.[117] In this format, an IgG–pNIPAAm conjugate is bound to the target biomarker in the sample. A secondary detection conjugate (e.g., AuNPs conjugated to IgG antibodies without smart polymers) is then added to the mixture, forming a full-stack immunosandwich. A droplet (~5–15 µL) of the reaction mixture can then be applied to a small piece of nylon membrane that is sitting atop a cellulose absorbent pad. The liquid is pulled through the nylon membrane and into the absorbent pad via capillary flow until the droplet at the surface of the membrane is consumed. When this type of capillary flow is performed through a membrane heated above the polymer LCST, the smart polymer–IgG conjugates exhibit affinity for the membrane based on hydrophobic interactions between collapsed pNIPAAm and the pNIPAAm-grafted or unmodified nylon membrane. The target biomarker and the associated colloidal gold label are thereby immobilized at the surface of the membrane and are unable to flow through the heated membrane. In the absence of the target, however, the AuNPs are not retained at the membrane surface and are free to flow into the absorbent pad. This assay format is functionally equivalent to what had been described in a microfluidic format previously[117]; however, the use of membrane-based capillary flow greatly simplified the infrastructure requirements by completely eliminating the need for a syringe pump or a controlled pressure/vacuum source.

2.5.3 Polylaminate Microfluidic Devices

The pNIPAAm-functionalized membranes developed by Golden et al.[117] were inserted into polylaminate microfluidic devices and were used for separation, enrichment, and detection of model proteins (e.g., streptavidin), as well as clinically relevant biomarkers (e.g., PfHRP2). The membrane capture region was oriented perpendicular to the flow stream to maximize contact with the antibody conjugate. Membranes were inserted between layers of a microfluidic card (Micronics, Inc.) constructed of PET and poly(methyl methacrylate). The channel inlet and outlet comprised a straight rectangular channel that opened into a circular well region, designed to hold a membrane piece between the adhesive layers.

A model system using an antistreptavidin IgG–pNIPAAm conjugate was used to characterize the efficiency of separation and concentration of a fluorescently labeled streptavidin as a model antigen. Antistreptavidin conjugates of pNIPAAm were found to bind fluorescently labeled streptavidin at the membrane under heated conditions, while fluorescently labeled streptavidin in a physical mixture with pNIPAAm flowed through the membrane and exited the channel as indicated by fluorescence of the flow-through solutions. Nylon membranes (1.2-μm pore) that were either unmodified or modified with 4100 and 8400 kDa pNIPAAm all showed greater than 80% capture efficiency. The 8400-molecular weight graft membrane showed the highest release efficiency and the sharpest release profile, with greater than 65% of loaded streptavidin released in the first 15 μL and an overall release efficiency of approximately 80%. The immunocomplex was found to release from unmodified membranes much more slowly and less efficiently than the pNIPAAm-grafted membranes, with only about 40% released in the first 15 μL of wash buffer flow-through. These results were consistent with those reported by Ebara et al.,[35,115] which showed slower release of pNIPAAm nanobeads from unmodified PDMS as compared with pNIPAAm-grafted PDMS.

Golden et al.[117] also demonstrated how the pNIPAAm-grafted membranes could be used for sample enrichment before reversing the temperature stimulus and releasing the captured immunoconjugates. The released antibody conjugates and antigens were enriched approximately 40-fold, from 0.2 to 8.5 nM in the first 50 μL of buffer flow-through below the LCST, with a total release efficiency of ~84% (total released/ total loaded). Capture of the dilute solution is not expected to be mediated by aggregate exclusion by the membrane pores (1.2 μm) since pNIPAAm at the concentration of the diluted solution (11.6 μg/mL) does not form particles above the nominal pore size of the membranes during the time frame of the capture phase, even in the absence of the antibody conjugate, which would likely favor smaller particles of pNIPAAm in solution.[42] This fact highlights a benefit of membrane separation over separation by a thermal precipitation. Much more dilute concentrations of antibody conjugate that could not be separated by thermal precipitation could be efficiently separated using a membrane capture system. The mechanism of capture is different in that the affinity between the membrane and the polymer is responsible for the capture, whereas it is a critical particle size that is responsible for precipitation in a thermal centrifugation process.

In the work by Golden et al.,[117] an anti-PfHRP2 IgG smart conjugate was also used to evaluate the separation of a full-stack sandwich immunocomplex that incorporated a horseradish peroxidase-linked secondary detection antibody. The quantity of released detection antibody was shown to be dependent on the PfHRP2 antigen concentration in the sample. The detection sensitivity of this assay was between 20 and 100 ng/mL of PfHRP2 antigen from a 50-μL sample, which is within the relevant range of antigen for patient samples and is comparable to the ranges detectable by standard ELISA of plasma samples.[151] The time for the completed membrane assay was under 10 minutes. The presence of a pNIPAAm-modified membrane in the microfluidic channel resulted in sharper release kinetics as compared to the unmodified nylon membrane.

2.5.4   Multilayer PDMS Smart Microfludic Devices

Multistep protocols performed within microfluidic devices often require that sample solutions be isolated within discrete volumes to prevent cross-contamination and side reactions. For such applications, multilayer PDMS devices have been designed with integrated valve components that can be controlled digitally. These valves make use of a thin flexible PDMS membrane that is used to seal fluidic channels and act as a valve. Applying a positive pressure to an actuation layer of channels causes the flexible membrane to deflect, sealing the fluidic channel at the point of overlap. Sequential activation of such valves can be used as a peristaltic micropump to manipulate fluids on the chip.

Such valves are also capable of serving as tunable mixers. The same membrane that deflects during actuation as a valve can also be partially deflected, resulting in topographical features being introduced into the channel that function as staggered groove mixers. Such staggered groove microfluidic mixers fold and stretch the fluid along the channel cross section, bringing molecules in the flow stream closer to the surface and reducing the distance a molecule must diffuse to reach the sidewall.

Hoffman et al.[116] developed a multilayer microfluidic device for the enrichment of pNIPAAm–streptavidin conjugates. The conjugates were reversibly bound to the pNIPAAM-grafted PDMS microchannel walls when the device was heated above the LCST. When the device was cooled below the LCST, the pNIPAAm–streptavidin conjugates were released back into solution. The device incorporated an isolatable recirculator that was equipped with transverse flow components capable of generating helical flow to drive mass transport of aggregated smart conjugates to and from the surface. The assay schematic is shown in Figure 2.11.

In the system described by Hoffman et al.,[116] an increase in mixing caused by the actuation of transverse topographical features in the channel assisted

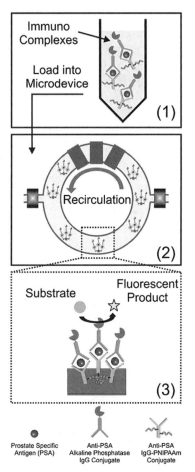

Figure 2.11 Schematic of smart immunoassay in a multilayer PDMS device. (1) IgG–pNIPAAm conjugates, IgG–enzyme conjugates, and antigen are mixed together and form immunocomplexes. (2) After 15 minutes, immunocomplexes are loaded into a microfluidic device heated to 39°C. The immunocomplexes are then mixed in an isolated recirculator, driving immobilization onto the PDMS surface. (3) After a brief wash to separate the immobilized immunocomplexes from the human plasma, substrate is loaded into the recirculator and mixed, allowing fluorescent product development. (See color insert.)

the conjugate capture by shortening the diffusion distance between the aggregates and the pNIPAAm-modified sidewall. Given the relatively large size of the aggregated pNIPAAm conjugates, the transverse flow was expected to be an important factor for achieving high capture and release efficiencies. Indeed, this condition was found to achieve the overall greatest level of capture. When 83 µM of free pNIPAAm polymer was used (forming larger aggregates), capture efficiency was ~56% with transverse flow mixing versus ~33% with diffusive mixing.

The kinetics of pNIPAAm–streptavidin release were measured from the pNIPAAm-grafted surface as the device was cooled to room temperature after the capture step. The effect of transverse mixing on conjugate release was measured as the temperature within the device fell below the phase transition temperature. When the device temperature was cooled to 25°C, the peristaltic recirculator was actuated at 5 Hz and the streptavidin conjugate was rapidly released from the surface. Due to recirculation with helical flow, the solution was quickly homogenized, resulting in a uniform distribution of the fluorescently labeled conjugate in the reactor. If the conjugate was allowed to desorb from the surface without activating the transverse flow components or the recirculator, the release rate was significantly slower. This effect was attributed to the enhanced rate and penetration of water to rehydrate the collapsed surface grafts and polymer–protein conjugates under transverse mixing.

By isolating the recirculator from the sample stream during a capture sequence, Hoffman et al.[116] were able to measure the capture/release efficiency and release kinetics from a finite conjugate volume under two different mass transport conditions: diffusion versus active mixing and recirculation. Using the results of these mechanistic experiments, they were able to demonstrate enrichment of conjugates by continuous flow of the conjugate through the preheated recirculator.

2.6 CONCLUSIONS

A multitude of smart reagents have been developed over the past two and a half decades for applications in bioassay and biodetection. Smart polymers have been conjugated to proteins, nucleotides, and nanoparticles to confer their conformational changes in response to a small change in the environment to the newly formed biosynthetic hybrid molecules. These biohybrids have been used in affinity thermoprecipitation immunoassays and other bioanalytical processing procedures to achieve capture, labeling, purification, enrichment, and detection of target biomarkers in clinical and spiked samples. More recently, smart conjugate-based detection systems have been adapted for use in POC detection applications by leveraging technologies that do not require electricity or advanced optical instrumentation yet still achieve sensitive detection. For example, smart magnetic particles can be separated upon application of a modest magnetic field afforded by a small bar magnet. Smart AuNPs have been used for detection, thereby eliminating the need for fluorescence readers or other optical instrumentation. Capillary-based fluid flow has been used to circumvent the need for microfluidic pumps or centrifugation. All of these adaptations of smart polymer-based bioassays to low-resource settings have potential to bring high-sensitivity detection to locations that are currently inaccessible to POC testing.

REFERENCES

1. Sorger, P.K. Microfluidics closes in on point-of-care assays. *Nature Biotechnology* **26**, 1345–1346 (2008).

2. Tudos, A.J., Besselink, G.A.J., & Schasfoort, R.B.M. Trends in miniaturized total analysis systems for point-of-care testing in clinical chemistry. *Lab on a Chip* **1**, 83–95 (2001).

3. Price, C.P. & Kricka, L.J. Improving healthcare accessibility through point-of-care technologies. *Clinical Chemistry* **53**, 1665–1675 (2007).

4. McDonnell, B., Hearty, S., Leonard, P., & O'Kennedy, R. Cardiac biomarkers and the case for point-of-care testing. *Clinical Biochemistry* **42**, 549–561 (2009).

5. Kaittanis, C., Santra, S., & Perez, J.M. Emerging nanotechnology-based strategies for the identification of microbial pathogenesis. *Advanced Drug Delivery Reviews* **62**, 408–423 (2010).

6. Lee, W.G., Kim, Y.-G., Chung, B.G., Demirci, U., & Khademhosseini, A. Nano/microfluidics for diagnosis of infectious diseases in developing countries. *Advanced Drug Delivery Reviews* **62**, 449–457 (2010).

7. Ndao, M. Diagnosis of parasitic diseases: old and new approaches. *Interdisciplinary Perspectives on Infectious Diseases*, 1–15 (2009).

8. Sanvicens, N., Pastells, C., Pascual, N., & Marco, M.P. Nanoparticle-based biosensors for detection of pathogenic bacteria. *Trends in Analytical Chemistry* **28**, 1243–1252 (2009).

9. Yager, P., Domingo, G.J., & Gerdes, J. Point-of-care diagnostics for global health. *Annual Review of Biomedical Engineering* **10**, 107–144 (2008).

10. Yager, P. et al. Microfluidic diagnostic technologies for global public health. *Nature* **442**, 412–418 (2006).

11. Rosen, S. Point of care diagnostics 2010 and beyond: Rapid testing at a crossroads. http://www.kaloramainformation.com (2009).

12. Ratsimbasoa, A. et al. Short report: evaluation of two new immunochromatographic assays for diagnosis of malaria. *American Journal of Tropical Medicine and Hygiene* **79**, 670–672 (2008).

13. Van den Broek, I. et al. Evaluation of three rapid tests for diagnosis of P-falciparum and P-vivax malaria in Colombia. *American Journal of Tropical Medicine and Hygiene* **75**, 1209–1215 (2006).

14. Playford, E.G. & Walker, J. Evaluation of the ICT malaria P.f/P.v and the OptiMal rapid diagnostic tests for malaria in febrile returned travellers. *Journal of Clinical Microbiology* **40**, 4166–4171 (2002).

15. Fogg, C. et al. Assessment of three new parasite lactate dehydrogenase (pan-pLDH) tests for diagnosis of uncomplicated malaria. *Transactions of the Royal Society of Tropical Medicine and Hygiene* **102**, 25–31 (2008).

16. Hopkins, H. et al. Rapid diagnostic tests for malaria at sites of varying transmission intensity in Uganda. *Journal of Infectious Diseases* **197**, 510–518 (2008).

17. Cunningham, D.D. Fluidics and sample handling in clinical chemical analysis. *Analytica Chimica Acta* **429**, 1–18 (2001).

18. Krishnan, M., Namasivayam, V., Lin, R.S., Pal, R., & Burns, M.A. Microfabricated reaction and separation systems. *Current Opinion in Biotechnology* **12**, 92–98 (2001).

19. Ocvirk, G., Verpoorte, E., Manz, A., Grasserbauer, M., & Widmer, H.M. High-performance liquid-chromatography partially integrated onto a silicon chip. *Analytical Methods and Instrumentation* **2**, 74–82 (1995).

20. Dineva, M.A., MahiLum-Tapay, L., & Lee, H. Sample preparation: a challenge in the development of point-of-care nucleic acid-based assays for resource-limited settings. *Analyst* **132**, 1193–1199 (2007).

21. Murray, C.K., Gasser, R.A., Magill, A.J., & Miller, R.S. Update on rapid diagnostic testing for malaria. *Clinical Microbiology Reviews* **21**, 97–110 (2008).

22. Moody, A. Rapid diagnostic tests for malaria parasites. *Clinical Microbiology Reviews* **15**, 66–78 (2002).

23. Cuatreca, P. & Anfinsen, C.B. Affinity chromatography. *Annual Review of Biochemistry* **40**, 259–278 (1971).

24. Lequin, R.M. Enzyme immunoassay (EIA)/enzyme-linked immunosorbent assay (ELISA). *Clinical Chemistry* **51**, 2415–2418 (2005).

25. Voller, A., Bartlett, A., & Bidwell, D.E. Enzyme immunoassays with special reference to ELISA techniques. *Journal of Clinical Pathology* **31**, 507–520 (1978).

26. Yolken, R.H. Enzyme immunoassays for the detection of infectious antigens in body-fluids—current limitations and future-prospects. *Reviews of Infectious Diseases* **4**, 35–68 (1982).

27. Auditore-Hargreaves, K. et al. Phase-separation immunoassays. *Clinical Chemistry* **33**, 1509–1516 (1987).

28. Bulmus, V., Ding, Z.L., Long, C.J., Stayton, P.S., & Hoffman, A.S. Site-specific polymer-streptavidin bioconjugate for pH-controlled binding and triggered release of biotin. *Bioconjugate Chemistry* **11**, 78–83 (2000).

29. Chen, G.H. & Hoffman, A.S. Preparation and properties of thermoreversible, phase-separating enzyme-oligo(N-isopropylacrylamide) conjugates. *Bioconjugate Chemistry* **4**, 509–514 (1993).

30. Chen, J.P. & Hoffman, A.S. Polymer protein conjugates .2. Affinity precipitation separation of human immuno-gamma-globulin by a poly(N-isopropylacrylamide)-protein-A conjugate. *Biomaterials* **11**, 631–634 (1990).

31. Chen, J.P., Yang, H.J., & Hoffman, A.S. Polymer protein conjugates .1. Effect of protein conjugation on the cloud point of poly(N-isopropylacrylamide). *Biomaterials* **11**, 625–630 (1990).

32. Ding, Z.L., Chen, G.H., & Hoffman, A.S. Synthesis and purification of thermally sensitive oligomer-enzyme conjugates of poly(N-isopropylacrylamide)-trypsin. *Bioconjugate Chemistry* **7**, 121–125 (1996).

33. Ding, Z.L., Fong, R.B., Long, C.J., Stayton, P.S., & Hoffman, A.S. Size-dependent control of the binding of biotinylated proteins to streptavidin using a polymer shield. *Nature* **411**, 59–62 (2001).

34. Ding, Z.L. et al. Temperature control of biotin binding and release with a streptavidin-poly(N-isopropylacrylamide) site-specific conjugate. *Bioconjugate Chemistry* **10**, 395–400 (1999).

35. Ebara, M., Hoffman, J.M., Hoffman, A.S., & Stayton, P.S. Switchable surface traps for injectable bead-based chromatography in PDMS microfluidic channels. *Lab on a Chip* **6**, 843–848 (2006).

36. Ebara, M., Hoffman, J.M., Stayton, P.S., & Hoffman, A.S. Surface modification of microfluidic channels by UV-mediated graft polymerization of non-fouling and "smart" polymers. *Radiation Physics and Chemistry* **76**, 1409–1413 (2007).

37. Fong, R.B., Ding, Z.L., Hoffman, A.S., & Stayton, P.S. Affinity separation using an Fv antibody fragment-"smart" polymer conjugate. *Biotechnology and Bioengineering* **79**, 271–276 (2002).

38. Fong, R.B., Ding, Z.L., Long, C.J., Hoffman, A.S., & Stayton, P.S. Thermoprecipitation of streptavidin via oligonucleotide-mediated self-assembly with poly (N-isopropylacrylamide). *Bioconjugate Chemistry* **10**, 720–725 (1999).

39. Hoffman, A.S. Bioconjugates of intelligent polymers and recognition proteins for use in diagnostics and affinity separations. *Clinical Chemistry* **46**, 1478–1486 (2000).

40. Hoffman, A.S. & Stayton, P.S. Conjugates of stimuli-responsive polymers and proteins. *Progress in Polymer Science* **32**, 922–932 (2007).

41. Kulkarni, S. et al. Controlling the aggregation of conjugates of streptavidin with smart block copolymers prepared via the RAFT copolymerization technique. *Biomacromolecules* **7**, 2736–2741 (2006).

42. Kulkarni, S., Schilli, C., Muller, A.H.E., Hoffman, A.S., & Stayton, P.S. Reversible meso-scale smart polymer-protein particles of controlled sizes. *Bioconjugate Chemistry* **15**, 747–753 (2004).

43. Lai, J.J. et al. Dual magnetic-/temperature-responsive nanoparticles for microfluidic separations and assays. *Langmuir* **23**, 7385–7391 (2007).

44. Lai, J.J. et al. Dynamic bioprocessing and microfluidic transport control with smart magnetic nanoparticles in laminar-flow devices. *Lab on a Chip* **9**, 1997–2002 (2009).

45. Malmstadt, N., Hoffman, A.S., & Stayton, P.S. "Smart" mobile affinity matrix for microfluidic immunoassays. *Lab on a Chip* **4**, 412–415 (2004).

46. Malmstadt, N., Hyre, D.E., Ding, Z.L., Hoffman, A.S., & Stayton, P.S. Affinity thermoprecipitation and recovery of biotinylated biomolecules via a mutant streptavidin—smart polymer conjugate. *Bioconjugate Chemistry* **14**, 575–580 (2003).

47. Malmstadt, N., Yager, P., Hoffman, A.S., & Stayton, P.S. A smart microfluidic affinity chromatography matrix composed of poly(N-isopropylacrylamide)-coated beads. *Analytical Chemistry* **75**, 2943–2949 (2003).

48. Monji, N., Cole, C.A., & Hoffman, A.S. Activated, N-substituted acrylamide polymers for antibody coupling- application to a novel membrane-based immunoassay. *Journal of Biomaterials Science. Polymer Edition* **5**, 407–420 (1994).

49. Monji, N. & Hoffman, A.S. A novel immunoassay system and bioseparation process based on thermal phase separating polymers. *Applied Biochemistry and Biotechnology* **14**, 107–120 (1987).

50. Narain, R., Gonzales, M., Hoffman, A.S., Stayton, P.S., & Krishnan, K.M. Synthesis of monodisperse biotinylated p(NIPAAm)-coated iron oxide magnetic nanoparticles and their bioconjugation to streptavidin. *Langmuir* **23**, 6299–6304 (2007).

51. Nash, M.A., Lai, J.J., Hoffman, A.S., Yager, P., & Stayton, P.S. "Smart" diblock copolymers as templates for magnetic-core gold-shell nanoparticle synthesis. *Nano Letters* **10**, 85–91 (2010).

52. Shimoboji, T., Ding, Z.L., Stayton, P.S., & Hoffman, A.S. Photoswitching of ligand association with a photoresponsive polymer-protein conjugate. *Bioconjugate Chemistry* **13**, 915–919 (2002).

53. Stayton, P.S. et al. Smart and biofunctional streptavidin. *Biomolecular Engineering* **16**, 93–99 (1999).

54. Stayton, P.S. et al. Control of protein-ligand recognition using a stimuli-responsive polymer. *Nature* **378**, 472–474 (1995).

55. Yin, X., Hoffman, A.S., & Stayton, P.S. Poly(N-isopropylacrylamide-co-propylacrylic acid) copolymers that respond sharply to temperature and pH. *Biomacromolecules* **7**, 1381–1385 (2006).

56. Hilbrig, F. & Freitag, R. Protein purification by affinity precipitation. *Journal of Chromatography. B, Analytical Technologies in the Biomedical and Life Sciences* **790**, 79–90 (2003).

57. Stocker, G., Dumoulin, D., Vandevyver, C., Hilbrig, F., & Freitag, R. Screening of a human antibody phage display library against a peptide antigen using stimuli-responsive bioconjugates. *Biotechnology Progress* **24**, 1314–1324 (2008).

58. Galaev, I.Y. & Mattiasson, B. Affinity thermoprecipitation—contribution of the efficiency of ligand protein-interaction and access of the ligand. *Biotechnology and Bioengineering* **41**, 1101–1106 (1993).

59. Mattiasson, B., Kumar, A., & Galaev, I.Y. Affinity precipitation of proteins: design criteria for an efficient polymer. *Journal of Molecular Recognition* **11**, 211–216 (1998).

60. Vaidya, A.A., Lele, B.S., Kulkarni, M.G., & Mashelkar, R.A. Enhancing ligand-protein binding in affinity thermoprecipitation: elucidation of spacer effects. *Biotechnology and Bioengineering* **64**, 418–425 (1999).

61. Kumar, A., Wahlund, P.O., Kepka, C., Galaev, I.Y., & Mattiasson, B. Purification of histidine-tagged single-chain Fv-antibody fragments by metal chelate affinity precipitation using thermoresponsive copolymers. *Biotechnology and Bioengineering* **84**, 494–503 (2003).

62. Garret-Flaudy, F. & Freitag, R. Use of the avidin (imino)biotin system as a general approach to affinity precipitation. *Biotechnology and Bioengineering* **71**, 223–234 (2001).

63. Vaidya, A.A., Lele, B.S., Kulkarni, M.G., & Mashelkar, R.A. Thermoprecipitation of lysozyme from egg white using copolymers of N-isopropylacrylamide and acidic monomers. *Journal of Biotechnology* **87**, 95–107 (2001).

64. Vaidya, A.A., Lele, B.S., Deshmukh, M.V., & Kulkarni, M.G. Design and evaluation of new ligands for lysozyme recovery by affinity thermoprecipitation. *Chemical Engineering Science* **56**, 5681–5692 (2001).

65. Mattiasson, B., Kumar, A., Ivanov, A.E., & Galaev, I.Y. Metal-chelate affinity precipitation of proteins using responsive polymers. *Nature Protocols* **2**, 213–220 (2007).

66. Monji, N. et al. Application of a thermally-reversible polymer-antibody conjugate in a novel membrane-based immunoassay. *Biochemical and Biophysical Research Communications* **172**, 652–660 (1990).

67. Takei, Y.G. et al. Temperature-responsive bioconjugates .3. Antibody poly(N-isopropylacrylamide) conjugates for temperature-modulated precipitations and affinity bioseparations. *Bioconjugate Chemistry* **5**, 577–582 (1994).

68. Gil, E.S. & Hudson, S.M. Stimuli-reponsive polymers and their bioconjugates. *Progress in Polymer Science* **29**, 1173–1222 (2004).

69. Rzaev, Z.M.O., Dincer, S., & Piskin, E. Functional copolymers of N-isopropylacrylamide for bioengineering applications. *Progress in Polymer Science* **32**, 534–595 (2007).

70. Lin, P. et al. Enzyme-linked fluorescence immunoassay for human IgG by using a pH-sensitive phase separating polymer as carrier. *Chemical Journal of Chinese Universities* **24**, 1198–1200 (2003).

71. Schild, H.G. Poly(N-isopropylacrylamide)—experiment, theory, and application. *Progress in Polymer Science* **17**, 163–249 (1992).

72. Yang, H.H. et al. Fluorescence immunoassay system based on the use of a pH-sensitive phase-separating polymer. *Analytical Biochemistry* **296**, 167–173 (2001).

73. Lin, P., Feng, J.J., Zheng, H., Yang, H.H., & Xu, J.G. Preparation of pH-sensitive polymer by thermal initiation polymerization and its application in fluorescence immunoassay. *Talanta* **65**, 430–436 (2005).

74. Lin, P., Zheng, H., & Xu, J.G. A novel pH-sensitive polymer phase-separating fluoroimmunoassay for the determination of immunoglobulin G in rabbit sera. *Chinese Journal of Analytical Chemistry* **33**, 1158–1160 (2005).

75. Lin, P., Zheng, H., Yang, H.H., Li, D.H., & Xu, J.G. A novel fluorescence immunoassay system based on pH-sensitive phase separating technique. *Chinese Journal of Chemistry* **23**, 285–290 (2005).

76. Lin, P. et al. Comparison of immobilization modes in pH-sensitive phase separation immunoassay. *Chinese Journal of Chemistry* **27**, 2190–2196 (2009).

77. Lin, P., Wang, S.H., & Wang, Y.L. Development of phase separation immunoassay. *Chinese Journal of Analytical Chemistry* **37**, 1839–1846 (2009).

78. Feil, H., Bae, Y.H., Feijen, J., & Kim, S.W. Effect of comonomer hydrophilicity and ionization on the lower critical solution temperature of N-isopropylacrylamide copolymers. *Macromolecules* **26**, 2496–2500 (1993).

79. Costioli, M.D., Fisch, I., Garret-Flaudy, F., Hilbrig, F., & Freitag, R. DNA purification by triple-helix affinity precipitation. *Biotechnology and Bioengineering* **81**, 535–545 (2003).

80. Safak, M., Alemdaroglu, F.E., Li, Y., Ergen, E., & Herrmann, A. Polymerase chain reaction as an efficient tool for the preparation of block copolymers. *Advanced Materials* **19**, 1499–1505 (2007).

81. Mori, T. & Maeda, M. Temperature-responsive formation of colloidal nanoparticles from poly(N-isopropylacrylamide) grafted with single-stranded DNA. *Langmuir* **20**, 313–319 (2004).

82. Jain, K.K. Nanodiagnostics: application of nanotechnology in molecular diagnostics. *Expert Review of Molecular Diagnostics* **3**, 153–161 (2003).

83. Jain, K.K. Nanotechnology in clinical laboratory diagnostics. *Clinica Chimica Acta; International Journal of Clinical Chemistry* **358**, 37–54 (2005).

84. Gao, L.Z. et al. Magnetite nanoparticle-linked immunosorbent assay. *Journal of Physical Chemistry C* **112**, 17357–17361 (2008).

85. Dittmer, W.U. et al. Rapid, high sensitivity, point-of-care test for cardiac troponin based on optomagnetic biosensor. *Clinica Chimica Acta; International Journal of Clinical Chemistry* **411**, 868–873 (2010).

86. Chen, G.D., Alberts, C.J., Rodriguez, W., & Toner, M. Concentration and purification of human immunodeficiency virus type 1 virions by microfluidic separation of superparamagnetic nanoparticles. *Analytical Chemistry* **82**, 723–728 (2010).

87. Jassam, N., Jones, C.M., Briscoe, T., & Horner, J.H. The hook effect: a need for constant vigilance. *Annals of Clinical Biochemistry* **43**, 314–317 (2006).

88. Tsai, H.Y., Hsu, C.F., Chiu, I.W., & Fuh, C.B. Detection of c-reactive protein based on immunoassay using antibody-conjugated magnetic nanoparticles. *Analytical Chemistry* **79**, 8416–8419 (2007).

89. Ahn, K.C. et al. High-throughput automated luminescent magnetic particle-based immunoassay to monitor human exposure to pyrethroid insecticides. *Analytical Chemistry* **79**, 8883–8890 (2007).

90. Furukawa, H., Shimojyo, R., Ohnishi, N., Fukuda, H., & Kondo, A. Affinity selection of target cells from cell surface displayed libraries: a novel procedure using thermo-responsive magnetic nanoparticles. *Applied Microbiology and Biotechnology* **62**, 478–483 (2003).

91. Sun, Y.B. et al. Magnetic separation of polymer hybrid iron oxide nanoparticles triggered by temperature. *Chemical Communications* **26**, 2765–2767 (2006).

92. Wakamatsu, H., Yamamoto, K., Nakao, A., & Aoyagi, T. Preparation and characterization of temperature-responsive magnetite nanoparticles conjugated with N-isopropylacrylamide-based functional copolymer. *Journal of Magnetism and Magnetic Materials* **302**, 327–333 (2006).

93. Wuang, S.C., Neoh, K.G., Kang, E.T., Pack, D.W., & Leckband, D.E. Heparinized magnetic nanoparticles: in vitro assessment for biomedical applications. *Advanced Functional Materials* **16**, 1723–1730 (2006).

94. Schmidt, A.M. Thermoresponsive magnetic colloids. *Colloid and Polymer Science* **285**, 953–966 (2007).

95. Shamim, N., Hong, L., Hidajat, K., & Uddin, M.S. Thermosensitive polymer coated nanomagnetic particles for separation of bio-molecules. *Separation and Purification Technology* **53**, 164–170 (2007).

96. Shamim, N., Hong, L., Hidajat, K., & Uddin, M.S. Thermosensitive polymer (N-isopropylacrylamide) coated nanomagnetic particles: preparation and characterization. *Colloids and Surfaces. B, Biointerfaces* **55**, 51–58 (2007).

97. Brazel, C.S. Magnetothermally-responsive nanomaterials: combining magnetic nanostructures and thermally-sensitive polymers for triggered drug release. *Pharmaceutical Research* **26**, 644–656 (2009).

98. Zhang, S.M., Zhang, L.N., He, B.F., & Wu, Z.S. Preparation and characterization of thermosensitive PNIPAA-coated iron oxide nanoparticles. *Nanotechnology* **19**, 325608 (2008).

99. Kneipp, K., Kneipp, H., & Moskovits, M. *Surface-Enhanced Raman Scattering Physics and Applications*. Berlin: Springer (2006).

100. Dou, X., Takama, T., Yamaguchi, Y., Yamamoto, H., & Ozaki, Y. Enzyme immunoassay utilizing surface-enhanced Raman scattering of the enzyme reaction product. *Analytical Chemistry* **69**, 1492–1495 (1997).

101. Xu, S.P. et al. Immunoassay using probe-labelling immunogold nanoparticles with silver staining enhancement via surface-enhanced Raman scattering. *Analyst* **129**, 63–68 (2004).

102. Anker, J.N. et al. Biosensing with plasmonic nanosensors. *Nature Materials* **7**, 442–453 (2008).

103. Yu, F., Yao, D.F., & Knoll, W. Surface plasmon field-enhanced fluorescence spectroscopy studies of the interaction between an antibody and its surface-coupled antigen. *Analytical Chemistry* **75**, 2610–2617 (2003).

104. Seydack, M. Nanoparticle labels in immunosensing using optical detection methods. *Biosensors & Bioelectronics* **20**, 2454–2469 (2005).

105. Attridge, J.W., Daniels, P.B., Deacon, J.K., Robinson, G.A., & Davidson, G.P. Sensitivity enhancement of optical immunosensors by the use of a surface-plasmon resonance fluoroimmunoassay. *Biosensors & Bioelectronics* **6**, 201–214 (1991).

106. Wilson, R. The use of gold nanoparticles in diagnostics and detection. *Chemical Society Reviews* **37**, 2028–2045 (2008).

107. Thaxton, C.S., Rosi, N.L., & Mirkin, C.A. Optically and chemically encoded nanoparticle materials for DNA and protein detection. *MRS Bulletin* **30**, 376–380 (2005).

108. Storhoff, J.J. et al. What controls the optical properties of DNA-linked gold nanoparticle assemblies? *Journal of the American Chemical Society* **122**, 4640–4650 (2000).

109. Zhu, M.Q., Wang, L.Q., Exarhos, G.J., & Li, A.D.Q. Thermosensitive gold nanoparticles. *Journal of the American Chemical Society* **126**, 2656–2657 (2004).

110. Yusa, S.I. et al. Salt effect on the heat-induced association behavior of gold nanoparticles coated with poly(N-isopropylacrylamide) prepared via reversible addition—fragmentation chain transfer (RAFT) radical polymerization. *Langmuir* **23**, 12842–12848 (2007).

111. Li, Y.T., Smith, A.E., Lokitz, B.S., & McCormick, C.L. In situ formation of gold-"decorated" vesicles from a RAFT-synthesized, thermally responsive block copolymer. *Macromolecules* **40**, 8524–8526 (2007).

112. Uehara, N., Ookubo, K., & Shimizu, T. Colorimetric assay of glutathione based on the spontaneous disassembly of aggregated gold nanocomposites conjugated with water-soluble polymer. *Langmuir* **26**, 6818–6825 (2010).

113. Honda, N., Lindberg, U., Andersson, P., Hoffman, S., & Takei, H. Simultaneous multiple immunoassays in a compact disc-shaped microfluidic device based on centrifugal force. *Clinical Chemistry* **51**, 1955–1961 (2005).

114. Lai, S. et al. Design of a compact disk-like microfluidic platform for enzyme-linked immunosorbent assay. *Analytical Chemistry* **76**, 1832–1837 (2004).

115. Ebara, M., Hoffman, J.M., Stayton, P.S., & Hoffman, A.S. Surface modification of microfluidic channels by UV-mediated graft polymerization of non-fouling and "smart" polymers. *Radiation Physics and Chemistry* **76**, 1409–1413 (2007).

116. Hoffman, J.M. et al. A helical flow, circular microreactor for separating and enriching "smart" polymer–antibody capture reagents. *Lab on a Chip* **10**, 3130–3138 (2010).

117. Golden, A.L., Lai, J.J., Fomban, N.T., Hoffman, J.H., Hoffman, A.S., & Stayton, P.S. A simple fluidic system for purifying and concentrating diagnostic biomarkers using stimuli-responsive antibody conjugates and membranes. *Bioconjugate Chemistry* **21**, 1820–1826 (2010).

118. Gonzalez-Buitrago, J.M. & Gonzalez, C. Present and future of the autoimmunity laboratory. *Clinica Chimica Acta* **365**, 50–57 (2006).

119. Wang, H. et al. Intact-protein-based high-resolution three-dimensional quantitative analysis system for proteome profiling of biological fluids. *Molecular & Cellular Proteomics* **4**, 618–625 (2005).

120. Lee, J.N., Park, C., & Whitesides, G.M. Solvent compatibility of poly(dimethylsiloxane)-based microfluidic devices. *Analytical Chemistry* **75**, 6544–6554 (2003).

121. Malmstadt, N., Nash, M.A., Purnell, R.F., & Schmidt, J.J. Automated formation of lipid-bilayer membranes in a microfluidic device. *Nano Letters* **6**, 1961–1965 (2006).

122. Friebe, A. & Ulbricht, M. Controlled pore functionalization of poly(ethylene terephthalate) track-etched membranes via surface-initiated atom transfer radical polymerization. *Langmuir* **23**, 10316–10322 (2007).

123. Geismann, C., Yaroshchuk, A., & Ulbricht, M. Permeability and electrokinetic characterization of poly(ethylene terephthalate) capillary pore membranes with grafted temperature-responsive polymers. *Langmuir* **23**, 76–83 (2007).

124. Wu, G.G., Li, Y.P., Han, M., & Liu, X.X. Novel thermo-sensitive membranes prepared by rapid bulk photo-grafting polymerization of N,N-diethylacrylamide onto the microfiltration membranes Nylon. *Journal of Membrane Science* **283**, 13–20 (2006).

125. Liang, L., Shi, M.K., Viswanathan, V.V., Peurrung, L.M., & Young, J.S. Temperature-sensitive polypropylene membranes prepared by plasma polymerization. *Journal of Membrane Science* **177**, 97–108 (2000).

126. Singh, N., Wang, J., Ulbricht, M., Wickramasinghe, S.R., & Husson, S.M. Surface-initiated atom transfer radical polymerization: a new method for preparation of polymeric membrane adsorbers. *Journal of Membrane Science* **309**, 64–72 (2008).

127. Ulbricht, M. Advanced functional polymer membranes. *Polymer* **47**, 2217–2262 (2006).

128. Yusof, A.H.M. & Ulbricht, M. Polypropylene-based membrane adsorbers via photo-initiated graft copolymerization: optimizing separation performance by preparation conditions. *Journal of Membrane Science* **311**, 294–305 (2008).

129. Nagase, K. et al. Effects of graft densities and chain lengths on separation of bioactive compounds by nanolayered thermoresponsive polymer brush surfaces. *Langmuir* **24**, 511–517 (2008).

130. Ying, L., Yu, W.H., Kang, E.T., & Neoh, K.G. Functional and surface-active membranes from poly(vinylidene fluoride)-graft-poly(acrylic acid) prepared via RAFT-mediated graft copolymerization. *Langmuir* **20**, 6032–6040 (2004).

131. Nagase, K. et al. Influence of graft interface polarity on hydration/dehydration of grafted thermoresponsive polymer brushes and steroid separation using all-aqueous chromatography. *Langmuir* **24**, 10981–10987 (2008).

132. Nash, M.A., Yager, P., Hoffman, A.S., & Stayton, P.S. Mixed stimuli-responsive magnetic and gold nanoparticle system for rapid purification, enrichment, and detection of biomarkers. *Bioconjugate Chemistry* **21**, 2197–2204 (2010).

133. Bracher, P.J., Gupta, M., & Whitesides, G.M. Patterning precipitates of reactions in paper. *Journal of Materials Chemistry* **20**, 5117–5122 (2010).

134. Carrilho, E., Martinez, A.W., & Whitesides, G.M. Understanding wax printing: a simple micropatterning process for paper-based microfluidics. *Analytical Chemistry* **81**, 7091–7095 (2009).

135. Klasner, S.A. et al. Paper-based microfluidic devices for analysis of clinically relevant analytes present in urine and saliva. *Analytical and Bioanalytical Chemistry* **397**, 1821–1829 (2010).

136. Leung, V., Shehata, A.A.M., Filipe, C.D.M., & Pelton, R. Streaming potential sensing in paper-based microfluidic channels. *Colloids and Surfaces. A, Physicochemical and Engineering Aspects* **364**, 16–18 (2010).

137. Lu, Y., Shi, W.W., Qin, J.H., & Lin, B.C. Fabrication and characterization of paper-based microfluidics prepared in nitrocellulose membrane by wax printing. *Analytical Chemistry* **82**, 329–335 (2010).

138. Kim, Y.M., Oh, S.W., Jeong, S.Y., Pyo, D.J., & Choi, E.Y. Development of an ultra-rapid one-step fluorescence immunochromatographic assay system for the quantification of microcystins. *Environmental Science & Technology* **37**, 1899–1904 (2003).

139. Lonnberg, M. & Carlsson, J. Quantitative detection in the attomole range for immunochromatographic tests by means of a flatbed scanner. *Analytical Biochemistry* **293**, 224–231 (2001).

140. Posthuma-Trumpie, G.A., Korf, J., & van Amerongen, A. Lateral flow (immuno) assay: its strengths, weaknesses, opportunities and threats. A literature survey. *Analytical and Bioanalytical Chemistry* **393**, 569–582 (2009).

141. van Dam, G.J. et al. Diagnosis of schistosomiasis by reagent strip test for detection of circulating cathodic antigen. *Journal of Clinical Microbiology* **42**, 5458–5461 (2004).

142. Zhu, Y.C. et al. Development of a rapid, simple dipstick dye immunoassay for schistosomiasis diagnosis. *Journal of Immunological Methods* **266**, 1–5 (2002).

143. Gussenhoven, G.C. et al. LEPTO dipstick, a dipstick assay for detection of Leptospira-specific immunoglobulin M antibodies in human sera. *Journal of Clinical Microbiology* **35**, 92–97 (1997).

144. Goldman, E.R. et al. Multiplexed toxin analysis using four colors of quantum dot fluororeagents. *Analytical Chemistry* **76**, 684–688 (2004).

145. Shyu, R.H., Shyu, H.F., Liu, H.W., & Tang, S.S. Colloidal gold-based immunochromatographic assay for detection of ricin. *Toxicon* **40**, 255–258 (2002).

146. Horton, J.K., Swinburne, S., & Osullivan, M.J. A novel, rapid, single-step immunochromatographic procedure for the detection of mouse immunoglobulin. *Journal of Immunological Methods* **140**, 131–134 (1991).

147. Zhou, P. et al. Nanocolloidal gold-based immunoassay for the detection of the N-methylcarbamate pesticide carbofuran. *Journal of Agricultural and Food Chemistry* **52**, 4355–4359 (2004).

148. Laitinen, M.P.A. & Vuento, M. Affinity immunosensor for milk progesterone: identification of critical parameters. *Biosensors & Bioelectronics* **11**, 1207–1214 (1996).

149. Henderson, K. & Stewart, J. Factors influencing the measurement of oestrone sulphate by dipstick particle capture immunoassay. *Journal of Immunological Methods* **270**, 77–84 (2002).

150. Aveyard, J., Mehrabi, M., Cossins, A., Braven, H., & Wilson, R. One step visual detection of PCR products with gold nanoparticles and a nucleic acid lateral flow (NALF) device. *Chemical Communications* **41**, 4251–4253 (2007).

151. Kifude, C.M. et al. Characterization of enzyme linked immunosorbent assay for plasmodium falciparum histidine-rich protein 2 in blood, plasma and serum. *Clinical and Vaccine Immunology: CVI* **15**, 1012–1018 (2008).

152. Howerton, D., Anderson, N., Bosse, D., Granade, S., & Westbrook, G. *Good Laboratory Practices for Waived Testing Sites. CDC Morbidity and Mortality Weekly Report, Recommendations and Reports* **54** (November 11, 2005).

CHAPTER 3

Design of Intelligent Surface Modifications and Optimal Liquid Handling for Nanoscale Bioanalytical Sensors

LAURENT FEUZ, FREDRIK HÖÖK, and ERIK REIMHULT

3.1 INTRODUCTION

One of the remaining challenges in the development of bioanalytical sensors is to improve the efficiency by which either low-molecular-weight compounds or biomolecules that are present at utterly low concentrations can be detected. Considerable efforts have therefore been put into increasing the sensitivity of the transducer principles utilized in different biosensing devices. Since the sensor signal is generally proportional to surface coverage, which for a certain surface functionalization is directly dependent on the affinity of the interaction and bulk concentration of target molecules, it is critical that the sensor concept is sufficiently sensitive to detect low coverage of adsorbed proteins within reasonable timescales, preferably from small sample volumes. This goal can be approached in different ways.

Perhaps the most efficient method is to use fluorescent labels as a signal enhancer.[1] However, attachment of chemical labels adds significant preparative steps, and for complex biological systems, inhomogeneous labeling is often an issue of great concern. In certain cases, external labels may also alter the nature of the interactions. For these reasons, but also because of their potential to extract detailed information on interaction kinetics, label-free surface-sensitive methods, such as the quartz crystal microbalance (QCM),[2] electrical impedance (EI),[3] and surface plasmon resonance (SPR)[4] have increased in popularity. To further improve the performance of surface-based sensors,

Intelligent Surfaces in Biotechnology: Scientific and Engineering Concepts, Enabling Technologies, and Translation to Bio-Oriented Applications, First Edition.
Edited by H. Michelle Grandin and Marcus Textor.
© 2012 John Wiley & Sons, Inc. Published 2012 by John Wiley & Sons, Inc.

significant efforts are today focused on miniaturized versions of such and related concepts, with the primary advantages of providing

(i) large-scale multiplexing via multiple sensor elements on the very same chip,

(ii) handling of minute sample volumes by integration with microfluidics, and possibly,

(iii) increased sensitivity and decreased limit of detection.

Promising miniaturized sensor principles include resonating or surface-stress sensitive cantilevers,[5–9] semiconducting nanowires,[10–13] and nanoplasmonics,[14,15] each of which in principle is analogous to QCM, EIS, and SPR, respectively, and is schematically shown in Figure 3.1.

These techniques have their own pros and cons, and the emerging consensus is that they are best suited for different types of applications. For example, semiconductor nanowires sense changes in interfacial charge,[12,13] which makes them best suited to probe highly charged molecules, such as DNA and RNA. Another of their advantages is the simplicity by which changes in the electrical resistance of the nanowires can be measured and translated into a change in interfacial charge induced by biomolecular binding reactions. However, for operation in high-sensitivity mode, they require aqueous solutions with low ionic strength, and thus nonphysiological conditions. This may limit their generic applicability but might make them well suited to probe, for example, membrane protein-controlled ion translocation reactions across supported lipid bilayers[11] being highly desirable in the search for new drug-screening assays. Small-scale cantilevers are primarily sensitive to changes in surface stress. Hence, in analogy with QCM, it is not obvious how to quantify the measured response in terms of number of bound molecules. This may, in certain cases, complicate the analysis of binding kinetics but may provide instead unique information about structural changes in the adsorbed film of biomolecules.[16] Nanoplasmonic sensors share most of their sensing features with conventional SPR, one of them being that the measured response is to a good approximation proportional to the number of bound molecules. This makes nanoplasmonic sensors well-suited for the analysis of binding kinetics. Combined with their relatively high sensitivity[17] and their compatibility with miniaturization,[15] this has led to the investment of significant resources into the development of this class of bioanalytical sensors.

There are numerous excellent reviews[3,10,18–21] and books[22,23] on these and additional types of transducer principles for label-free sensors available, and on how to apply them in different configurations, from macro to nano, to obtain maximum biosensor sensitivity. In general, these transducer principles are based on converting different physical contrasts induced upon a biomolecular recognition reaction, such as molecular mass, optical refractive index, electrical resistance, and electrical charge to a recorded time-resolved quantitative response. It is important to keep in mind for the discussion in this

(a)

(b)

(c)

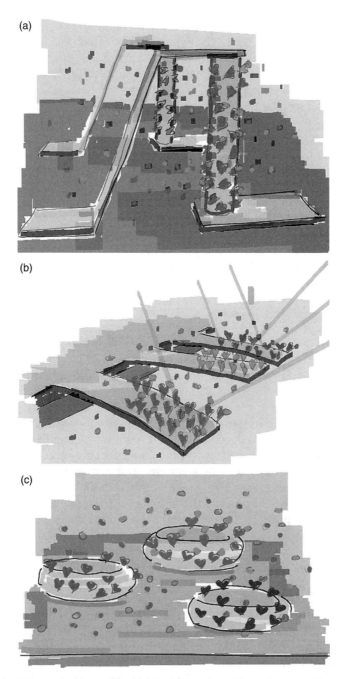

Figure 3.1 Schematic illustration of (a) small-scale surface-stress sensitive cantilevers, (b) semiconductor nanowires, and (c) nanoplasmonically active gold disks designed with immobilized probe molecules for selective detection of suspended analyte molecules. The different colors represent capture agents for different molecules immobilized on the respective sensors. (See color insert.)

chapter that macroscopic sensor elements typically can be approximated as having uniformly distributed sensitivity thanks to their much larger physical extension relative to their nanoscale sensing depth and the molecular dimensions. However, as sensors are miniaturized to nanoscale dimensions, the transducer becomes susceptible to edge effects, from the finite lateral extension of the sensor element, and the sensitivity across the sensor element can vary by orders of magnitude.[24] Not uncommonly, the sensitivity is highest at the edges and corners of a sensor element.

While the transducer principle is the most commonly discussed aspect of biosensors in the literature, in this chapter, we will discuss two more rarely considered but equally important aspects that must be considered to optimize the performance of surface-based bioanalytical sensors: proper surface modification and optimal liquid handling. The importance of optimizing these two aspects apply to all sensor designs, but become especially important in the detection of low-abundant biomolecules present in a complex background of other biomolecules in biological fluids. This is the case in, for example, biomarker identification[25–27] and disease diagnostics.[28–31] The importance of optimizing with respect to this particular challenge for miniaturized sensor formats can be detailed as the following:

(i) The target molecules of interest must bind specifically and selectively with recognition elements on the sensor surfaces. The specificity of the immobilized recognition element to the suspended target should be sufficiently high to yield selective recognition from a complex mixture. This requires a selection of probes such that cross-reactivity is low, but it is also important that the immobilization preserves the three-dimensional (3-D) structure of the recognition element as specific interactions for biological molecules are strongly dependent on 3-D conformation and binding geometry. This requirement can be met by suitable *surface chemistry* on the sensor, as discussed in the first part of this chapter. Selectivity of the interaction requires that only the target molecule binds to the surface; that is, the sensor surface must be designed such that it is inert for all other proteins present in the sample. It is worthwhile to emphasize the importance of keeping all surfaces other than the actual sensor surface (i.e., the walls of liquid reservoirs, tubings, and measurement chambers) inert toward protein adsorption since nonspecific protein adsorption on these regions will lead to reduced bulk concentrations. The importance of intelligent surface-modification schemes that ensure creation of defined nanoscale areas for biospecific detection on the sensitive regions of the measurement system while suppressing sample loss elsewhere on the sensor is discussed in Sections 3.2 and 3.3 of this chapter.

(ii) The target molecules must also be brought in sufficiently close proximity to the surface such that binding to recognition elements on the biosensor surface can occur. Efficient *transport* of the molecules from the bulk of the solution to the sensor surface is thus a key factor, especially when working with low-abundant compounds. Transport efficiency highly depends on the device geometry and the handling of liquid flow. As shown in a theoretical exposé in Section 3.4 of this chapter, channel dimensions and sensor size are relevant parameters when optimizing transport to the surface.

In Sections 3.2 and 3.3, we address intelligent surface modification (criterion i) being compatible not only with homogeneous macroscopic sensors but also with small (nano) scale sensors, and different means of generating functional surface patterns for specific and efficient recognition of analytes on nanoscale sensor elements. In contrast to macroscopic sensors, miniaturized sensors are generally composed of two or more materials, of which only one acts as the actual sensor element. For example, the sensitive part of semiconducting nanowire sensors is typically an oxidized semiconductor substrate. In contrast, small-scale cantilevers are compatible with essentially all substrate materials that can be deposited as a sufficiently thin film, which means that one can, in this case, be relatively flexible with respect to the choice of surface modification. Nanoplasmonic sensors are instead restricted to metals, most often gold, which makes thiol-based surface-modification strategies the most natural choice. This may seem relatively straightforward, but unfortunately it is not. The prime aim of the two first sections is to address this particular challenge and to guide the reader to follow as rational approaches as possible in order to functionalize the sensor element, while surrounding areas are made inert. This also has important implications for efficient sample handling discussed in Section 3.4, in which we address the challenge of optimizing liquid handling (criterion ii) in order to reach the surface coverage that corresponds to the detection limit of the sensor within a sufficiently short timescale even in the case of small sample volumes containing low analyte concentrations. Particular focus is put on the challenge of balancing the sensor dimension with suitable liquid handling and the total amount of analyte available in small volumes of dilute samples.

3.2 ORTHOGONAL SMALL (NANO)-SCALE SURFACE MODIFICATION USING MOLECULAR SELF-ASSEMBLY

A prerequisite when aiming for selective and specific sensing of biomolecules is to render all surfaces inert toward the adsorption of molecules that are of no interest. Both the sensor element itself as well as the surrounding surfaces should be rendered nonfouling such that binding of target molecules becomes restricted to the sensitive areas of the sensor. In short, the ideal biosensor consists of bioactive areas coinciding with the sensitive areas of the sensor and inert areas everywhere else to ensure minimum sample consumption and the highest specificity and selectivity. To meet this challenge, an intelligent functionalization scheme has to be developed that makes use of molecular patterning over the sensor. This challenge is especially demanding in the case of small-scale sensors, in which case dimensions of the molecules used for passivation and capture as well as the analytes of interest are on the same length scale as those of the sensor element.

In deciding on a strategy to modify a particular sensor surface, one must consider the substrate surface properties, the environmental conditions under which the coating must be stable (time frame, pH, storage conditions, etc.), and the degree of passivation to nonspecific biomolecular interactions required. While the environmental conditions for application and storage might not differ greatly for biosensors, the materials that have to be functionalized, as well as the sensor geometry and the complexity of the analyte solution (ranging from controlled laboratory conditions with single analytes present to blood samples or sea water samples in which many species are present), can vary greatly. The requirement to block all surfaces to nonspecific binding is common, but the challenge varies with respect to how difficult this is to achieve in different applications. When considering the creation of the prerequisite nonfouling interface, it is instructive to divide the design of the molecular interface into three mostly independently designable parts: surface anchor, spacer, and functional unit (recognition element). The role and strategy of choice for each component will be discussed next, with particular focus on the design criteria required to generate a biofunctional pattern (see Fig. 3.2).

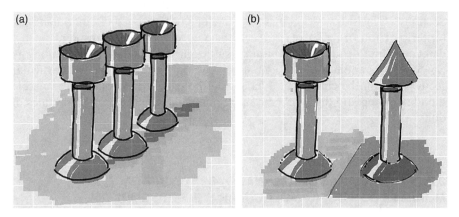

Figure 3.2   Schematic illustration of the different molecular components required to create a biosensor surface. The surface anchor ensures the binding to the underlying substrate material; the spacer's role is to screen all interactions of the target with the substrate; and the optional functional unit (recognition element) is used to selectively capture the target. (a) A surface-modification scheme on a single substrate material, representative for macroscale biosensors. (b) A biosensor surface consisting of two different substrate materials, as often encountered in small (nano) scale sensors. Two different anchors, each specific to one of the substrate materials, are required to modify the substrate. (See color insert.)

3.2.1   Surface Anchor: How to Define and Retain a Molecular Pattern

The surface anchor is perhaps the most decisive choice to create a proper interface for both macroscopic and nanoscale biosensors. The choice of anchor strategy determines the stability of the molecular interface, for example, how strongly attached the molecules will be, under the various conditions the sensor might be subject to, if they enable ordered transitions at the interface coupled to the sensor, and/or how mobile the functional units will be. The choice of anchor can also, together with the spacer, determine the achievable packing density of both spacers and recognition elements. The choice of anchor cannot be discussed separately from the materials chemistry of the sensor itself. This holds particularly true for nanoscale sensors, in which case the sensor element will be made of a different material than the surrounding surface. This, in turn, requires the use of material-specific molecular binding groups as anchors to exclusively assemble certain types of molecules to different parts of the sensor. Examples are nanoplasmonic gold sensors on a glass (SiO_2) background,[32] metal nanowires, or carbon nanotubes suspended over silicon oxide or silicon nitride.[21,33] Often the material contrast is between a metal and an oxide (typically silicon oxide) background, but a sensor element can also itself be an oxide or coated with an oxide such as TiO_2 or ITO.[34,35] The material contrast between the sensor element and the background makes it possible, for example, to only express recognition units on the sensor element by assembling them using anchors that bind specifically to the material of the sensor element but not to the background. A second anchor group specific to the surrounding surface chemistry can then be used to backfill the surface with a molecular coating, which preferably suppresses binding of additional molecules completely. The use of anchors with such orthogonal binding properties to produce molecular patterns by molecular self-assembly was first demonstrated by Whitesides et al.[36] and has since been repeatedly used in numerous incarnations.

Strategies for anchoring can be discussed from several different starting points, but one suitable starting point is whether the anchor attaches strongly enough to approach chemisorption or whether weaker physical interactions like electrostatic or dipolar interactions are used.

3.2.1.1 Weak Anchors: "Physisorption"   If weak interactions are used, the spacer unit, which most often is a polymer, has to be attached by multiple anchoring units to remain at the sensor interface. Per definition, an anchor consisting of only a single or a few charges will lead to reversible adsorption of the spacers. This, in turn, will allow nonspecific adsorption to the sensor area when defects in the coating are created as well as an undefined number of active functional groups at the interface. A commonly used strategy is therefore to increase the anchor size in order to allow multiple coupled but weakly adhering anchor units to bind to the sensor substrate simultaneously. If one unit reversibly comes off, it will remain in the vicinity of the interface by restriction of the remaining units still bound to the substrate for a sufficiently

long time to rebind. A dramatic increase in the binding affinity of macromolecules can thus be achieved.[37] The simplest example of this strategy is the use of proteins like albumins to render surfaces nonfouling. The single amino acid affinity to the surface is very low, but the multiple contacts of peptide sequences on the protein, for practical purposes, result in irreversible protein affinity to the surface through a very large number of attractive, mainly van der Waals, interactions. Naturally, more advanced concepts have evolved that allow a higher degree of interfacial control and even substrate-specific adhesion.

The most well-established such strategy is the poly(L-lysine)-*graft*-poly (ethylene glycol) (PLL-*g*-PEG) platform.[38,39] Multiple poly(ethylene glycol) (PEG) spacer chains are grafted along the backbone of a highly charged poly-lysine chain. This anchor architecture allows many weak attachment points through the backbone onto which a desired density of spacer side chains can be added. The properties in terms of spacer and functional units can thus also be varied by synthesis and can be incorporated into a single macromolecule at a desired ratio.[39] These macromolecules can then be adsorbed on negatively charged surfaces, that is, most oxides used for biosensors, and can be used to assemble the same ratio of spacers and functional units on the surface. Other examples of this strategy are, for instance, the poly(styrene sulfonate)–poly(ethylene glycol) (PSS–PEG)[40], poly(ethylene imine)-*graft*-poly(ethylene glycol) (PEI-*g*-PEG)[41,42] and poly(L-lysine)-*graft*-poly(methyl oxazoline) (PLL-*g*-PMOXA),[43,44] which also rely on charge interactions, or poly(ethylene oxide)–poly(propylene oxide)–poly(ethylene oxide) (Pluronics),[45] which relies on hydrophobic affinity to hydrophobic interfaces.

After great efforts invested into the optimal relation between the anchor unit density along the backbone and the spacer (grafting) density and molecular weight, the use of such anchor strategies to render surfaces nonfouling or to give them specific functionality has been very successful. The suppression of nonspecific binding of proteins from, for example, serum and other protein solutions have suggested that a very high surface density of spacer units and low density of defects can be achieved.[46,47] A possible reason for this good performance is that the reversibility of binding of individual segments along the backbone chain due to weak anchoring allows rearrangement and high packing of the anchored units on the surface. This intelligent design allows both high overall surface affinity and some lateral surface mobility to increase the packing density. A chain of multiple anchors with high affinity to the surface will instead freeze the system in a nondensely packed conformation with loops, thus exposing a high degree of the average surface area to nonspecific binding.[48]

However, some limitations also derive from the strategy of using multiple low-affinity anchors per macromolecule, namely, that when a sufficient density of charged functional groups with similar affinity to the substrate is used, they might also adsorb to the interface and disrupt the desired orientation of the layered coating. Similarly, hydrophobic functional groups can lead to micelle formation in the bulk, and the weak subunit surface affinity might not be sufficient to break up the micelles during surface assembly to form a well-oriented molecular interface. Finally, since it is sufficient to have part of the backbone adsorbing to the surface to ensure strong adhesion of a macromolecule to the sensor surface, remaining parts of the backbone that are not bound, for example, due to space constriction from neighboring macromolecules can then be kinetically trapped and extend out into solution. Such exposed backbones are likely to occur, but the resulting defects are not dense enough or are not providing sufficient binding affinity for noticeable fouling of typical small extracellular proteins. However, their presence has been indicated, for example, through binding of larger objects, for example, by low fouling of negatively charged liposomes (~100 nm in diameter) to PLL-g-PEG, while zwitterionic liposomes did not bind.[49,50]

In the typical example of PLL-g-PEG, the adsorption is achieved through electrostatic interaction of a positively charged backbone with a negatively charged substrate surface. The total charge interaction overcomes the entropic and other energy contributions that drive the macromolecule to desorb into solution again. It also ensures the directionality of the anchor–spacer–functional group, which is necessary to control the interfacial properties. While charge is not a material-specific interaction, it can nonetheless be used with success for patterning of sensors and other substrates. This can be achieved by direct self-assembly if a material contrast exists between, for example, a strongly charged oxide and a metal. Metal oxides and semimetal oxides for biosensor applications mostly produce surfaces with a strongly negative surface potential at physiological pH, while gold, a common sensor metal, which lacks a thick and stable surface oxide, mainly produces mirror charge interaction. Sufficiently strong binding will then only be achieved to the highly charged oxide, while weakly anchored macromolecules can be washed off or replaced by more strongly adsorbing species to the non-oxide-forming metal surfaces on the sensor.[51] Alternatively, material-specific chemisorption to, for example, gold is used prior to backfilling using, for example, PLL-g-PEG[52] (see below).

3.2.1.2 Strong Anchors: "Chemisorption"

Although anchor strategies making use of stronger chemical interactions are typically referred to as chemisorption in the field of surface functionalization, this term in practice has tended to include anchor strategies that produce bonds of lower strength than typically acknowledged as a chemical bond. However, a binding strength sufficiently high to irreversibly bind a spacer to the surface over the life span of a sensor at ambient conditions allows tethering of spacer and functional units using single-anchor moieties. The most prominent examples of such anchors are silanes ($-Si(OH)_3$), which bind to, for example, silicon dioxide, and thiols (-SH), which bind strongly to certain metals, such as gold, silver, and copper. Historically, these binding mechanisms have been explored in the context of the development of self-assembled hydrocarbon monolayers (self-assembled monolayer [SAM]) in the 1980s,[53,54] but they have been later amply applied to modify sensor surfaces and nanoparticles with longer and bulkier polymers such as PEG[55,56] and DNA[57]. The same holds for phosphate ($-OPO(OH)_2$) and phosphonate ($-PO(OH)_2$), which bind, for example, to TiO_2 and iron oxides.[58–60] Recently, bioinspired anchors such as catechol derivatives have also been used as high-affinity anchors.[61] More examples exist, but in relation to the large number of possibilities for (bioinspired) chemical coupling, the number of well-characterized anchor systems for molecular coating of common sensor materials must be considered rather limited.

The question of characterization of the quality and of the coating process as well as the durability of the formed coating becomes particularly important for patterning applications. Patterning through molecular assembly of chemisorbing anchors to the material contrast of the sensor elements and surrounding areas requires that anchors with orthogonal binding affinities to the respective materials can be found; that is, one anchor should bind to one material with high enough affinity to ensure irreversible tethering of spacers and functional elements, while its affinity to other areas should remain sufficiently low to be replaced by another anchor with irreversible affinity to that surface material. Since the interactions are chemical in nature, such orthogonality is expected to be found. For example, while thiols bind strongly to gold, they have very low affinity to oxides.[36] Silanes, on the other hand, have very low affinity to gold. Sequential adsorption of different species tagged with the respective anchors would therefore translate the underlying sensor material contrast into molecular patterns at the interface.

This game can be taken to even higher complexity by using some of the other mentioned anchors. Phosphate and phosphonates are, for example, highly specific for binding to TiO_2 over SiO_2, which has been demonstrated for molecular patterning down to the nanoscale of SAMs and proteins on a PEG background.[62] However, although this selectivity is good, the affinity of phosphonates to TiO_2 is low and is therefore not sufficient to tether, for example, typical nonfouling polymer brushes such as PEG. More useful in this respect are, for example, catechol derivatives such as the well-known dopamine[63,64] and DOPA[64–66], or the more novel nitrodopamine,[64,66,67] nitroDOPA[64,66,67] and anacat.[64] These anchors have recently been investigated and found to yield very high affinities to oxides such as TiO_2 and Fe_3O_4, but low affinities, for example, to SiO_2, oxidized gold, and Fe_2O_3.[60,64,67] Therefore, they are suitable candidates to be used for orthogonal patterning of intelligent surface patterns on the nanoscale compared to phosphonates (too-low affinity) and silanes (difficult due to sensitivity to trace amounts of water and low specificity).

3.2.1.3   *Weak versus Strong Anchors for Nanoscale Sensors*   Which anchor strategy should be chosen for patterning nanostructured sensors in order to maximize the capture efficiency of analytes at the part of the sensor with the highest sensitivity? It is safe to say that the still preliminary literature on the subject of nanoscale sensor functionalization is not able to deliver a final verdict on the subject. It is likely that the answer will depend on the specific material and geometric requirements of the sensor. A few consider-

TABLE 3.1   Compatibility of Weak and Strong Anchors to Different Surface Materials

		Anchor Examples	Surface Materials
Weak anchors (physisorption)		Amino acids, proteins	Flexible but nonspecific
		Polyelectrolytes	Metal oxides, charged surfaces
		Hydrophobic chains	Hydrophobic surfaces
		Hydrophilic lipid head group	Hydrophilic surfaces
Strong anchors (chemisorption)		Silanes	SiO_2 (metal and nonmetal oxides/ hydroxides)
		Thiols	Au, Ag, Cu, Pt, ITO
		Phosph(on)ates	TiO_2, Al_2O_3, and many other transition metal oxides
		Catechols	TiO_2, Fe_3O_4 (metal oxides)

ations based on comparing the differences between "chemisorbed" single anchors and "physisorbed" multiple anchors, however, can be enlightening for further investigations into this subject (see Table 3.1).

Many nanoscale biosensors, for example, nanoplasmonic sensors,[24] have high sensitivity at the border region between the sensor element and the surrounding substrate. Depending on the fabrication method, this region can also show some interdiffusion of the different substrate materials. Furthermore, often adhesion layers are used to make metals adhere to oxides. These nonideal conditions lead to specific problems with the respective functionalization strategy. In principle, chemisorbed single anchors will, for nonintermixing sensor substrate materials, allow for a perfect definition of the sensing element and the background using orthogonally binding anchors. However, if there is intermixing of two or more materials in the substrate, for example, Ti in the adhesion layer diffusing into the gold, then thiols used to specifically functionalize the gold sensor might show reduced affinity in the border region (where the sensitivity of the sensor is high), while, for example, nitrocatechols with high affinity to a TiO_2 surrounding background might bind also to the edge part of the sensor. For instance, the nonspecific binding could be reduced by almost one order of magnitude (from a few percent to less than 1%) for nanoplasmonic gold hole sensors entirely surrounded by the same material as used for adhesion of gold, that is, TiO_2[68], compared to the same sensor design with the gold adhered to SiO_2 using Cr as the adhesion layer to a SiO_2 background.[52]

Flexible and reversibly adsorbing macromolecules such as PLL-*g*-PEG might, however, bridge areas of undefined surface chemistry. They will display some affinity to an intermixed-materials region and, due to their size, they might extend over it with sufficient attachment points to the oxide to which they adhere well. However, the large size also means that they can extend onto, for example, an electrode or plasmonic sensor area from the passivated background even when this is *not* desired. It is still unclear what form such physisorbed molecules take on at the edge between materials to which they strongly adhere and those to which they do not. In contrast to, for example, single high-affinity anchors, it is unlikely that a well-defined boundary can be created, and it is possible that some underlying substrate area or part of the charged or hydrophobic backbone is exposed to the solution. This can lead to nonspecific interactions as discussed earlier. Thus, it is not clear that any of the outlined orthogonal patterning methods will generally lead to the desired definition and suppression of nonspecific binding at the edge of a nanoscale sensor, possibly causing significant background response.

In terms of flexibility of adding functionality to the surface, the two anchor strategies also differ. Using macromolecules with multiple anchors of low affinity allows synthesis of molecules that have multiple spacers and functional groups per molecule. Thus, the ratio of functional groups to spacers can be precisely defined and characterized before the assembly through chemical synthesis and analysis. The same ratio will be obtained after self-assembly on the sensor. However, for each newly desired ratio or functional mixture, new macromolecules have to be synthesized and characterized since the method is not modular in the assembly stage. Due to the typical many-nanometer size of these molecules and the weak interactions used for the assembly, a simple mixing of differently functionalized macromolecules will lead to nanoscale heterogeneity in the coverage of functional groups on the sensor. The consequences of this are difficult to predict. On a nanoscale sensor, the sensitivity is typically also unevenly distributed over the sensor, and distribution of, for example, capture groups over the sensor therefore can strongly influence both the timing and the absolute magnitude of the response.

Libraries of different spacers and functional groups can be created in advance using chemisorbing single anchors.[60] If their molecular weights and solubility are reasonably similar, a simple mix-and-match approach can be employed by which the molar ratios of interest are mixed in the bulk to self-assemble into a similar ratio on the surface.[69] While phase segregation is well-known in SAMs,[70,71] this problem is generally believed to be minor for the assembly of differently functionalized polymer brushes. However, in practice, deviations of the surface molar ration from the molar ration in the bulk molar ratio can be observed and replication of bulk ratios cannot be taken for granted.[69,72]

3.2.2   Spacer: How to Suppress Binding

Anchors are key to the creation of patterns and the stability of the sensor architecture, but the choice of properties of the spacer unit will determine the effectiveness of the interface in controlling nonspecific biomolecular interactions with the sensor. Additionally, the choice of strategy to attach the spacer to the anchor will influence the binding and assembly of the anchors to the surface. Simple, biologically derived spacers such as proteins and lipids can be used, as well as SAMs, but hydrophilic polymer spacers, for example, PEG, are most common in biosensor design and best suited to pattern a substrate (see Table 3.2 for an overview of different passivation strategies). The goal of the spacer is to completely screen the interactions of the analytes with the underlying sensor substrate without introducing any new attractive or long-range repulsive interactions. The waterlike hydrogen bonding ability of PEG ensures low affinity of water-soluble biological compounds, and the entropic contributions of the polymer coil upon compression ensure a high energy penalty for any molecule trying to approach the substrate surface.[73,74] Thus, nonspecific biomolecular adsorption due to short-range van der Waals interactions and longer-range electrostatic interactions can be prevented if the attached polymer brush is sufficiently thicker than the Debye screening length.[60,74] The thickness of a film of tethered linear polymer chains is predominantly determined by the Kuhn length (monomer volume length constant), the molecular weight, and the grafting density of the polymer.[75] For a given spacer polymer this can typically be translated into a "universal curve" for monomer area density, for which nonspecific adsorption is suppressed when the combination of molecular weight and grafting density is chosen to produce a monomer area density over a threshold value.[39,44] Thus, a thicker spacer layer, in general, can be considered advantageous to suppress nonspecific binding; however, for surface-sensitive sensors and, in particular, nanoscale sensors such as nanoplasmonic devices, a thicker layer sacrifices sensitivity. The sensitivity of a surface-based sensor decays, often in an exponential fashion, with distance from the substrate. The spacer layer is not part of the sensor element and constitutes a dead volume where sensing does not occur. For example, nanoplasmonic devices and capacitive sensors are sensitive over a length scale on the order of most commonly used spacer modifications. Minimization of the spacer thickness with retained suppression of nonspecific adsorption is thus desirable.

There are two main strategies to form the spacer film typically referred to as "grafting from" and "grafting to." The most straightforward strategy to produce large-area films is the "grafting-from" technique, by which selected anchors are first immobilized on the surface with initiators attached. The brush polymer spacer is then grown from the surface by an *in situ* surface-initiated polymerization reaction. Monomers present in the solution get polymerized onto the surface by, for example, radical chain polymerization,[76] living cationic

TABLE 3.2 Combinations of Anchors and Spacers to Render Substrates Inert to Nonspecific Biomolecular Binding

		Advantages	Disadvantages	Surface Materials	Examples
Proteins		Easy to handle General Biocompatible	Unspecific to surface material, surface patches exposed, nonspecific binding and orientation	Relatively general	Bovine serum albumin, fibrinoge Milk proteins
Self-assembled monolayers		Applicable to many surface materials Receptor exposure good	Small substrate defects alter function, low resistance to fouling	Au, Ag, SiO₂, TiO₂, Al₂O₃	oligo(ethylene glycol)–thiols oligo(ethylene glycol)–silanes
Surface-grafted polymer brushes		Surface chemistry specific grafting Grafting from of any spacer Mix-and-match functionality by grafting to	Difficult-to-control surface density, low availability of functional group	Au, Ag, SiO₂, TiO₂, Al₂O₃, Fe₃O₄, Fe₂O₃	PEG–thiols PEG–silanes PEG–DOPA₃ PEG–nitrocatech
Physisorbed graft copolymer brushes		Applicable to many surface materials Low defect intensity Known density of functional groups	Large surface area per macromolecule, low availability of functional group, nonspecific surface attachment	Au, Ag, SiO₂, TiO₂, Nb₂O₅, Si₃N₄, Al₂O₃	PLL-g-PEG PLL-g-PMOXA Pluronics™
Amphiphilic membranes		Cell membrane mimic Multivalency through lateral mobility	Cannot be dried, limited to certain surface materials	SiO₂, TiO₂, ITO, hydrophobic surfaces	Lipids Block copolymers

polymerization,[77] or controlled living polymerization such as atom transfer radical polymerization (ATRP).[78] Both thin and thick films can be produced by these methods. It should be noted that patterning with this method requires either patterning of the anchors in several steps with the polymerization on one part of the pattern in between each anchoring step and killing of all radical or living groups before the start of the next patterning step, or to find orthogonal sets of initiators where one initiator survives the polymer growth conditions for the first initiator. The latter is a challenge. Additionally, it is difficult to tune the fraction of functional units on the pattern by *in situ* growth of the spacer since every spacer will be identical and therefore the functionalization of the spacers is also typically 100%. Therefore, despite its advantage over the "grafting-to" technique in terms of achieving dense polymer brushes (density determined by the initial initiator density in turn defined by the anchor foot print), it is not preferred for functionalization and patterning of sensors for which, as described, the distribution and density of functional groups is of prime importance.

In the "grafting-to" approach, the spacer (and functional group) is attached to the anchor before the latter is adsorbed onto the sensor surface. Therefore, the discussion of anchor patterning is possible to translate directly into the patterning of spacers and functional groups with the "grafting-to" approach and the same levels of definition can be obtained. However, if a bulky spacer like a polymer brush is to be formed, the physical extension of the spacer and mutual exclusion interactions will determine the grafting density on the surface. This leads to a grafting density significantly below the polymer brush regime and therefore below the monomer density per unit area necessary to suppress nonspecific adsorption of most biomolecules. This drawback can mostly be circumvented by either adsorbing macromolecules like PLL-*g*-PEG for which the spacer grafting density is already sufficiently high from synthesis or adsorbing the anchor–spacer complex in a poor solvent for the spacer.[60,64,69,79,80] In the latter approach, the spacer will collapse to a fraction of its well-solubilized volume in water and therefore allows a higher density to be achieved on the surface. In this way, the density can mostly be made sufficient to suppress nonspecific binding.[64,74,79] However, having to take spacer solubility into account during the anchor patterning stage is an additional complication during assembly and patterning since the chemical reaction leading to chemisorption has to be characterized and feasible under the poor solvent conditions of the spacer.

In summary, the "grafting-to" approach is more advantageous for the most well-described and versatile strategy of using polymer brushes as spacers for biosensor surface modification applied to patterning of nanoscale biosensor structures, since it allows tailoring of the pattern exclusively through anchor orthogonality or distribution as discussed previously. Furthermore, and importantly, it offers mixing of anchor–spacer molecules through self-assembly to control the density and distribution of functional groups over the sensor surface.

3.2.3 Recognizing and Capturing Analytes on an Intelligent Nanostructure

We have so far discussed how to successfully pattern a functionality onto a miniaturized biosensor and to embed it in a noninteracting background, which only leaves the remaining task of designing the functionality such that it performs the desired purpose. Although a review of different recognition elements is not a focus of this chapter, a few points on important considerations when designing the recognition element of a sensor will be given. A number of reviews already exist that address different techniques to couple biological recognition elements to solid substrates, and we refer the interested reader to some of these for detailed knowledge on specific surface functionalization strategies.[81–83]

The *first criterion* is general for all biosensors making use of capturing of targets, and that is that the *specificity* of the recognition has to be very high. High specificity in the biomolecular realm typically requires conservation of a 3-D structure of the immobilized probe complementary to the biomolecule (target) of interest. Since such recognition elements are synthetically beyond current state of the art in chemistry, recognition elements are usually collected from libraries of existing or evolved biological compounds performing recognition functions in biological systems. Choosing recognition elements that already exist in biological systems also aids, but does not guarantee, that the *second important criterion, selectivity*, is fulfilled. Selectivity is assured by avoiding both specific and nonspecific attractive interactions with other species that are present in the analyte solution.

The most commonly discussed, and used, biologically derived recognition elements are antibodies, which increasingly are being replaced by engineered fragments of antibodies. Simpler peptides are also often discussed as recognition elements but are mainly used for targeting since their affinity is low and therefore not ideal for nanoscale sensors developed to detect analytes at low abundance. In recent years, aptamers have received a lot of interest as an alternative to creating specific recognition elements with a defined 3-D structure. We will briefly introduce these common systems and then discuss, in more general terms, important design criteria for adding recognition elements to biosensor surface functionalization schemes.

3.2.3.1 Antibodies Antibodies are widely used because of the high specificity of antibody–antigen binding. However, they are also very sensitive to their environment, meaning that the way they are immobilized should carefully consider proper conformation and orientation. Immunoglobulin G (IgG) is the most commonly encountered antibody in biosensing. Like typical antibodies, it consists of one Fc and two Fab' binding sites and requires that at least one of the Fab' fragments are exposed to solution.[84] Immobilization techniques have included microcontact printing,[85] biotin–streptavidin binding utilizing biotin-modified IgGs,[86–89] direct spotting,[86] and covalent binding.[90]

3.2.3.2 Antibody Fragments

Antibody fragments provide the same specificity as whole antibodies, but by having a large part of the antibody omitted, they are much smaller. In the context of sensors whose sensitivity is highly confined to the surface, such as semiconductor nanowires and nanoplasmonic sensors, this can be a key advantage. As for antibodies, the orientation of an antibody fragment to expose its binding site is essential but somewhat more demanding. Up to a threefold increase in activation has been reported[84] when the orientation has been controlled. Common immobilization strategies that have been explored include binding to streptavidin-coated surfaces by biotinylation[87] and direct coupling to gold using cystein residues.[91]

3.2.3.3 Aptamers

Aptamers are single-stranded DNA or RNA oligonucleotide sequences folded into a 3-D structure capable of binding specifically to a target molecule. They are generated in the systematic evolution of ligands by exponential enrichment (SELEX) process, which was first reported by Ellington and Szostak [92] and Tuerk and Gold[93] in 1990. In this approach, suitable binding sequences are first isolated from large oligonucleotide libraries and are subsequently amplified.[94,95] As antibodies, they are characterized by both their high affinity and specificity to their targets[94,95] but are more resource intensive to develop. Despite being similar to antibodies in function, their quasi-synthetic origin offers several advantages such as easier immobilization on sensing surfaces, higher reproducibility, longer shelf life, easier regeneration, and a higher resistance to denaturation. However, they typically provide lower affinity than antibodies.

3.2.3.4 General Considerations for Recognition Element Immobilization

Needless to say, immobilization of a recognition element to the spacer layer has to be irreversible and thus preferably involves a chemical bond. Density and conservation of active conformation and optimum orientation of recognition units such as proteins/antibodies or enzymes are other particular challenges.[96,97] Although the density of recognition elements will determine the maximum attainable sensor signal, simple maximization of the density is not advisable; steric hindrance as well as denaturation due to mutual strong interactions between recognition elements can occur and can lead to inactivity.[84]

Proper immobilization onto the designated part of the pattern is important to achieve both specificity and selectivity. The structure of the recognition element has to be preserved to ensure specificity. Denaturation of the specific conformation also risks causing reduced selectivity by exposing nonspecific binding domains. Doing the functionalization from, for example, a polymer surface designed to reduce nonspecific binding (see above) typically ensures that the surface does not strongly affect the 3-D structure of the recognition element. However, the orientation of the recognition element also has to be such that binding can occur.[98] Orientation of molecules at biosensor interfaces, especially at nanostructured interfaces, is difficult to infer, and mostly, one has to rely on the knowledge that the coupling elements have been designed such that the correct orientation is preferred.

As mentioned earlier for antibodies, a common coupling strategy, due to its ease of use, is biotin–avidin coupling. A biotinylated nonfouling surface such as PLL-*g*-PEG-biotin is exposed to an avidin derivative with low nonspecific binding, such as streptavidin or neutravidin, to form a layer on top, which can bind additional biotinylated ligands.[98,99] Although, for example, neutravidin is water soluble, engineered to be zwitterionic, and neutral, and thus does not cause massive nonspecific binding under most biosensor experiments, it is known that this coupling strategy significantly reduces the circulation times of nanoparticles *in vivo*.[60] This is likely due to opsonization; a surface fully covered with neutravidin can thus not be expected to be equally nonfouling as the unfunctionalized interface.

The use of biotin–avidin as a coupling strategy is also illustrative from another point of view, in terms of ensuring specific coupling and orientation. Biotinylation of ligands for proteins and peptides is mostly carried out with biotinylation kits, which will add a biotin to, for example, surface-exposed amine groups. Only rarely can it be ensured that there will only be one biotin per ligand with this approach. This has negative consequences such that biotin modifications might also occur to the binding domain, leading to reduced specificity and selectivity, and that a range of orientations are possible for the immobilized ligand. Furthermore, each ligand, depending on the density of biotin groups and surface-bound avidin, can bind to more than one site on the surface, increasing the risk for denaturation of the structure and lowering the overall density of recognition elements. Therefore, it is possible that every immobilized ligand might be rendered inactive. While we discussed the problem of multiple functional groups for the attachment of each ligand in the framework of biotin–avidin, the described limitations can be generalized, and are also valid, for example, for common chemical immobilization strategies making use of peptide surface functional groups, such as the most common chemical coupling strategies through amine and carboxyl groups.

It is also important to point out that specificity does not automatically mean as high affinity, as for the biotin–avidin binding that is often used to demonstrate the proof of principle for new recognition biosensor. For example, antibodies, which can be highly specific, have typical affinities in the range of 0.1 to 10.0 nM. The affinity can effectively be reduced by partial denaturation and suboptimal orientation at a biosensor interface. A nanoscale sensor trying to detect low-abundant analytes (sub-nanomolar concentration) therefore has to take into account that a certain sensing site might only be populated with a single analyte molecule for a short time before the molecule desorbs again. Related to this point is that a recognition interaction can indeed be so weak that multivalent binding is required for detection. As discussed in a separate section below, multivalent interactions are common in real biological systems, which is a motivation to design biosensors that can explore and use such interactions. However, when multivalent binding is required for the capture of an analyte, a sufficient number of closely spaced recognition elements in the correct geometrical configuration must be present on the sensing element. A sensor surface is typically two-dimensional, which puts further geometrical constraints on the art of multivalency that can be applied. Using flexible spacers for the attachment of recognition elements can help in circumventing this constraint.

In summary, a range of well-established recognition elements, mostly recruited from already existing biological molecular systems, exist and have been adapted to surface-based sensor surface modifications. However, their proper function as recognition elements is crucially dependent on how they are linked to the surface both in terms of chemistry and geometry. The latter aspect is more crucial when designing intelligent surface modifications for nanoscalse sensors than for traditional macroscale biosensors. So far, most work is concentrated on evaluating the applicability of existing surface modifications, designed for macroscopic sensors, followed by selection based on performance. There is thus significant room for improvement with respect to optimizing the surface anchor, the spacer, and possibly also the functional unit for optimally designed nanoscale sensors.

3.3   ALTERNATIVE SURFACE PATTERNING STRATEGIES

As an alternative to the use of material selective (orthogonal) surface modifications, which relies strictly on careful selection of the anchor groups, various printing methods can also be used in order to generate small-scale patterns suitable for different types of biosensor applications. Below follows a brief description of some of these, focusing on the challenges of generating multifunctional small-scale patterned surfaces.

3.3.1   Lithographic Patterning of Physisorbed Macromolecules

A patterning concept that has been applied successfully to macromolecules anchored by physisorption is lithographic patterning. This was first described for large areas using photolithographically defined patterns of resist and liftoff, and molecular assembly patterning by liftoff (MAPL).[100] In this approach, areas on the substrate that should first be functionalized with, for example, a functional version of PLL-g-PEG are exposed, while the remaining surface is covered by developed resist. Assembly of the PLL-g-PEG might occur everywhere, but when the photoresist is subsequently lifted off, the PLL-g-PEG in these areas is lifted off with the resist. The free areas can then be exposed to differently functionalized (or typically unfunctionalized) macromolecules like PLL-g-PEG, which will adsorb strongly to the now exposed areas. It is advisable to create the functional part of the pattern first and to backfill with a purely nonfouling species since any defects in the functional coating caused by the multistep processing will then be "healed" by adsorption of the non-functional molecules in the defects. With the reverse process functional binding sites might instead end up in what should be nonfouling areas of the pattern.

The standard MAPL strategy cannot be applied to nanoscale sensor applications due to the fact that sufficiently high resolution photolithographic patterning cannot be achieved. However, by combining the MAPL approach with nanoimprint lithography (NIL), patterns with feature sizes of 100 nm have been produced[100] and with extreme ultraviolet interference lithography even down to 50 nm[101]. Furthermore, a polymer resist-free alternative patterning approach, built on the MAPL principle, was recently developed. A popular strategy to produce nanostructures, especially high-aspect-ratio sensor nanostructures, is to etch substrates with several films of materials deposited on top of each other. Reactive ion etching is preferably performed through metal masks of, for example, chrome, which are inert to the etch gases. It was recently demonstrated that chrome etch masks can be used also as lift-off masks for patterning of PLL-*g*-PEG after the etching step.[102] With this method, the mask is left in place after reactive etching of the structure. Then, the molecular assembly by physisorption of PLL-*g*-PEG is performed; the chrome mask is removed by a short acid etch, which is nondestructive to the polymer, but which removes the polymer on top of the chrome structure. The free, previously masked surface is then backfilled with another macromolecule. Thus, the MAPL concept has been extended down to the true nanoscale necessary for small-scale sensors such as nanoplasmonic or nanopore electrochemical sensors[100,102]

3.3.2   Nanoscale Molecular Surface Modification through Printing

Microcontact printing is a hugely successful method to create molecular patterns on the micron scale. The technique makes use of soft stamps, typically of PDMS, with a topography that is the mirror image of the pattern that should be created on a substrate.[103–105] The stamp is inked with a solution of the molecule that should be deposited onto the pattern, and the stamp is then applied with pressure to ensure a conformal contact to the substrate. Molecules on the stamp transfer to the substrate during the direct contact. In contact with the surface, both physisorption and chemisorption can occur depending on what molecular attachment strategy is preferred. SAM[104], functional PEG brush,[106,107] lipid bilayer,[108] and protein[107,109,110] patterns have all been created in this way. Application of contact printing and related methodologies to molecular patterning on nanoscale sensors, however, awaits further developments, and we will therefore only briefly describe the challenges that need to be addressed to reach this goal.

First, the demands on the stamp material design increases as patterns have to be created that are smaller than the current typical micron or submicron replicas used today. Since conformal contact has to be achieved, both the pillars creating the contact as well as the stamp body have to be soft. However, slender or high-aspect-ratio nanoscale polymeric structures tend to collapse laterally or bundle due to capillary forces and other surface effects,[105] which put limits on their softness relative to their aspect ratio and spacing. Similarly, for nanoscale sensor objects that are well spaced (low aspect ratio), the inverse problem of sagging can occur,[105] in which case contact of the stamp body leads to molecular transfer to undesired areas of the sensor substrate.

Second, the molecular transfer has to occur onto already fabricated sensor substrates. This requires alignment of the stamp with a precision of a few nanometers onto the sensor unless the use of a stamp is combined with orthogonally binding anchors as discussed for the orthogonal molecular self-assembly approach. Using soft stamps and current alignment methods, such precision is beyond today's standard methodology, with the exception of that in combination with direct writing as will be described below. Misalignment will lead to, at the very least, severe edge effects from missing or overlapping functionalization and passivation of the sensor elements. Such defects in the passivation and functional layers will significantly compromise the specificity of the biosensor signal.

Third, for polymer, biomolecule, and other surface modifications relevant for biosensor modification, the molecules have to transfer in sufficient amounts in the correct conformation and self-assemble on the contacted surface. The density has to be sufficient to meet all the requirements discussed earlier for spacer and functional groups. This requires that the molecules are applied in a solvent. Pressing a solvent-containing stamp tends to produce wetting of the printing solution also in the vicinity of the contacting pillar, which limits the pattern definition by molecular diffusion.[105,111,112] These effects are irrelevant on the micron scale but become increasingly relevant when pattern definition has to be defined on the nanometer scale.[112]

Fourth, many geometries that take advantage of the unique aspects of nanoscale sensors to minimize, for example, sample consumption or to produce directional sensing make use of an inherently 3-D nanoscale design of the sensor elements. Since contact printing on these length scales is an inherently two-dimensional method that cannot guarantee a homogeneous distribution of the patterned molecules into, for example, nanopores, the application of contact printing might be limited to planar sensor configurations even if molecular printing on the nanoscale would become routine.

3.3.3 Nanoscale Molecular Surface Modification through Direct Writing

Until recently, molecular patterning on the nanoscale was only practically feasible by either vacuum physical deposition methods, which are not suitable for biological compounds, or molecular self-assembly as described earlier. However, the advent and continuous improvement of dip-pen lithography[113,114] and related methods have opened up the possibility to write molecular patterns with nanometer precision. Using an inked, nanosized tip, in advanced designs connected to a reservoir for continuous writing, and the control principles of scanning probe microscopy, molecules can be deposited by nanometer precision onto a substrate.[113,114] Massive parallelization making use of a thousand, or more, tips writing on the surface simultaneously has significantly reduced the time for molecular pattern deposition over the large areas typically employed for nanoscale biosensors.[115]

Application of direct writing to nanoscale biosensor functionalization has the advantage over, for example, contact printing that the structure can be imaged and individually aligned with the inking tip. Also, in the case of direct writing, the goal is to transfer the functionalized spacer molecules or reacting a ligand to a functionalized spacer in the defined area of writing.[114] Therefore, the correct environmental conditions have to be met for those reactions, and the surface density of the surface functionality has to be controlled similarly to what was discussed for self-assembly patterning. This is a bigger challenge when working with small rather than large volumes of solutes, but it is somewhat offset by the opportunity to confine the functionalization to only the region of interest. Successful demonstrations of polymer surface modifications suitable for biosensor functionalization using versions of direct tip-assisted writing of nanoscale patterns have been demonstrated through patterning approaches using combinations of "nanoshaving," "nanografting," and grafting from of polymer brushes from deposited or activated initiators.[116] Combined with backfilling of initiators or polymers adhering to surrounding areas, these techniques could be used to achieve functionalization of nanoscale sensors without the need for orthogonal sets of anchor chemistry. Despite adding an additional and quasi-serial processing step to the surface-modification process, this constitutes a significant simplification.

In contrast to printing, inking has also been proven to be applicable to 3-D nanoscale structures. By using tips that can dispose larger amounts of liquid than a traditional hard-tip dip pen, cavities can be filled to functionalize surfaces on a structure for which the tip cannot contact directly.[117] Versions of dip-pen lithography using soft or hydrogel tips have also recently been demonstrated, which make use of soft tips in order to channel larger volumes to the surface under conformal contact on the nanoscale.[114,117,118] However, writing on topographically patterned substrates and substrates with material contrast poses additional challenges in terms of controlling the wetting as the molecular sample is ejected in a solvent. When the solvent is ejected, it must wet the substrate surface sufficiently better than the ejecting tip in order to transfer to the substrate, but it cannot wet the substrate so well that it spreads over a larger than designed area or preferentially spreads over adjacent surface areas with a different surface chemistry. The presence of molecules for patterning acting as detergents in the solvent increases the complexity of being able to control wetting, deposition, and chemical reactivity simultaneously.

3.3.4   Multivalency and the Intelligent Fluid Biointerface

Discussions on biosensor detection often implicitly assume that a surface-bound capture agent binds to the analyte with sufficient affinity to allow the detection of its presence at the sensor element over the measurement time-scale. Therefore, surface-modification schemes are generally based on the recognition units being immobilized at the biosensor interface at a sufficient or optimal density for detection, as discussed for all the sensor functionalization concepts presented earlier. However, in nature, most recognition processes are of low affinity. Multivalent interactions to boost the total affinity are more the rule than the exception for many important processes.[37] This is especially true for interactions occurring at cell membranes where fluidity enables the lateral diffusion of several ligands in the membrane to be recognized as the local concentration becomes sufficient. Thus, many recognition phenomena such as transcription factor binding to DNA[119], phosphoinositide-mediated protein binding,[120] or carbohydrate–protein binding[121] are the integral of many simultaneously occurring, polyvalent low-affinity events occurring in the necessary geometrical and sequential constellation, where each single binding event is essentially transient. Such events can in the best case only very inefficiently be probed by the conventional surface-modification schemes discussed so far.

To mimic multivalent recognition processes, the intelligent surface design that regulate these events in biological systems have to be implemented as surface modifications on miniaturized sensors. The key to this in biological systems is the fluidity of recognition elements or the scaffold to which they are attached. Fluidity of the surface coating implies that it has to consist of a liquid or liquid crystalline system. The most well-known and frequently implemented liquid crystalline surface modification is the lipid bilayer, which is inspired by biological membranes and has been assembled onto biosensors as well as for other applications in many different incarnations.[122–124] As a reductionist version of cell membranes, phospholipid molecules self-assemble into surface-adhering membranes with the hydrophilic head oriented toward the liquid environment and the hydrophobic tails facing each other by a variety of methods.[122,123]

By a popular method, lipid vesicles of the desired composition are first spontaneously formed and homogenized to a diameter in the 100-nm range in solution, and thereafter adsorbed onto the solid surface of the biosensor. The liposomes fuse together into a planar supported lipid bilayer under suitable conditions of pH, temperature, and counterions for the combination of lipid composition and surface material.[49,125–129] Although this method is popular, it mainly works directly on a set of oxide surfaces (e.g., SiO_2, TiO_2, ITO), but it has been complemented with other surface modifications such as tethering of lipids into a monolayer and similar strategies to promote fusion also to metal surfaces,[130–133] as well as being applied to nanoscale porous surfaces.[134–136] A supported lipid membrane conforms to surface features larger than ca. 20 nm or smaller than a few nanometers[137] and retains fluidity similar to a biological membrane.[123] This can be achieved when the interaction of the individual lipid with the substrate is very weak, but the internal cohesion of the membrane is very strong due to the hydrophobic core, allowing the membrane as a whole to be robustly attached and able to span areas that are even macroscopically large. By design of nature, commonly used phospholipid membranes can be regarded as nonfouling to most biological fluids free from specifically lipid degrading lipases due to a combination of stable hydration of the head-group region, predominantly zwitterionic charge of the head groups, the low number of defects, the ability to self-heal, and fluidity.[138,139] Supported lipid bilayers have already been implemented for numerous sensing applications in the laboratory setting,[123,124,134] although their mechanical fragility has prevented use in field applications. Multivalent binding has also recently been inferred from binding events taking place to lipid membrane functionalized biosensors.[120,140–142]

Despite their promise to functionalize biosensors to probe biorecognition processes occurring with membrane-bound species and general sensing of multivalent binding, implementation of lipid membrane functionalization schemes for nanoscale sensor surfaces is rare. Assembly of planar lipid bilayers by liposome fusion and other means is restricted on the nanoscale due to the very high energy associated with exposing the edges of a membrane. An energy gain from opening up of a liposome to exposing the edges thus has to be compensated by greater reduction in energy from the increased surface adhesion.[143] However, if such high adhesion energy is achieved, it is likely to strongly affect membrane properties such as fluidity. The edges of lipid membranes are also by nature more hydrophobic and therefore both pinning points for large membrane molecules and sites of high binding energy for molecules in solution. Thus, one risks having an ill-defined surface modification at the edges of the sensing areas where nanoscale biosensors are often most sensitive. Furthermore, the nanoscale sensor area has to incorporate a sufficient number of tethered recognition elements to perform multivalent binding. An obvious way to circumvent the nanoscale restriction is to expand the allowable area of lipid surface modification to a greater surface than the sensor element.[144,145] When the recognition element is mobile, recognition can, in principle, occur anywhere on the surface by multiple ligands and be transported by diffusion within the membrane to the sensing site. This requires homogenization of the surface chemistry, for example, by covering the entire surface with an oxide film suitable for lipid membrane assembly. A major drawback with this approach, though, is that some of the advantages of nanoscale sensors are not utilized. In fact, the functionalization of the recognition element is not patterned and is therefore identical to that of a macroscale sensor. Homogeneous surface modifications additionally tend to reduce the sensitivity of nanoscale transducers. Not patterning the capture of analytes to the nanoscale sensor area voids the chance of improving on the sensitivity of a nanoscale sensor by designing functional areas to optimize the transport of analytes only to the areas of sensitivity, as will be discussed in a separate section.

Given the severe practical obstacles to implement planar or supported lipid membranes as intelligent surface modifications on the nanoscale, other membrane geometries should be considered. As described, lipid membranes including peptides, glycolipids, and other suitable recognition elements are preferably assembled in liposomes, which can be controlled in composition and size in a relatively straightforward manner. At a size of 100 nm in diameter, a liposome has roughly the extension of the sensing element of most nanoscale sensors. Direct assembly of liposomes by a tether to a nanoscale sensor that has first been passivated to nonspecific binding by a spacer layer and patterned to capture the liposomes thus allows placing a stable, functional lipid membrane recognition element patterned exclusively on the sensor elements.[24] However, potential drawbacks to consider are the highly curved geometry, the often restricted space in the most sensitive tethering region, and that many nanoscale sensors, for example, nanoplamonic sensors, have a low penetration depth and might be insensitive to a recognition event occurring at the far side of the liposome.[24]

3.3.5 Summary Functionalization of Nanoscale Biosensors

In summary, there exist today a multitude of different surface functionalization strategies compatible with small-scale sensors. However, their application to nanoscale sensors requires additional consideration of the geometrical constraints that are imposed, and the optimal design depends critically on the specific application. In general, modular approaches to functionalization exploiting self-assembly of the molecular coatings to the material contrast offered by small-scale sensors are advantageous. This allows rapid retailoring of the molecular structure to meet the demands of new application areas and is also a way to characterize surface-modification strategies in detail. In the following section, we will discuss how different means to control the actual transport of analytes to nanoscale sensing areas, keeping the possible ways to functionalize small-scale sensors in mind, can provide additional improvement of the overall performance of bioanalytical sensors. We will focus, in particular, on the handling of small sample volumes with low concentrations of analytes.

3.4 THE CHALLENGE OF ANALYTE TRANSPORT

As outlined in the introduction, a decisively important but seldom considered design criterion for biosensors, especially nanoscale biosensors, is the transport of the analyte to the active sensing area. In this section, we will explore this design criterion, with the aim to provide an understanding of the suitable geometries for optimal use of nanoscale biosensors. This has further implications for both patterning strategies and choice of transducer principles. Several examples will be given and explored analytically.

Irrespective of whether binding is occuring on the sensitive regions of a small-scale sensor or not, the rate of molecular transport from the bulk solution to the sensor surface is a key design parameter, especially with respect to the detection of low-abundance analytes. In the scope of detecting low-abundant proteins (or any suspended biomolecule), it is worth considering some basic aspects and asking the following questions:

(1) How many molecules must bind to the sensor surface in order to get a detectable signal?
(2) What is the minimum bulk concentration required to reach (at equilibrium) a coverage corresponding to the detection limit?
(3) For a certain bulk concentration, what minimal sample volume is required to have enough molecules available in solution?
(4) How are molecules most efficiently transported to the sensor surface?
(5) How long will it take and how much sample will be consumed until the detection limit is reached?

While points 1–3 are often discussed and can be answered directly by knowing the saturated surface coverage of the analyte, the signal-to-noise ratio (S/N) of the detection system and the equilibrium dissociation constant of the ligand–receptor system, the answers to points 4 and 5 depend on the flow cell design and flow conditions during the experiment and require a more elaborate analysis. The latter is the main focus of this section.

Point 1: For a protein with a molecular mass of $M_W = 50,000$ g/mol (50 kDa) that saturates a sensor surface at a coverage, Γ_{sat}, of 200 ng/cm^2 (corresponding to around 50% of full surface coverage*[146]), there are $\Gamma_{sat}/M_W = 24,000$ proteins/μm^2 on the surface at saturated coverage. If the S/N of the sensor at saturated coverage is 100 (i.e., a detection limit x corresponding to a coverage of $x = 0.01$), there will be 240 proteins/μm^2 bound at the detection limit. Although a higher S/N has been reported,[147–149] this number is in good agreement with typical values obtained using conventional surface-based techniques, such as SPR, QCM, and impedance spectroscopy.

Point 2: The equilibrium coverage of a protein system, x_{eq}, is connected to the bulk concentration c_0 in the following way:

$$x_{eq} = (1 + K_D / c_0)^{-1}, \qquad (3.1)$$

where K_D is the equilibrium dissociation constant. For $K_D = 1$ nM, which is a typical value for many antigen–antibody pairs, and with the equilibrium coverage set to the detection limit ($x_{eq} = 0.01$), the lowest detectable bulk concentration is 10 pM. This means that for all concentrations <10 pM, the coverage will *never* be high enough to yield a measurable signal.

---

* Assuming that binding occurs according to the random sequential adsorption (RSA) model.

Point 3: In a 10 pM solution, there are 600,000 proteins/μL. Thus, the volume that contains 24,000 molecules (corresponding to the detection limit for a sensor with an active area of 100 μm^2) is 40 nL. However, 40 nL of a 10 pM solution will never be enough to reach the detection limit since proteins bound on a surface are always in equilibrium with molecules in solution. Hence, this value just serves as a rough indication of the ultimate limit regarding sample volume, which in a practical situation must be at least one order of magnitude higher. It is also worthwhile noting that conventional surface-based sensors often have active areas with orders of magnitude larger than 100 μm^2.

Points 4 and 5: Transport of molecules to the sensor surface is a key element in sensor design and is surprisingly seldom discussed explicitly in biosensor literature, in spite of some noteworthy exceptions.[150–152] On a sensor surface in contact with an analyte solution, molecules close to the surface will bind to the receptors. Hence, the region adjacent to the sensor surface will become depleted from target molecules, thus forming a so-called depletion layer and generating a concentration gradient. This, in turn, triggers a flux of molecules toward the surface, which is the main transport mechanism for target molecules to reach the surface. There are three fluxes (i.e., number of molecules per time per area) that are relevant in the following considerations:

Convective Flux, j_C: amount of molecules that are constantly delivered to the system, usually by means of a flow. It depends on the parameters

Q	bulk flow (m^3/s)
c_0	target bulk concentration (M)
H	channel height (m)
W	channel width (m)

Diffusive Flux, j_D: amount of molecules that reach the sensor surface. It depends on the parameters

D	diffusion coefficient (m^2/s)
c_0	target bulk concentration (M)
δ	depletion layer (m)

Reactive Flux, j_R: amount of molecules that the surface receptors can bind. It depends on the parameters

k_{on}	association rate constant (M/s)
ρ_R	surface receptor density (mol/m^2)
c_S	target surface concentration (M)

In biosensing, the binding rate of target molecules is often limited by the number of molecules transported to the vicinity of the surface. This corresponds to the situation when $j_D \ll j_R$; that is, the capacity of the surface receptors to bind target molecules is much higher than the number of molecules that reach the surface. This means that the surface-immobilized receptors can instantly bind every molecule that hits the surface, making the binding kinetics mass transport (or diffusion) limited (MTL). If instead $j_D \gg j_R$, more molecules are transported to the surface than the receptors on the surface can bind. The binding rate is then limited by the actual reaction between binding partners, and binding occurs in the reaction controlled (RC) regime. A binding rate can never be higher than in this case and is strictly determined by the nature of the molecular interaction (quantified by the actual rate of association, k_{on}, and dissociation, k_{off}, which yield to the equilibrium dissociation constant, $K_D = k_{off}/k_{on}$).

Before addressing the relation between diffusive flux (j_D) and reactive flux (j_R), we shall look at how j_D can be maximized. We therefore assume MTL binding conditions and investigate how j_D evolves with respect to different convective fluxes, j_C.

3.4.1 Convective versus Diffusive Flux (j_C vs. j_D)

In the following, we distinguish between three different scenarios (Fig. 3.3) and assume MTL conditions:

(A) *Stagnant Analyte Solution* ($j_C = 0$) The depletion zone grows infinitely.

(B) *Slow* Flow Conditions* ($j_C = j_D$) The depletion zone grows across the whole channel height but is halted at a distance, δ_s, under steady-state equilibrium conditions due to the convective flux. The capture efficiency is 100%, but the molecular flux to the surface is low.

(C) *Fast* Flow Conditions* ($j_C > j_D$) The convective flux is always higher than the diffusive flux so that the depletion zone remains smaller than

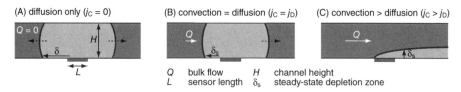

(A) diffusion only ($j_C = 0$)	(B) convection = diffusion ($j_C = j_D$)	(C) convection > diffusion ($j_C > j_D$)

Q bulk flow H channel height
L sensor length δ_s steady-state depletion zone

Figure 3.3 Three different scenarios around a sensor surface of length L: (A) stagnant conditions without flow, where the depletion zone δ grows infinitely into the channel; (B) the convective flux j_C is matched by the diffusive flux j_D, leading to a halt of the depletion zone at a distance, δ_s, from the sensor surface; and (C) the convective flux is higher than the diffusive flux so that the depletion zone develops only close to the sensor surface.

---

* The transition from "slow" to "fast" flow is in this case determined by j_C becoming larger than j_D under steady-state conditions. The absolute values for the flow depend on the channel dimensions.

the channel height. This leads to an increased flux to the surface, but many molecules will flow past the sensor without having a chance to interact with the surface, thereby lowering the capture efficiency.

3.4.1.1 Scenario A ($j_c = 0$)

Considering the simplest case, that is, a sensor with a finite (length L in Fig. 3.3A) area in contact with a stagnant analyte solution, the depletion zone will grow infinitely since no new target molecules supply the depleted region. Although highly dependent on the relative size of the sensor area and channel dimensions, the depletion zone will initially be dominated by growth parallel to the sensor surface, until the upper wall of the channel is reached, after which the growth of the depletion zone will be dominated by further expansion into the channel. To a good approximation, the size of the depletion zone, δ, will grow according to

$$\delta \sim \sqrt{Dt}, \tag{3.2}$$

where D is the diffusion coefficient of the target molecule and t is time. Although this equation only yields a scaling relation (and thus can only be stated in orders of magnitude), Equation 3.2 shows that (for a D of 10^{-6} cm^2/s, which is a typical value for proteins, and under the assumption that every molecule that hits the surface binds) a depletion layer of around 10 µm forms within 1 second and further expands to 100 µm after about 2 minutes and to 600 µm after about 1 hour (Fig. 3.4a). The size of the depletion zone can also be used to give a rough estimation of the molecular flux to the surface j_D according to

$$j_D \sim \frac{Dc_0}{\delta} \sim c_0 \left(\frac{D}{t} \right)^{1/2}, \tag{3.3}$$

where the concentration gradient has been approximated by the bulk concentration c_0 divided by the distance that the molecules have to diffuse to reach the surface (i.e. δ).

It becomes obvious from Fig. 3.4a that the flux j_D decreases by an order of magnitude within the first 2 minutes. Within this time, a couple of hundred thousands of molecules will reach a surface of 100 µm^2 (resulting in a surface coverage of around 25%) for a 100 nM solution, while it will only be a couple of thousands (coverage < 1%) for a 1 nM solution and less than 100 molecules for a 10 pM solution. Integrating Equation 3.3 over time yields a general expression for the surface coverage Γ_{sat}:

$$\Gamma_{sat} / M_W \sim c_0 \sqrt{Dt}, \tag{3.4}$$

which further allows the estimation of the time t_x needed to reach the detection limit x of the system:

$$t_x \sim \frac{1}{D} \left(\frac{x \Gamma_{sat} / M_W}{c_0} \right)^2 \tag{3.5}$$

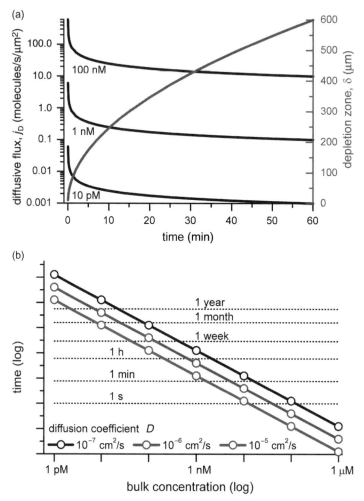

Figure 3.4 (a) Diffusive flux j_D and development of the depletion zone δ from a sensor surface over time under stagnant (i.e., no flow) conditions. $D = 10^{-6}$ cm^2/s (b), time required to reach a coverage corresponding to a detection limit of 1% of the saturated coverage (according to Eq. 3.5). Note that the absolute values given on the y-axis are not strictly correct since they have been calculated from scaling relations (Eqs. 3.2, 3.3, and 3.5) and are thus missing an unknown prefactor. (See color insert.)

For a 10 pM solution, the time required to reach the detection limit (set to $x = 0.01$) is in the range of months to years, while it takes minutes to hours to get a detectable signal from a 1 nM solution and less than a second from a 100 nM solution (Fig. 3.4b).

In general, molecular adsorption from a stagnant solution is only a valuable approach if high bulk concentrations are probed. For low-abundant target molecules (<nM), the times required to obtain a detectable signal are too long

for such a system to be of practical use. A common way to increase the molecular flux of molecules toward a sensor surface and thereby to reduce the time required for detection is by applying a flow in the channel, which may eventually lead to RC binding kinetics.

3.4.1.2 Scenario B ($j_C = j_D$)

If a flow Q in the channel supplies the system with additional target molecules, this convective flux of molecules, j_C, will bring the expansion of the depletion zone in the channel to a halt, thus leading to a constant molecular flux to the surface rather than a temporally decreasing flux as in scenario A. In scenario B, (Fig. 3.3B), the convective flux is so low that the depletion layer can still expand across the whole channel height and into the channel. The convective flux j_C in the channel is

$$j_C \sim \frac{c_0 Q}{HW} \qquad (3.6)$$

Steady-state conditions are reached if $j_D = j_C$; that is,

$$\frac{D c_0}{\delta} \sim \frac{c_0 Q}{HW}. \qquad (3.7)$$

From there, the size of the depletion zone under *steady-state* conditions can be derived:

$$\delta_s \sim HWD/Q. \qquad (3.8)$$

It becomes evident from Figure 3.5 that only for extremely low flows (well below 1 nL/min for a $100 \times 100 \ \mu m^2$ channel), the depletion zone extends

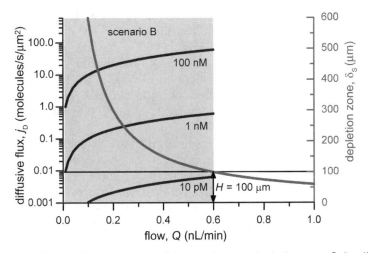

Figure 3.5 Diffusive flux j_D and size of the steady-state depletion zone δ_s for different flows Q for a channel height H of 100 μm. The channel width W is 100 μm, $D = 10^{-6} \ cm^2/s$. Scenario B (depletion zone expanding across the whole channel height) only occurs for flows <0.6 nL/min (gray shaded area). (See color insert.)

across the entire channel. For a flow of $Q = 0.5$ nL/min and a bulk concentration $c_0 = 1$ nM, the steady-state flux toward the surface is 0.5 molecules/s/μm^2, which means that a coverage of 240 molecules/μm^2 (= detection limit) is reached after roughly 8 minutes, that is, about a factor of 3 faster than for stagnant conditions. Even though the initial flux in scenario A (6 molecules/(sμm^2) for a 1 nM solution) is higher than the steady-state flux of scenario B, the former decays rapidly in time and becomes smaller than 0.5 molecules/(sμm^2) after 2.5 minutes. This means that the steady-state flux will determine the time required to reach the detection limit. While the gain compared to scenario A is even more considerable for lower concentrations (10 pM: 13 hours vs. half a year), there is no profit in the case of high concentrations. The steady-state flux for a 100 nM solution is around 50 molecules/(sμm^2), which is considerably lower than the initial flux under stagnant conditions (several hundred molecules/(sμm^2)), and the detection limit is reached within 1 second.

Note that in scenario B, the capture efficiency is essentially 100%, meaning that every molecule that enters the channel will bind to the sensor surface. Although this might sound attractive from a sample consumption perspective, this approach is usually not suitable when working with low bulk concentrations since the time required to reach the detection limit is still very long. Further, the flux toward the surface presented here holds only for the part of the sensor area that is closest to the nondepleted solution. The sensor area further downstream will be reached by even lower fluxes. Since the readout signal of a sensor often averages over the whole sensor surface, the overall recorded response will be yet slower than predicted earlier.

3.4.1.3 *Scenario C* ($j_C > j_D$)   If the convective flux is chosen such that it is under all circumstances higher than the diffusive flux, the depletion zone will be smaller than the channel height (Fig. 3.3C). For instance, a 1 nM bulk solution under stagnant conditions has an initial (and maximal) diffusive flux to the surface of about $j_D = 6$ molecules/(sμm^2) (Fig. 3.4a). In a channel with dimensions of 100×100 μm^2, a flow of 1 μL/min of a 1 nM solution will provide the system with $j_C = 1000$ molecules/(sμm^2), thus ensuring that the conditions of scenario C are fulfilled.

The depletion zone in this case is smaller than the channel height. Here, the size of the steady depletion zone δ_s can be estimated by asking what the maximum distance from the surface is at which a molecule has enough time to diffuse the distance δ_s to the surface before having convected past the sensor of length L. Close to the surface, it is safe to approximate the flow profile by a linear shear flow, so that the velocity of a molecule at a distance δ_s from the surface is

$$v \sim \delta_s \frac{Q}{H^2 W}. \tag{3.9}$$

The time required to convect past the sensor of length L at a height δ_s over the sensor surface is

$$\tau_C \sim \frac{L}{v} \sim \frac{LH^2W}{Q\delta_s}. \tag{3.10}$$

The time to diffuse the distance δ_s is

$$\tau_D \sim \frac{\delta_s^2}{D}. \tag{3.11}$$

By matching these two times, one gets a steady-state depletion zone of size

$$\delta_s \sim \left(\frac{DH^2WL}{Q} \right)^{1/3}. \tag{3.12}$$

Implementing this result in the equation for diffusive flux, one gets

$$j_D \sim \frac{Dc_0}{\delta_s} \sim c_0 \left(\frac{D^2Q}{H^2WL} \right)^{1/3}. \tag{3.13}$$

Only for extremely low flows (e.g., 1 nL/min), the depletion zone expands over almost the whole channel height (Fig. 3.6). Already for a flow of 1 μL/min, the depletion zone does not grow larger than 10 μm. The magnitude of the depletion zone depends not only on the channel dimensions and the flow but also varies along the sensor, as illustrated in Figure 3.6b. Consequently, the average flux to the surface varies with the sensor length L, with higher fluxes for short sensors. This effect is most pronounced for very short (a few micrometers) sensors.

3.4.1.4 Summary of Scenarios A, B, and C
The diffusive fluxes and times to reach the detection limit for the three scenarios introduced earlier are presented in Table 3.3.

For high concentrations (100 nM in the above-mentioned example), reaching the detection limit within short times is never a problem. In all presented scenarios, the sensor response time is below 1 second. Measuring under flow becomes more important when working with low-concentration solutions. In scenario B, where full collection of molecules is ensured by having a low flow such that the depletion zone expands across the channel, times are considerably reduced compared to the stagnant solution case (scenario A). However, times can be further reduced with higher flows (scenario C), where a small depletion zone shortens the diffusion path lengths for the molecules. In addition, decreasing the sensor length from 100 to 2 μm increases the average flux to the surface by factors of 3–4 for the cases presented.

With recent developments in nanofabrication, channels with dimensions in the nanometer range are becoming readily available. This reduction in dimensions has dramatic influence on the transport of molecules to the surface simply because the diffusion path lengths are reduced by orders of magnitudes.

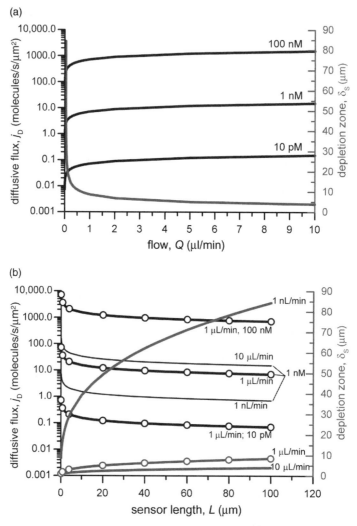

Figure 3.6 Diffusive flux j_D and size of the steady-state depletion zone δ_s in a channel with a height of 100 μm (a) for varying flows Q and different bulk concentrations for a sensor length $L = 100$ μm and (b) for varying sensor length L and different bulk concentrations and flow conditions. (See color insert.)

In Table 3.4, the results for a 100-nm-high and -wide channel are presented. The volumetric flow Q has been adapted such that the average flow *velocity* matches the situation of the macrochannel in Table 3.3. The times to reach the detection limit are decreased by one order of magnitude compared to the macrochannel case. Further comparisons between the macro- and the nano-channel are discussed in the following sections.

TABLE 3.3 Summary of Diffusive Fluxes j_D and Times to Reach the Detection Limit of a Sensor with S/N = 100 in a Microchannel for the Three Scenarios Depicted in Figure 3.3

Bulk concentration c_0	Scenario A ($j_C = 0$)		Scenario B ($j_C = j_D$) H = 100 μm	Scenario C ($j_C > j_D$) H = 100 μm Q = 1 μL/min		
	$t = 1$ s $\delta \approx 10$ μm	$t = 10$ min $\delta \approx 250$ μm	Q = 0.5 nL/min $\delta_s \approx 120$ μm	L = 100 μm $\delta_s \approx 8$ μm	20 μm $\delta_s \approx 5$ μm	2 μm $\delta_s \approx 2$ μm
Diffusive flux j_D [molecules/(s μm²)]						
10 pM	0.06	0.0025	0.005	0.07	0.12	0.25
1 nM	6	0.25	0.5	7	12	25
100 nM	600	25	50	700	1200	2500
Time to reach detection limit						
10 pM	0.5 year		12 h	1 h	30 min	15 min
1 nM	30 min		10 min	30 s	20 s	10 s
100 nM	<1 s		(5 s)*	<1 s	<1 s	<1 s

*In this case, the initial diffusive flux (600 molecules/s/μm², from scenario A) is higher than the steady state flux of scenario B (50 molecules/s/μm²) so that A is the dominating scenario. The detection limit is thus reached in <1 s.

TABLE 3.4 Diffusive Fluxes j_D and Times to Reach the Detection Limit of a Sensor with S/N = 100 in a Nanochannel for Scenarios B and C

Bulk concentration c_0	Scenario B ($j_C = j_D$) H = W = 100 nm Q = 0.5 pL/min	Scenario C ($j_C > j_D$) H = W = 100 nm Q = 1 pL/min
		L = 100 nm
	$\delta_s \approx 120$ nm	$\delta_s \approx 40$ nm
	Diffusive flux j_D [molecules/(s µm²)]	
10 pM	5	9
1 nM	500	900
100 nM	50,000	90,000
	Time to reach detection limit	
10 pM	50 s	30 s
1 nM	<1 s	<1 s
100 nM	<1 s	<1 s

3.4.2 Reactive versus Diffusive Flux (j_R vs. j_D)

So far, we have only considered the flux of molecules toward the surface. What has not yet been analyzed is how fast molecules will actually bind to the surface. This will depend on the relation between the diffusive flux j_D (which determines how many molecules reach the surface) and the reactive flux j_R (which determines how quickly receptors on the surface can bind target molecules). Above, we discussed the situation when $j_D \ll j_R$, that is, the MTL case. Here, we will discuss design criteria that increase the probability to reach the RC regime (i.e., $j_D \gg j_R$). In addition to rapid detection, operation under these conditions also helps unravel kinetic and thermodynamic data about the molecular interactions.

In the MTL case, the analyte concentration close to the surface, c_s, is almost zero, so that the diffusive flux can be defined as

$$j_D \sim \frac{D(c_0 - c_s)}{\delta_s} \sim \frac{Dc_0}{\delta_s}. \tag{3.14}$$

In the RC case, the analyte concentration close to the surface is instead on the same order as the bulk concentration, and the reactive flux is defined as

$$j_R \sim k_{on}\rho_R c_s \sim k_{on}\rho_R c_0, \tag{3.15}$$

where k_{on} is the association rate constant and ρ_R is the receptor density on the surface.

The Damköhler number Da is used to compare these two fluxes and allows estimating in which regime binding occurs:

$$Da = \frac{j_R}{j_D} = \frac{k_{on}\rho_R\delta_s}{D}. \tag{3.16}$$

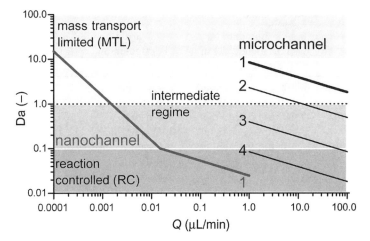

Figure 3.7   The Damköhler number Da is plotted versus the flow Q for both a microchannel (100×100 μm², $Q > 1$μL/min) and a nanochannel (100×100 nm², $Q < 1$μL/min). For the nanochannel, Q corresponds to the total flow through an experimentally relevant system, that is, an array of nanopores with 10 pores/μm² and a total area of 50×50 μm² (i.e., 25,000 pores in total). The average flow velocity in both the micro- and the nanochannels are of comparable magnitude. 1, "standard" conditions; 2, shorter sensor; 3, faster diffusion; 4, slower binding kinetics or lower receptor density. Absolute values for the parameters used in 1–4 can be found in Table 3.5.

For Da $\gg$ 1, binding is diffusion limited, while for Da $\ll$ 1, binding is RC.

Figure 3.7 shows Damköhler numbers for varying flow rates. Since in reality the transition from the MTL regime to the RC regime is smooth, an intermediate regime for $0.1 <$ Da < 10 is indicated in Figure 3.7. For a microchannel under "standard" conditions ($1 \, Q > 1$μL/min; see Table 3.5), binding occurs in the MTL regime. Decreasing the sensor length (2) is beneficial to get closer to the RC regime but is not entirely sufficient in the presented case. Working with smaller target molecules (i.e., having a higher diffusion coefficient, 3) is likewise beneficial. It is only with either a system with slower association kinetics or a sensor surface with lower receptor density (4) that RC binding occurs. Also, if the channel dimensions are reduced to nanometric size ($1 \, Q < 1$μL/min), RC binding can be established for flows greater than 0.01 μL/min* under standard conditions. The kink in the curve for nanochannels illustrates the crossover from scenario B (full collection of target molecules) to scenario C (thin depletion zone over the sensor surface).

---

* To compare nanochannels with microchannels, an array of nanopores with 10 pores/μm² and a total area of 50×50 μm² (i.e., 25,000 pores in total) is assumed. The flows correspond to the total flow through such an array, with the average flow *velocities* in the nano- and microchannels being of comparable magnitude.

TABLE 3.5   Parameters Used to Produce the Curves in Figures 3.7–3.9

	"Standard" Parameters (1) in Figures 3.7–3.9	Varied Parameters in Figure 3.7	Varied Parameters in Figures 3.8 and 3.9
Channel height, H	100 µm (µ-channel) 100 nm (n-channel)	2: $L = 2$ µm (shorter sensor)	2: $L = 2$ µm (shorter sensor)
Channel width, W	100 µm (µ-channel) 100 nm (n-channel)	3: $D = 10^{-8}$ m²/s (faster diffusion)	3: $D = 10^{-8}$ m²/s (faster diffusion)
Sensor length, L	100 µm (µ-channel) 100 nm (n-channel)		or $\rho_R = 10^{-9}$ mol/m² (lower receptor density)
Association rate constant, k_{on}	10^6 M/s	4: $k_{on} = 10^4$ M/s (slower binding kinetics)	4: $k_{on} = 10^4$ M/s and $k_{off} = 10^{-5}$ s⁻¹ (slower binding kinetics)
Dissociation rate constant, k_{off}	10^{-3}/s	or $\rho_R = 10^{-9}$ mol/ m² (lower receptor density)	
Diffusion coefficient, D	10^{-10} m²/s		5: $x = 0.001$ (lower detection limit)
Surface receptor density, ρ_R	10^{-7} mol/m²		
Bulk concentration, c_0	1 nM		
Detection limit, x^*	0.01		

*Fraction of monolayer coverage of a 50-kDa protein.

3.4.3   Design and Operation Criteria for Efficient Mass Transport

We are now in a position to answer question 5 posed at the beginning of this section: "How long will it take and how much sample will be consumed until the detection limit is reached?" We first look at how long it takes to reach either the detection limit of the system or equilibrium conditions. In the RC case, the binding follows a single exponential curve, and the time to reach equilibrium is thus

$$t_{R,eq} \sim (k_{on}c_0 + k_{off})^{-1}. \tag{3.17}$$

The time to reach the detection limit x is

$$t_{R,x} \sim \frac{x t_{R,eq}}{x_{eq}}, \tag{3.18}$$

where x_{eq} is the equilibrium coverage defined in Equation 3.1. In the MTL case, this time is prolonged by the factor Da:

$$t_{D,x} \sim \mathrm{Da}\, \frac{x t_{R,eq}}{x_{eq}}. \tag{3.19}$$

Figure 3.8a shows the time required to reach the detection limit of a sensor under different conditions. (See also the color version in the color insert.) Cases where binding reactions occur in the MTL regime are identified by dependence on the flow rate (e.g., 5), while RC binding does not depend on the flow rate (e.g., 4). We stress at this point that in reality, the change from one regime to the other is not abrupt but rather a smooth transition. For simplicity, this fact has been omitted in the figures and the transitions here are sharp.

When comparing with standard conditions (1 blue, Fig. 3.8a), it becomes clear that a short sensor (2) is beneficial and decreases t_x by a factor of almost 4 in the presented case. Working with smaller molecules (larger diffusion coefficient D, 3) not only facilitates moving toward RC conditions but also shortens the response time. It also becomes evident why a popular approach to measure under RC conditions is to decrease the receptor density ρ_R on the surface (3 as well). Having a system with slow "on" kinetics (4) also promotes reaching RC conditions, however, at a rather high price with respect to time. It is efficient to lower the detection limit x of the sensor (5), which results in a linear decrease in detection time. Decreasing channel dimensions to the nanometric length scale (1 red) allows for binding under RC conditions for flows larger than a few nanoliters per minute, and thus a reduced detection time compared to the microchannel standard conditions (1 blue). The difference in slopes for MTL conditions in the nanochannel ($\mathrm{MTL_B}$) and the microchannel ($\mathrm{MTL_C}$) originates from the fact that binding in the nanochannels occurs under full collection of target molecules (scenario B) while scenario C is present in the microchannel.

It is then straightforward to calculate the volume consumption required to reach the detection limit of the system by multiplying the time required t_x with the flow Q shown in Figure 3.8b. The main message from this plot is that volume consumption is smaller for the nanochannels (red) than for the microchannel (blue). In general, a lower time to reach the detection limit is connected to lower sample consumption. In the case of $\mathrm{MTL_B}$ (i.e., full collection of target molecules; see nanochannel for $Q < 0.001$ µL/min), the increase in flow is exactly compensated by the gain in time so that the total volume consumption does not depend on flow.

Since both the time (Fig. 3.8a) and the volume consumption required to reach the detection limit (Fig. 3.8b) are parameters that one would like to minimize in many practical situations, the overall performance of a sensor can be summarized by plotting the product of these two parameters versus the volumetric flow rate (Fig. 3.9). We deliberately weigh time and volume consumption equally in this example, being aware that depending on the application, minimizing time (e.g., in diagnostics) or volume consumption (e.g., expensive and/or low availability of target molecules) might be prioritized.

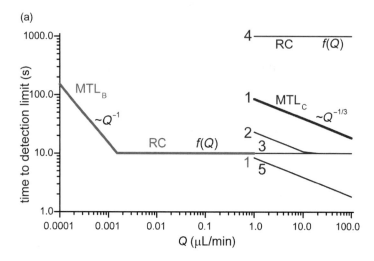

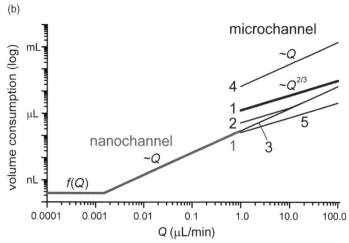

Figure 3.8 The time t_x required to reach the detection limit x (a) and the total volume consumption until the detection limit is reached (b) are plotted versus the flow Q for both a microchannel ($100 \times 100 \ \mu m^2$, blue) and a nanochannel ($100 \times 100 \ nm^2$, red). For the nanochannel, Q corresponds to the total flow through an experimentally relevant system, that is, an array of nanopores with 10 pores/μm^2 and a total area of $50 \times 50 \ \mu m^2$ (i.e., 25,000 pores in total). The average flow velocity in both the micro- and the nanochannels are of comparable magnitude. 1, "standard" conditions; 2, shorter sensor; 3, faster diffusion or lower receptor density; 4, slower binding kinetics; 5, lower detection limit. Absolute values for the parameters used in 1–5 can be found in Table 3.5. Subscript B stands for the case of full collection efficiency of target molecules (i.e., the depletion zone spans over the whole channel height and grows laterally into the channel), and subscript C stands for the case where the depletion zone is much smaller than the channel height. RC, reaction controlled regime; MTL, mass transport limited regime. (See color insert.)

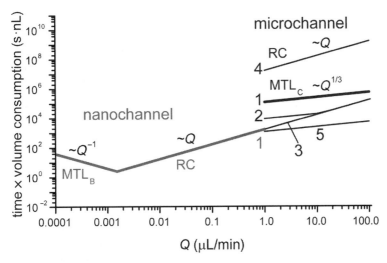

Figure 3.9 The product of the time to reach the detection limit and the sample volume consumed in that time is plotted versus the flow Q. Such a master curve can be used to assess the overall performance of a biosensor. 1, "standard" conditions; 2, shorter sensor; 3, faster diffusion or lower receptor density; 4; slower binding kinetics; 5, lower detection limit. Absolute values for the parameters used in 1–5 can be found in Table 3.5. (See color insert.)

The slopes that are obtained for the RC and the MTL_B regimes are generic since one of the two parameters (time and volume consumption, respectively) is flow independent. In the case of MTL_C, the slope depends on how the importance of the respective parameters is weighted. A compilation of all the slopes in Figures 3.8 and 3.9 can be found in Table 3.6. Based on these master curves, some general guidelines when operating a biosensor under constant flow can be drawn:

- Under RC conditions (e.g., 3, 4, 1 red for higher flows), it is always beneficial to decrease the flow. Since the time to reach a certain coverage under RC conditions is flow independent, there is no gain in using high flow.
- Under MTL conditions where the depletion zone spans over the whole channel height (MTL_B, e.g., 1 red for low flows), it is always beneficial to increase the flow. While the sample consumption remains constant in doing so, one reaches a certain coverage faster.
- Under MTL conditions where the depletion zone is much smaller than the channel height (MTL_C, e.g., 1 blue, 2 for low flows, 5), the choice of the flow rate depends on one's priorities. In our example, where time and volume consumption are regarded as equally important, it is beneficial to use a low flow. The reduction in sample consumption outweighs the longer time one has to wait to reach a certain coverage.

TABLE 3.6 Summary of the Slopes in Figures 3.8 and 3.9

		Reaction Controlled (RC)	Mass Transport Limited, MTL$_B$ (Full Collection)	Mass Transport Limited, MTL$_C$ (Thin Depletion Zone)
Time, t	Figure 3.8a	$\neq f(Q)$	$\sim Q^{-1}$	$\sim Q^{-1/3}$
Volume consumption, tQ	Figure 3.8a,b	$\sim Q$	$\neq f(Q)$	$\sim Q^{2/3}$
Master curve, $t \times tQ$	Figure 3.9	$\sim Q$	$\sim Q^{-1}$	$\sim Q^{1/3}$

From the considerations discussed earlier, the advantage of using sensors with channel and sensor dimensions on the nanometer scale becomes apparent from an analyte transport point of view. Not only time efficiency (Fig. 3.8a) and low sample consumption (Fig. 3.8b) are strong arguments for small sensors, but also improved access to more relevant and information-rich reaction-limited binding conditions (Fig. 3.7).

3.5 CONCLUDING REMARKS

From the analysis presented in the last section, it is obvious that analyte trans-port alone is a strong argument for pushing the development of miniaturized sensors forward. However, as specifically addressed in this chapter, what these sensors have in common is that the small sensitive regions generally exist in close proximity to larger, insensitive regions. Hence, if the surrounding regions are not made inert by suitable surface-modification schemes, the majority of the target molecules will bind to regions outside the sensitive part of the sensor and thus will be lost from a sensing point of view. The future development in this line of research thus relies heavily on further development and under-standing of surface functionalization strategies that allow binding of target molecules to the sensitive regions only, by keeping the surrounding regions inert and patterning highly specific and selective recognition elements on the sensitive areas. As previously treated theoretically[153] and experimen-tally,[68,154] such functionalizations can concentrate the adsorbing analyte mol-ecules on small biofunctional areas. Proteins reaching the inert regions are repelled, allowing them to diffuse or convect to the bioactive areas where they correspondingly bind at a considerably higher rate than if binding occurs over the entire surface. Given that the sensitivity in terms of surface coverage is the same for nanoscale and macroscopic sensors, this provides a real advan-tage of nanoscale sensors compared to conventional techniques such as QCM, SPR, and EI, where the entire surface is sensitive. However, the fact that the dimension of nanoscale sensors coincides with the dimension of the molecular building blocks makes precise control over the spatial distribution of the molecular binding events extremely demanding. Further development of the different patterning approaches, including improvement in selectively binding anchor chemistry, nanolithography, immobilization methods for recognition elements, and approaches to address also multivalent recognition events, is currently being addressed in many labs. Improved nanofabrication schemes are likely to help reduce the uncertainty imposed by ill-defined material compositions at the boundary between different materials. Furthermore, an interesting approach is to use the actual transducer elements as active elements to aid the selective patterning of these areas; for instance, the surface potential, temperature, and magnetic fields can locally be manipulated to improve certain surface-modification schemes. In a variation on that principle, the lateral mobility of supported lipid bilayers can be used not only to aid multivalent interactions but also to position probe elements by exerting external electrical[155–157] or hydrodynamic[158] forces to concentrate membrane-bound components at surface-based sensor elements. Despite the enormous work on nanoscale sensors and the tremendous attention they have attracted in the scientific community over the last 10 years, one can say that the design of intelligent surface coatings and flow geometries adapted to the realization of the full potential of such sensors is still only at the early stage of development.

REFERENCES

1. Ciruela, F. Fluorescence-based methods in the study of protein-protein interactions in living cells. *Current Opinion in Biotechnology* **19**, 338–343 (2008).

2. Cooper, M.A. & Singleton, V.T. A survey of the 2001 to 2005 quartz crystal microbalance biosensor literature: applications of acoustic physics to the analysis of biomolecular interactions. *Journal of Molecular Recognition* **20**, 154–184 (2007).

3. Daniels, J.S. & Pourmand, N. Label-free impedance biosensors: opportunities and challenges. *Electroanalysis* **19**, 1239–1257 (2007).

4. Homola, J. Surface plasmon resonance sensors for detection of chemical and biological species. *Chemical Reviews* **108**, 462–493 (2008).

5. Waggoner, P.S. & Craighead, H.G. Micro- and nanomechanical sensors for environmental, chemical, and biological detection. *Lab on a Chip* **7**, 1238–1255 (2007).

6. Braun, T. et al. Quantitative time-resolved measurement of membrane protein-ligand interactions using microcantilever array sensors. *Nature Nanotechnology* **4**, 179–185 (2009).

7. Burg, T.P. et al. Weighing of biomolecules, single cells and single nanoparticles in fluid. *Nature* **446**, 1066–1069 (2007).

8. Zhang, J. et al. Rapid and label-free nanomechanical detection of biomarker transcripts in human RNA. *Nature Nanotechnology* **1**, 214–220 (2006).

9. Shekhawat, G., Tark, S.H., & Dravid, V.P. MOSFET-embedded microcantilevers for measuring deflection in biomolecular sensors. *Science* **311**, 1592–1595 (2006).

10. Patolsky, F., Zheng, G., & Lieber, C.M. Nanowire-based biosensors. *Analytical Chemistry* **78**, 4260–4269 (2006).

11. Misra, N. et al. Bioelectronic silicon nanowire devices using functional membrane proteins. *Proceedings of the National Academy of Sciences of the United States of America* **106**, 13780–13784 (2009).

12. Stern, E. et al. Label-free immunodetection with CMOS-compatible semiconducting nanowires. *Nature* **445**, 519–522 (2007).

13. Zheng, G.F., Patolsky, F., Cui, Y., Wang, W.U., & Lieber, C.M. Multiplexed electrical detection of cancer markers with nanowire sensor arrays. *Nature Biotechnology* **23**, 1294–1301 (2005).

14. Anker, J.N. et al. Biosensing with plasmonic nanosensors. *Nature Materials* **7**, 442–453 (2008).

15. Stewart, M.E. et al. Nanostructured plasmonic sensors. *Chemical Reviews* **108**, 494–521 (2008).

16. Ji, H.F. et al. Microcantilever biosensors based on conformational change of proteins. *Analyst* **133**, 434–443 (2008).

17. Svedendahl, M., Chen, S., Dmitriev, A., & Kall, M. Refractometric sensing using propagating versus localized surface plasmons: a direct comparison. *Nano Letters* **9**, 4428–4433 (2009).

18. Arlett, J.L., Myers, E.B., & Roukes, M.L. Comparative advantages of mechanical biosensors. *Nature Nanotechnology* **6**, 203–215 (2011).

19. Jonsson, M.P., Dahlin, A.B., Jonsson, P., & Hook, F. Nanoplasmonic biosensing with focus on short-range ordered nanoholes in thin metal films. *Biointerphases* **3**, FD30–FD40 (2008).

20. Noy, A. Bionanoelectronics. *Advanced Materials* **23**, 807–820 (2011).

21. Ramgir, N.S., Yang, Y., & Zacharias, M. Nanowire-based sensors. *Small* **6**, 1705–1722 (2010).

22. Cooper, M.A. *Label-Free Biosensors: Techniques and Applications.* New York, NY: Cambridge University Press (2009).

23. Schultz, J. et al. *Biosensing: International Research and Development.* Dordrecht, The Netherlands: Springer (2006).

24. Dahlin, A.B., Jonsson, M.P., & Hook, F. Specific self-assembly of single lipid vesicles in nanoplasmonic apertures in gold. *Advanced Materials* **20**, 1436–1442 (2008).

25. Rifai, N., Gillette, M.A., & Carr, S.A. Protein biomarker discovery and validation: the long and uncertain path to clinical utility. *Nature Biotechnology* **24**, 971–983 (2006).

26. Kulasingam, V. & Diamandis, E.P. Strategies for discovering novel cancer biomarkers through utilization of emerging technologies. *Nature Clinical Practice Oncology* **5**, 588–599 (2008).

27. Sawyers, C.L. The cancer biomarker problem. *Nature* **452**, 548–552 (2008).

28. Soto, C. Diagnosing prion diseases: needs, challenges and hopes. *Nature Reviews Microbiology* **2**, 809–819 (2004).

29. Bell, J. Predicting disease using genomics. *Nature* **429**, 453–456 (2004).

30. Anderson, N.L. & Anderson, N.G. The human plasma proteome—history, character, and diagnostic prospects. *Molecular & Cellular Proteomics* **1**, 845–867 (2002).

31. Reichlin, T. et al. Early diagnosis of myocardial infarction with sensitive cardiac troponin assays. *New England Journal of Medicine* **361**, 858–867 (2009).

32. Sepúlveda, B., Angelomé, P.C., Lechuga, L.M., & Liz-Marzán, L.M. LSPR-based nanobiosensors. *Nano Today* **4**, 244–251 (2009).

33. Wang, J. Carbon-nanotube based electrochemical biosensors: a review. *Electroanalysis* **17**, 7–14 (2005).

34. Mun, K.S., Alvarez, S.D., Choi, W.Y., & Sailor, M.J.A. Stable, label-free optical interferometric biosensor based on TiO_2 nanotube arrays. *ACS Nano* **4**, 2070–2076 (2010).

35. Sannomiya, T., Dermutz, H., Hafner, C., Voros, J., & Dahlin, A.B. Electrochemistry on a localized surface plasmon resonance sensor. *Langmuir* **26**, 7619–7626 (2010).

36. Laibinis, P.E., Hickman, J.J., Wrighton, M.S., & Whitesides, G.M. Orthogonal self-assembled monolayers—alkanethiols on gold and alkane carboxylic-acids on alumina. *Science* **245**, 845–847 (1989).

37. Mammen, M., Choi, S.K., & Whitesides, G.M. Polyvalent interactions in biological systems: implications for design and use of multivalent ligands and inhibitors. *Angewandte Chemie (International ed.)* **37**, 2755–2794 (1998).

38. Kenausis, G.L. et al. Poly(L-lysine)-g-poly(ethylene glycol) layers on metal oxide surfaces: attachment mechanism and effects of polymer architecture on resistance to protein adsorption. *Journal of Physical Chemistry B* **104**, 3298–3309 (2000).

39. Pasche, S., De Paul, S.M., Voros, J., Spencer, N.D., & Textor, M. Poly(L-lysine)-graft-poly(ethylene glycol) assembled monolayers on niobium oxide surfaces: a quantitative study of the influence of polymer interfacial architecture on resistance to protein adsorption by ToF-SIMS and in situ OWLS. *Langmuir* **19**, 9216–9225 (2003).

40. Feller, L.M., Cerritelli, S., Textor, M., Hubbell, J.A., & Tosatti, S.G.P. Influence of poly(propylene sulfide-block-ethylene glycol) di-and triblock copolymer architecture on the formation of molecular adlayers on gold surfaces and their effect on protein resistance: a candidate for surface modification in biosensor research. *Macromolecules* **38**, 10503–10510 (2005).

41. Brink, C., Osterberg, E., Holmberg, K., & Tiberg, F. Using poly(ethylene imine) to graft poly(ethylene glycol) or polysaccharide to polystyrene. *Colloids and Surfaces* **66**, 149–156 (1992).

42. Malmsten, M., Emoto, K., & Van Alstine, J.M. Effect of chain density on inhibition of protein adsorption by poly(ethylene glycol) based coatings. *Journal of Colloid and Interface Science* **202**, 507–517 (1998).

43. Konradi, R., Pidhatika, B., Muhlebach, A., & Textort, M. Poly-2-methyl-2-oxazoline: a peptide-like polymer for protein-repellent surfaces. *Langmuir* **24**, 613–616 (2008).

44. Pidhatika, B., Moller, J., Vogel, V., & Konradi, R. Nonfouling surface coatings based on poly(2-methyl-2-oxazoline). *Chimia* **62**, 264–269 (2008).

45. Lee, J.H., Kopecek, J., & Andrade, J.D. Protein-resistant surfaces prepared by peo-containing block copolymer surfactants. *Journal of Biomedical Materials Research* **23**, 351–368 (1989).

46. Pasche, S., Textor, M., Meagher, L., Spencer, N.D., & Griesser, H.J. Relationship between interfacial forces measured by colloid-probe atomic force microscopy and protein resistance of poly(ethylene glycol)-grafted poly(L-lysine) adlayers on niobia surfaces. *Langmuir* **21**, 6508–6520 (2005).

47. Pasche, S., Vörös, J., Griesser, H.J., Spencer, N.D., & Textor, M. Effects of ionic strength and surface charge on protein adsorption at PEGylated surfaces. *Journal of Physical Chemistry B* **109**, 17545–17552 (2005).

48. Saxer, S. et al. Surface assembly of catechol-functionalized poly(L-lysine)-graft-poly(ethylene glycol) copolymer on titanium exploiting combined electrostatically driven self-organization and biomimetic strong adhesion. *Macromolecules* **43**, 1050–1060 (2009).

49. Kumar, K. et al. Formation of supported lipid bilayers on indium tin oxide for dynamically- patterned membrane-functionalized microelectrode arrays. *Lab on a Chip* **9**, 718–725 (2009).

50. Andreasson-Ochsner, M., Romano, G., Hakanson, M., et al. Single cell 3-D platform to study ligand mobility in cell-cell. *Lab on a Chip* **11**(17), 2876–2883 (2011).

51. Agheli, H., Malmstrom, J., Larsson, E.M., Textor, M., & Sutherland, D.S. Large area protein nanopatterning for biological applications. *Nano Letters* **6**, 1165–1171 (2006).

52. Marie, R., Dahlin, A.B., Tegenfeldt, J.O., & Hook, F. Generic surface modification strategy for sensing applications based on Au/SiO₂ nanostructures. *Biointerphases* **2**, 49–55 (2007).

53. Sagiv, J. Organized monolayers by adsorption.1. Formation and structure of oleophobic mixed monolayers on solid-surfaces. *Journal of the American Chemical Society* **102**, 92–98 (1980).

54. Nuzzo, R.G. & Allara, D.L. Adsorption of bifunctional organic disulfides on gold surfaces. *Journal of the American Chemical Society* **105**, 4481–4483 (1983).

55. Unsworth, L.D., Tun, Z., Sheardown, H., & Brash, J.L. Chemisorption of thiolated poly(ethylene oxide) to gold: surface chain densities measured by ellipsometry and neutron reflectometry. *Journal of Colloid and Interface Science* **281**, 112–121 (2005).

56. Schwendel, D. et al. Temperature dependence of the protein resistance of poly- and oligo(ethylene glycol)-terminated alkanethiolate monolayers. *Langmuir* **17**, 5717–5720 (2001).

57. Herne, T.M. & Tarlov, M.J. Characterization of DNA probes immobilized on gold surfaces. *Journal of the American Chemical Society* **119**, 8916–8920 (1997).

58. Tosatti, S., Michel, R., Textor, M., & Spencer, N.D. Self-assembled monolayers of dodecyl and hydroxy-dodecyl phosphates on both smooth and rough titanium and titanium oxide surfaces. *Langmuir* **18**, 3537–3548 (2002).

59. Zoulalian, V. et al. Self-assembly of poly(ethylene glycol)-poly(alkyl phosphonate) terpolymers on titanium oxide surfaces: synthesis, interface characterization, investigation of nonfouling properties, and long-term stability. *Langmuir* **26**, 74–82 (2010).

60. Amstad, A., Textor, M., & Reimhult, E. Stabilization and functionalization of iron oxide nanoparticles for biomedical applications. *Nanoscale* (2011) DOI: 10.1039/C1NR10173K.

61. Lee, H., Dellatore, S.M., Miller, W.M., & Messersmith, P.B. Mussel-inspired surface chemistry for multifunctional coatings. *Science* **318**, 426–430 (2007).

62. Michel, R. et al. Selective molecular assembly patterning: a new approach to micro- and nanochemical patterning of surfaces for biological applications. *Langmuir* **18**, 3281–3287 (2002).

63. Xu, C.J. et al. Dopamine as a robust anchor to immobilize functional molecules on the iron oxide shell of magnetic nanoparticles. *Journal of the American Chemical Society* **126**, 9938–9939 (2004).

64. Malisova, B., Tosatti, S., Textor, M., Gademann, K., & Zurcher, S. Poly(ethylene glycol) adlayers immobilized to metal oxide substrates through catechol derivatives: influence of assembly conditions on formation and stability. *Langmuir* **26**, 4018–4026 (2010).

65. Dalsin, J.L., Hu, B.H., Lee, B.P., & Messersmith, P.B. Mussel adhesive protein mimetic polymers for the preparation of nonfouling surfaces. *Journal of the American Chemical Society* **125**, 4253–4258 (2003).

66. Amstad, E., Gillich, T., Bilecka, I., Textor, M., & Reimhult, E. Ultrastable iron oxide nanoparticle colloidal suspensions using dispersants with catechol-derived anchor groups. *Nano Letters* **9**, 4042–4048 (2009).

67. Amstad, E. et al. Influence of electronegative substituents on the binding affinity of catechol-derived anchors to Fe3O4 nanoparticles. *Journal of Physical Chemistry C* **115**, 683–691 (2011).

68. Feuz, L., Jonsson, P., Jonsson, M.P., & Hook, F. Improving the limit of detection of nanoscale sensors by directed binding to high-sensitivity areas. *ACS Nano* **4**, 2167–2177 (2010).

69. Amstad, E. et al. Surface functionalization of single superparamagnetic iron oxide nanoparticles for targeted magnetic resonance imaging. *Small* **5**, 1334–1342 (2009).

70. Folkers, J.P., Laibinis, P.E., & Whitesides, G.M. Self-assembled monolayers of alkanethiols on gold—comparisons of monolayers containing mixtures of short-chain and long-chain constituents with CH3 and ch2oh terminal groups. *Langmuir* **8**, 1330–1341 (1992).

71. Tamada, K., Hara, M., Sasabe, H., & Knoll, W. Surface phase behavior of n-alkanethiol self-assembled monolayers adsorbed on Au(111): an atomic force microscope study. *Langmuir* **13**, 1558–1566 (1997).

72. Benetti, E.M. et al. Poly(methacrylic acid) grafts grown from designer surfaces: the effect of initiator coverage on polymerization kinetics, morphology, and properties. *Macromolecules* **42**, 1640–1647 (2009).

73. Heuberger, M., Drobek, T., & Spencer, N.D. Interaction forces and morphology of a protein-resistant poly(ethylene glycol) layer. *Biophysical Journal* **88**, 495–504 (2005).

74. Vermette, P. & Meagher, L. Interactions of phospholipid- and poly(ethylene glycol)-modified surfaces with biological systems: relation to physico-chemical properties and mechanisms. *Colloids and Surfaces. B, Biointerfaces* **28**, 153–198 (2003).

75. de Gennes, P.G. Polymers at an interface; a simplified view. *Advances in Colloid and Interface Science* **27**, 189–209 (1987).

76. Prucker, O. & Rühe, J. Mechanism of radical chain polymerizations initiated by azo compounds covalently bound to the surface of spherical particles. *Macromolecules* **31**, 602–613 (1998).

77. Jordan, R., West, N., Ulman, A., Chou, Y.M., & Nuyken, O. Nanocomposites by surface-initiated living cationic polymerization of 2-oxazolines on functionalized gold nanoparticles. *Macromolecules* **34**, 1606–1611 (2001).

78. Ejaz, M., Tsujii, Y., & Fukuda, T. Controlled grafting of a well-defined polymer on a porous glass filter by surface-initiated atom transfer radical polymerization. *Polymer* **42**, 6811–6815 (2001).

79. Golander, C. et al. Protein adsorption on PEG surfaces. In: Harris, J. (ed.), *Poly(Ethylene Glycol) Chemistry: Biotechnical and Biomedical Applications*, pp. 221–245. New York: Plenum Press (1992).

80. Kingshott, P., Thissen, H., & Griesser, H.J. Effects of cloud-point grafting, chain length, and density of PEG layers on competitive adsorption of ocular proteins. *Biomaterials* **23**, 2043–2056 (2002).

81. Kalia, J. & Raines, R. T. Advances in Bioconjugation. *Current Organic Chemistry* **14**, 138–147 (2010).

82. Knopp, D., Tang, D.P., & Niessner, R. Bioanalytical applications of biomolecule-functionalized nanometer-sized doped silica particles. *Analytica Chimica Acta* **647**, 14–30 (2009).

83. Camarero, J.A. Recent developments in the site-specific immobilization of proteins onto solid supports. *Biopolymers* **90**, 450–458 (2008).

84. Lu, B., Smyth, M.R., & Okennedy, R. Oriented immobilization of antibodies and its applications in immunoassays and immunosensors. *Analyst* **121**, R29–R32 (1996).

85. LaGraff, J.R. & Chu-LaGraff, Q. Scanning force microscopy and fluorescence microscopy of microcontact printed antibodies and antibody fragments. *Langmuir* **22**, 4685–4693 (2006).

86. Wacker, R., Schroder, H., & Niemeyer, C.M. Performance of antibody microarrays fabricated by either DNA-directed immobilization, direct spotting, or streptavidin-biotin attachment: a comparative study. *Analytical Biochemistry* **330**, 281–287 (2004).

87. Peluso, P. et al. Optimizing antibody immobilization strategies for the construction of protein microarrays. *Analytical Biochemistry* **312**, 113–124 (2003).

88. Padeste, C., Grubelnik, A., Steiger, B., Hefti, J., & Tiefenauer, L. *Molecular architectures for enzyme sensors*. PSI Annual Report 2001 (2001).

89. Zacco, E., Pividori, M.I., & Alegret, S. Electrochemical biosensing based on universal affinity biocomposite platforms. *Biosensors & Bioelectronics* **21**, 1291–1301 (2006).

90. Danczyk, R. et al. Comparison of antibody functionality using different immobilization methods. *Biotechnology and Bioengineering* **84**, 215–223 (2003).

91. Ros, R. et al. Antigen binding forces of individually addressed single-chain Fv antibody molecules. *Proceedings of the National Academy of Sciences of the United States of America* **95**, 7402–7405 (1998).

92. Ellington, A.D. & Szostak, J.W. In vitro selection of rna molecules that bind specific ligands. *Nature* **346**, 818–822 (1990).

93. Tuerk, C. & Gold, L. Systematic evolution of ligands by exponential enrichment—RNA ligands to bacteriophage-T4 DNA-polymerase. *Science* **249**, 505–510 (1990).

94. Luppa, P.B., Sokoll, L.J., & Chan, D.W. Immunosensors—principles and applications to clinical chemistry. *Clinica Chimica Acta* **314**, 1–26 (2001).

95. Tombelli, S., Minunni, A., & Mascini, A. Analytical applications of aptamers. *Biosensors & Bioelectronics* **20**, 2424–2434 (2005).

96. Yu, Q.M. & Golden, G. Probing the protein orientation on charged self-assembled monolayers on gold nanohole arrays by SERS. *Langmuir* **23**, 8659–8662 (2007).

97. Vallieres, K., Chevallier, P., Sarra-Bournett, C., Turgeon, S., & Laroche, G. AFM Imaging of immobilized fibronectin: does the surface conjugation scheme affect the protein orientation/conformation? *Langmuir* **23**, 9745–9751 (2007).

98. Zhen, G.L. et al. Immobilization of the enzyme beta-lactamase on biotin-derivatized poly(L-lysine)-g-poly(ethylene glycol)-coated sensor chips: a study on oriented attachment and surface activity by enzyme kinetics and in situ optical sensing. *Langmuir* **20**, 10464–10473 (2004).

99. Huang, N.P., Voros, J., De Paul, S.M., Textor, M., & Spencer, N.D. Biotin-derivatized poly(L-lysine)-g-poly(ethylene glycol): a novel polymeric interface for bioaffinity sensing. *Langmuir* **18**, 220–230 (2002).

100. Falconnet, D., Koenig, A., Assi, T., & Textor, M. A combined photolithographic and molecular-assembly approach to produce functional micropatterns for applications in the biosciences. *Advanced Functional Materials* **14**, 749–756 (2004).

101. Blattler, T. et al. Nanopatterns with biological functions. *Journal of Nanoscience and Nanotechnology* **6**, 2237–2264 (2006).

102. Pla-Roca, M., Isa, L., Kumar, K., Textor, M., & Reimhult, E. Selective functionalization of nanopores and nanowells with polymer brushes using by metallic chromium lift-off. In preparation (unpublished data).

103. Qin, D., Xia, Y.N., & Whitesides, G.M. Soft lithography for micro- and nanoscale patterning. *Nature Protocols* **5**, 491–502 (2010).

104. Wilbur, J.L., Kumar, A., Kim, E., & Whitesides, G.M. Microfabrication by microcontact printing of self-assembled monolayers. *Advanced Materials* **6**, 600–604 (1994).

105. Perl, A., Reinhoudt, D.N., & Huskens, J. Microcontact printing: limitations and achievements. *Advanced Materials* **21**, 2257–2268 (2009).

106. Csucs, G., Michel, R., Lussi, J.W., Textor, M., & Danuser, G. Microcontact printing of novel co-polymers in combination with proteins for cell-biological applications. *Biomaterials* **24**, 1713–1720 (2003).

107. Saravia, V. et al. Bacterial protein patterning by micro-contact printing of PLL-g-PEG. *Journal of Biotechnology* **130**, 247–252 (2007).

108. Hovis, J.S. & Boxer, S.G. Patterning and composition arrays of supported lipid bilayers by microcontact printing. *Langmuir* **17**, 3400–3405 (2001).

109. Bernard, A. et al. Printing patterns of proteins. *Langmuir* **14**, 2225–2229 (1998).

110. James, C.D. et al. Patterned protein layers on solid substrates by thin stamp microcontact printing. *Langmuir* **14**, 741–744 (1998).

111. Xia, Y.N. & Whitesides, G.M. Use of controlled reactive spreading of liquid alkanethiol on the surface of gold to modify the size of features produced by microcontact printing. *Journal of the American Chemical Society* **117**, 3274–3275 (1995).

112. Delamarche, E. et al. Transport mechanisms of alkanethiols during microcontact printing on gold. *Journal of Physical Chemistry B* **102**, 3324–3334 (1998).

113. Wu, C.C., Reinhoudt, D.N., Otto, C., Subramaniam, V., & Velders, A.H. Strategies for patterning biomolecules with dip-pen nanolithography. *Small* **7**, 989–1002 (2011).

114. Braunschweig, A.B., Huo, F.W., & Mirkin, C.A. Molecular printing. *Nature Chemistry* **1**, 353–358 (2009).

115. Salaita, K. et al. Massively parallel dip-pen nanolithography with 55000-pen two-dimensional arrays. *Angewandte Chemie (International ed. in English)* **45**, 7220–7223 (2006).

116. Ducker, R., Garcia, A., Zhang, J.M., Chen, T., & Zauscher, S. Polymeric and bio-macromolecular brush nanostructures: progress in synthesis, patterning and characterization. *Soft Matter* **4**, 1774–1786 (2008).

117. Senesi, A.J., Rozkiewicz, D.I., Reinhoudt, D.N., & Mirkin, C.A. Agarose-assisted dip-pen nanolithography of oligonucleotides and proteins. *ACS Nano* **3**, 2394–2402 (2009).

118. Huo, F.W. et al. Polymer pen lithography. *Science* **321**, 1658–1660 (2008).

119. Chen, H.W. & Privalsky, M.L. Cooperative formation of high-order oligomers by retinoid-x receptors—an unexpected mode of dna recognition. *Proceedings of the National Academy of Sciences of the United States of America* **92**, 422–426 (1995).

120. Baumann, M., Textor, M., & Reimhult, E. Binding kinetics of pleckstrin homology domain PLCδ1 to PIP$_2$ containing supported lipid bilayers analyzed by dual polarization interferometry (2011), submitted.

121. Jayaraman, N. Multivalent ligand presentation as a central concept to study intricate carbohydrate-protein interactions. *Chemical Society Reviews* **38**, 3463–3483 (2009).

122. Reimhult, E., Baumann, M.K., Kaufmann, S., Kumar, K., & Spycher, P.R. Advances in nanopatterned and nanostructured supported lipid membranes and their applications. *Biotechnology and Genetic Engineering Reviews* **27**, 185–216 (2010).

123. Castellana, E.T. & Cremer, P.S. Solid supported lipid bilayers: from biophysical studies to sensor design. *Surface Science Reports* **61**, 429–444 (2006).

124. Janshoff, A. & Steinem, C. Transport across artificial membranes—an analytical perspective. *Analytical and Bioanalytical Chemistry* **385**, 433–451 (2006).

125. Merz, C., Knoll, W., Textor, M., & Reimhult, E. Formation of supported bacterial lipid membrane mimics. *Biointerphases* **3**, FA41–FA50 (2008).

126. Reimhult, E., Hook, F., & Kasemo, B. Temperature dependence of formation of a supported phospholipid bilayer from vesicles on SiO$_2$. *Physical Review E* **66**, 051905 (2002).

127. Reimhult, E., Hook, F., & Kasemo, B. Intact vesicle adsorption and supported biomembrane formation from vesicles in solution: influence of surface chemistry, vesicle size, temperature, and osmotic pressure. *Langmuir* **19**, 1681–1691 (2003).

128. Seantier, B. & Kasemo, B. Influence of mono- and divalent ions on the formation of supported phospholipid bilayers via vesicle adsorption. *Langmuir* **25**, 5767–5772 (2009).

129. Rossetti, F.F., Bally, M., Michel, R., Textor, M., & Reviakine, I. Interactions between titanium dioxide and phosphatidyl serine-containing liposomes: formation and patterning of supported phospholipid bilayers on the surface of a medically relevant material. *Langmuir* **21**, 6443–6450 (2005).

130. Sinner, E.K. & Knoll, W. Functional tethered membranes. *Current Opinion in Chemical Biology* **5**, 705–711 (2001).

131. Achalkumar, A.S., Bushby, R.J., & Evans, S.D. Cholesterol-based anchors and tethers for phospholipid bilayers and for model biological membranes. *Soft Matter* **6**, 6036–6051 (2010).

132. Ye, Q., Konradi, R., Textor, M., & Reimhult, E. Liposomes tethered to omega-functional peg brushes and induced formation of PEG brush supported planar lipid bilayers. *Langmuir* **25**, 13534–13539 (2009).

133. Tanaka, M. & Sackmann, E. Polymer-supported membranes as models of the cell surface. *Nature* **437**, 656–663 (2005).

134. Reimhult, E. & Kumar, K. Membrane biosensor platforms using nano- and micro-porous supports. *Trends in Biotechnology* **26**, 82–89 (2008).

135. Jonsson, P., Jonsson, M.P., & Hook, F. Sealing of submicrometer wells by a shear-driven lipid bilayer. *Nano Letters* **10**, 1900–1906 (2010).

136. Sugihara, K., Voros, J., & Zambelli, T. A gigaseal obtained with a self-assembled long-lifetime lipid bilayer on a single polyelectrolyte multilayer-filled nanopore. *ACS Nano* **4**, 5047–5054 (2010).

137. Roiter, Y. et al. Interaction of lipid membrane with nanostructured surfaces. *Langmuir* **25**, 6287–6299 (2009).

138. Glasmastar, K., Larsson, C., Hook, F., & Kasemo, B. Protein adsorption on supported phospholipid bilayers. *Journal of Colloid and Interface Science* **246**, 40–47 (2002).

139. Ross, E.E. et al. Planar supported lipid bilayer polymers formed by vesicle fusion. 2. Adsorption of bovine serum albumin. *Langmuir* **19**, 1766–1774 (2003).

140. Yang, T.L., Jung, S.Y., Mao, H.B., & Cremer, P.S. Fabrication of phospholipid bilayer-coated microchannels for on-chip immunoassays. *Analytical Chemistry* **73**, 165–169 (2001).

141. Reimhult, E., Kasemo, B., & Hook, F. Rupture pathway of phosphatidylcholine liposomes on silicon dioxide. *International Journal of Molecular Sciences* **10**, 1683–1696 (2009).

142. Jung, H., Robison, A.D., & Cremer, P.S. Multivalent ligand-receptor binding on supported lipid bilayers. *Journal of Structural Biology* **168**, 90–94 (2009).

143. Seifert, U. Configurations of fluid membranes and vesicles. *Advances in Physics* **46**, 13–137 (1997).

144. Jonsson, M.P., Jonsson, P., Dahlin, A.B., & Hook, F. Supported lipid bilayer formation and lipid-membrane-mediated biorecognition reactions studied with a new nanoplasmonic sensor template. *Nano Letters* **7**, 3462–3468 (2007).

145. Han, X.J. et al. Nanopore arrays for stable and functional free-standing lipid bilayers. *Advanced Materials* **19**, 4466–4470 (2007).

146. Luthgens, E. & Janshoff, A. Equilibrium coverage fluctuations: a new approach to quantify reversible adsorption of proteins. *ChemPhysChem* **6**, 444–448 (2005).

147. Armani, A.M., Kulkarni, R.P., Fraser, S.E., Flagan, R.C., & Vahala, K.J. Label-free, single-molecule detection with optical microcavities. *Science* **317**, 783–787 (2007).

148. Dahlin, A.B., Tegenfeldt, J.O., & Hook, F. Improving the instrumental resolution of sensors based on localized surface plasmon resonance. *Analytical Chemistry* **78**, 4416–4423 (2006).

149. Guo, Y.B. et al. Real-time biomolecular binding detection using a sensitive photonic crystal biosensor. *Analytical Chemistry* **82**, 5211–5218 (2010).

150. Squires, T.M., Messinger, R.J., & Manalis, S.R. Making it stick: convection, reaction and diffusion in surface-based biosensors. *Nature Biotechnology* **26**, 417–426 (2008).

151. Escobedo, C., Brolo, A.G., Gordon, R., & Sinton, D. Flow-through vs flow-over: analysis of transport and binding in nanohole array plasmonic biosensors. *Analytical Chemistry* **82**, 10015–10020 (2010).

152. Lebedev, K., Mafe, S., & Stroeve, P. Convection, diffusion and reaction in a surface-based biosensor: modeling of cooperativity and binding site competition on the surface and in the hydrogel. *Journal of Colloid and Interface Science* **296**, 527–537 (2006).

153. Kim, D.R. & Zheng, X.L. Numerical characterization and optimization of the microfluidics for nanowire biosensors. *Nano Letters* **8**, 3233–3237 (2008).

154. Jonsson, M.P., Dahlin, A., Feuz, L., Petronis, S., & Hook, F. Locally functionalized short-range ordered nanoplasmonic pores for bioanalytical sensing. *Analytical Chemistry ASAP* (2010) **82**, 2087–2094.

155. Cheetham, M.R. et al. Concentrating membrane proteins using asymmetric traps and AC electric fields. *Journal of the American Chemical Society* **133**, 6521–6524 (2011).

156. Groves, J.T., Boxer, S.G., & McConnell, H.M. Electric field-induced critical demixing in lipid bilayer membranes. *Proceedings of the National Academy of Sciences of the United States of America* **95**, 935–938 (1998).

157. Yoshina-Ishii, C. & Boxer, S.G. Controlling two-dimensional tethered vesicle motion using an electric field: interplay of electrophoresis and electro-osmosis. *Langmuir* **22**, 2384–2391 (2006).

158. Jonsson, P., Gunnarsson, A., & Hook, F. Accumulation and separation of membrane-bound proteins using hydrodynamic forces. *Analytical Chemistry* **83**, 604–611 (2011).

CHAPTER 4

Intelligent Surfaces for Field-Effect Transistor-Based Nanobiosensing

AKIRA MATSUMOTO, YUJI MIYAHARA, and KAZUNORI KATAOKA

4.1 INTRODUCTION

Tremendous advancements have been achieved during the last several decades in the field of micro-/nanoelectronics. Meanwhile, an ever-increasing knowledge of medicine and biology has continuously stimulated efforts to devote these technologies to the frontier of bio- and nanotechnologies. These fusion technologies have already provided a number of brilliant benchmark tools for parallel processing of information, miniaturization of analytical systems, and elucidation of the molecular mechanisms of life. Biosensors may best exemplify the fruitful achievement and, at the same time, further potential of such collaborative approaches between micro-/nanoelectronics and medicine/biology. Biosensors, in general, consist of a transducer, a function that is primarily played by electronics, and a membrane component bearing biologically active substances. Biosensor-related research is literally multidisciplinary. Controls over the aforementioned operations, that is, the transducer and membrane, involve many aspects of science including electrochemistry, biochemistry, surface chemistry, solid-state physics, integrated circuit silicon technology, and so on. From the standpoint of surface and materials engineering, a major challenge seems to stem from an essential disparity in the properties of the two materials in (direct or indirect) contact forming the detection interface, namely, the solid-state electronics (typically made of metals or semiconductors) and the wet-phase biological targets. This feature brings about a unique challenge and necessity in this area of the research to deal with somewhat unusual physicochemistry, which is concomitantly very much characteristic of such heterogeneous interfaces and material structures.

In this chapter, we provide an overview of recent progress and trends in the research of field-effect transistor (FET)-based biosensors, so-called

Intelligent Surfaces in Biotechnology: Scientific and Engineering Concepts, Enabling Technologies, and Translation to Bio-Oriented Applications, First Edition.
Edited by H. Michelle Grandin and Marcus Textor.
© 2012 John Wiley & Sons, Inc. Published 2012 by John Wiley & Sons, Inc.

biologically coupled field-effect transistors (bio-FETs). Bio-FETs are an emerging class of label-free sensors applicable to a wide range of biological targets, which can also be miniaturized and integrated by virtue of advanced semiconductor processing technology. The focus of the chapter is on a comprehension of the intelligent surfaces so far explored to cope with requirements for the design of bio-FETs, including carbon nanotube (CNT), self-assembled monolayers (SAMs), and stimulus-responsive gel-modified surfaces, among others. The fundamental principles and various conventionally studied types of bio-FETs are first introduced. Some recent approaches exploiting intelligent surfaces for the facilitation of signal transduction and amplification will follow. Then, examples of new targets of bio-FETs, which are currently under active investigation, will also be summarized. At the end of these listings, a future perspective is provided.

4.2   FET-BASED BIOSENSORS

4.2.1   Metal–Insulator–Semiconductor (MIS) Capacitors

The MIS structure provides a good basis for understanding the operation of the bio-FET. The MIS structure is simply a capacitor in which the insulator is placed between the metal and the semiconductor electrodes as shown in Figure 4.1. When a voltage is applied across the metal and the semiconductor electrodes, the electronic state of the semiconductor is modified depending on the pattern and magnitude of the applied voltage. When a p-type silicon is used as the substrate, a majority of carriers are positive charges or "holes." When no voltage is applied on the metal electrode, the charge distribution in the silicon is uniform, thereby achieving a perfect electrical balance between holes and immobile ions called "acceptors." When a negative voltage is applied on the metal electrode, additional holes are attracted to the insulator–silicon interface due to the Coulomb force, as schematically depicted in Figure 4.1a. As a result, the electric field is induced in the insulator. This condition is called accumulation, since a majority of carriers (holes) are accumulated at the surface of the silicon. The number of holes attracted to the insulator–silicon interface decreases with increase of the applied voltage. In contrast, when the applied voltage is positive, holes are expelled from the silicon surface, leaving behind negatively charged immobile acceptors, a situation illustrated in Figure 4.1b. This state is called depletion, since mobile charged carriers (holes) are depleted in the surface region. In this situation the electric field is induced both in the insulator and the depletion layer. With a further increase of the voltage in the positive direction, negatively charged mobile carriers or electrons are induced at the insulator–silicon interface as shown in Figure 4.1c. This state is called inversion, where the number of electrons, which are minor carriers in the p-type silicon, exceeds that of holes, and thus the surface is inverted to n-type. This thin layer of electrons at the interface, called the

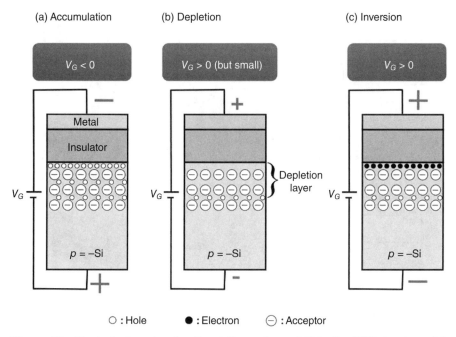

O : Hole   ● : Electron   ⊖ : Acceptor

Figure 4.1 Control of carrier density at the surface of Si in the MIS structure: (a) accumulation, where the majority carriers, holes, are accumulated at the surface of the silicon substrate; (b) depletion, where the carriers are depleted at the surface of the silicon substrate; and (c) inversion, where the minority carriers, electrons, are induced at the surface of the silicon substrate.

inversion layer, plays an important role in the operation of the metal–insulator–semiconductor field-effect transistor (MISFET) and also the bio-FET.

4.2.2 Principles of bio-FETs

The operational structure of the bio-FET is essentially analogous to that of the MISFET except that the metal gate electrode is replaced by an aqueous solution in which a reference electrode (in most cases Ag/AgCl) is also installed for fixing the potential of the gate insulator surface (Fig. 4.2). When a sufficiently positive voltage is applied to the gate (through the reference electrode), an n-type inversion layer is generated in the vicinity of the silicon/insulator interface across the region called "channel" between the source and drain. Herein, the electrical resistance of the channel is variable depending on (inversely proportional to) the electron density of itself. Therefore, alternation of the electron density in the channel can give rise to the change in the source–drain voltage–current (VDS-ID) characteristics. Such a change can actively be induced by introducing additional charges onto the gate surface, which either electrostatically attract or expel the carrier electrons in silicon, leading to the

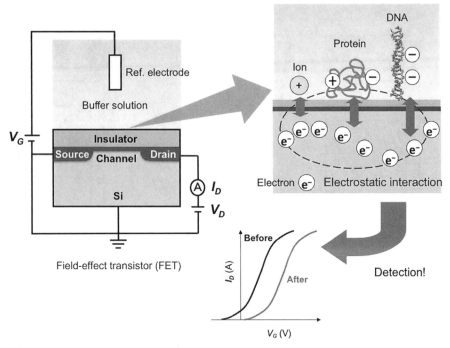

Figure 4.2   Schematic representation of the structure and principles of bio-FETs. Molecular events of interest involving charge density changes arranged on the gate surface can be detected as a mode of modified characteristics of the FET as a result of electrostatic interactions between intrinsic molecular charges and the thin-insulator-segregated silicon electrons.

shift of VDS-ID characteristics. In other words, any "designed" charge density changes on the gate surface can be detected as a mode of the modified VDS-ID characteristics as a result of electrostatic interactions between these charges and the thin-insulator-segregated silicon electrons. Such a detection scheme, particularly when coupled with biochemical reactions or biorecognition events, is called a bio-FET.

Importantly, the bio-FET provides a label-free detection platform applicable to a wide range of biological targets. With no costly instrumentation such as laser and optical assistance, it can also be miniaturized and integrated by virtue of advanced semiconductor processing technology.

4.2.3   Ion-Sensitive Field-Effect Transistors (ISFETs) and Their Direct Coupling with Various Biorecognition Elements as a Conventional Approach to bio-FETs

The ion-selective FET (ISFET) is the most basic and prevailed form of the bio-FET.[1,2] The gate insulator of an ISFET is usually a double layer composed of SiO_2 and another material on top such as Si_3N_4, Al_2O_3, and Ta_2O_5, which serves as a pH-sensitive element.[3] The mechanism for the pH-dependent charge alternations that occur in these materials has been explained by the so-called site-binding model, taking into account a pH-dependent protonation (or deprotonation) of the surface-elaborated hydoxyl groups.[4,5] By additional surface modification of the top layer with other ion-sensitive components such as ionophores and crown ethers, one can also obtain FETs that are specific to various other ions.[3]

ISFETs also provide an important operational basis for many other conventional types of bio-FETs.[1,3] Enzymatic reaction-coupled field-effect transistors (En-FETs) have emerged as the second generation of bio-FETs whose operational principle is heavily dependent on the ISFET. En-FETs can be prepared by immobilizing enzymes onto the gate surface of an ISFET. A criterion for the operation of an En-FET is that either reaction products or consumed reactants during the enzymatic reactions (between enzyme and the substrate) are of charged species that can be quantified by the function of the ISFET. The analytes successfully detected based on the En-FET principle includes a series of saccharides, urea, penicillin, ascorbic acid, acethylcoline, and creatinine.[3,6]

Immunoreaction-coupled field-effect transistors (Immuno-FETs) are another example of protein-based bio-FETs.[7] The detection strategy of Immuno-FETs is based on the premise that antibody–antigen binding designed on the gate surface can lead to an altered charge distribution (redistribution) across the direction perpendicular to the gate surface, a change theoretically detectable by an ISFET. This approach is usually challenging mainly due to an issue related to the electrical double layer or the Debye length; that is to say, FET-based charge detection is inherently permitted only within a short distance corresponding to the Debye length, which is no greater than a few nanometers under the physiological ionic strength conditions, although typical sizes of proteins (including antibodies) are in the order of 10 nm. Beyond this length, counterions' screening effect predominates and the charge detection is severely hampered. To overcome this difficulty, some recent works are focused on dynamic assays (rather than static methods) either by conducting stepwise additions of target compounds or by kinetic analysis.[8–10] These approaches are to some extent successful.

One of the most recent versions of the bio-FET that capitalized on direct ISFET-target coupling structures is a genetic field-effect transistor (Gen-FET).[3,11] There is no debate on the importance of the development of massive and parallel methods enabling genetic analysis, for which the current standards are DNA chips and microarrays. Since DNA molecules are negatively charged in an aqueous solution, hybridization events can be detected by measuring a shift of the electrical characteristic such as the *VDS-ID* characteristics of the threshold gate voltage (V_T). Several independent groups have demonstrated the feasibility of such a way of detection. Our recent work has shown that a primer extension reaction could also be detected based on the Gen-FET format. Furthermore, combined with the sequential addition of each deoxy-nucleotide (dCTP, dATP, dGTP, or dTTP) in the presence of DNA polymerase, this could be monitored with a single base-level resolution, leading to the ability to report on single-nucleotide polymorphisms (SNPs)[12] as well as to read the sequence (sequencing).[13] These relatively new approaches draw increasing attention for their potential to have a revolutionary impact on medical and diagnostic applications.

Another extensively studied class of bio-FETs, with a relatively long history, is that for analyzing cell functions or "cell-FETs." There are two common approaches in this area. The first type focuses on the analysis of metabolic activities of cells.[14] Since the metabolic activity of cells can be correlated to the rate and state of various cellular events such as growth, development, and mortality, their kinetics can be indirectly monitored as a mode of the change in the intracellular pH. The other type of the cell-FET capitalizes on gaining contact with electrogenic cells such as neuronal, muscle, and cardiac cells both on single and cultured cell formats.[15–17] The electrogenic cells generate spontaneous or stimuli-triggered action potentials that can be measured by the ISFET. Myocardiac cells represent a major cell type with electrogenicity so far attracting a great deal of research interest.[18,19] The beating frequency of the cultured myocardiac cells is sensitive to the addition of cardiac stimulants and relaxants. Therefore, one of the ultimate goals in this area of the research is to develop a new basis for drug screening applications. For a similar purpose, we have recently employed the cell-FET for monitoring transporter–substrate interactions at the cell membrane.[20] A *Xenopus laevis* oocyte was utilized for this purpose as its expression system is a prevailing platform for *in vitro* pharmaceutical assays such as drug disposition and clearance. In general, these assays require target molecules to be labeled by radioisotopes and the oocytes to be lysed before measurement. An important advantage of the FET-based method is that it does not require cell-lethal procedures and is free from labels. It has been demonstrated that, by simply placing a single oocyte onto the gate, the extracelluar potential change at the interface between the cell membrane and the gate insulator could be monitored during the uptake of a substrate, presumably mediated by the transporter. Moreover, it was revealed that discrimination between wild and mutant types was feasible owing to discrepancy in their transport kinetics.

4.3 INTELLIGENT SURFACES FOR SIGNAL TRANSDUCTION AND AMPLIFICATION OF BIO-FETs

4.3.1 CNT-Mediated Signal Transduction

CNTs possess many unique properties that are potentially useful in electronics. Owing to mechanically as well as electrically excellent characteristics, there has been an increasing interest in utilizing CNTs for biosensor applications.[21,22]

The high surface area of single-walled carbon nanotubes (SWNTs), which has been estimated to be 1600 m^2/g, is of particular interest as it can provide a route to obtain an impressively high density of biomolecules at the detection interface. Since the first appearance of the single-walled carbon nanotube-based field-effect transistors (SWNT-FETs),[23,24] a large number of attempts have emerged aiming to apply the SWNT-FET to a range of biomolecular targets.

To fabricate the SWNT-FET, a semiconducting SWNT must be selectively (out of a mixture of metallic SWNTs) manipulated to ensure its contact against and bridge between the source and the drain materials. SWNT-FETs are composed of either individual SWNTs or dispersed networks of multiple numbers of SWNTs. The chemical vapor deposition (CVD) growth method is typically employed for the fabrication of dispersed SWNT networks on the gate surface, while microlithography and electron beam (e-beam) lithography are common techniques to pattern source and drain contacts.[21]

From the viewpoint of the role at the detection interface, the SWNT not only provides dense surface area for immobilization of biological receptors but also serves as an electrical modulator of the (SWNT-bridged) source–drain channel. The main factor causing changes in the channel conductance is still under debate, for which at least four possible mechanisms have been proposed so far. These include electrostatic gating, capacitance modulation, Schottky barrier effects, and carrier mobility change.[22,25,26] A variety of biological targets have been successfully detected based on the SWNT-FET format, including small molecules such as H+ (protons), NH_3, and NO_2,[27] as well as relatively large targets such as DNA (hybridization) and proteins.[28,29]

4.3.2 SAM-Assisted Detection

Utilization of SAMs, which are ordered molecular assemblies formed by the adsorption of an active surfactant on a solid surface, has prevailed as a benchmark methodology for the preparation and manipulation of interfaces with molecular-level precision. The SAM-derived techniques provide unique opportunities to obtain surfaces with chemical complexity with remarkable ease of manipulation, where the property of the surface can also be tailored by the control of the terminal functionalities.[30]

In the preparation of Gen-FETs, immobilization of probe DNA is usually conducted onto the surface of a metal oxide gate, which typically involves a complex chemistry of organosilane coupling reagents, a procedure known as silanization.[11] A recent work has shown that Gen-FETs can also be prepared by forming a SAM of DNA probes on a gold electrode surface that serves as an extended gate for the FET. A 20-mer probe DNA modified with a thiol function, 6-amino-1-hexanethiol (at its 5′ terminus), was utilized for the attachment of the probe to the gold electrode surface. The interaction between the thiol (SH-) group (typically, alkanethiols) and gold is the mode that has been most intensively investigated and utilized for the preparation of SAMs.[31] In this configuration, it was demonstrated that, with optimized surface density of the probe DNA and with the help of the superimposed high-frequency voltage (effective in stabilizing the surface potential of the gold surface), the target DNA hybridization as well as the extension reactions were detectable.

The same group has further exploited the thiol–gold interaction for the design of an enzyme immunoassay (also by using a gold electrode as an extended gate for the FET under superimposed high-frequency voltage). In this case, the enzyme chemistry of acetylcholinesterase (AChE) was combined for the generation of a thiol compound. Its adsorption rate onto the gold gate electrode was found to be linearly dependent on the concentration, thereby giving a basis for a label-free immunoassay.[9,10]

4.3.3 Stimuli-Responsive Polymer Gel-Based Interfaces for "Debye Length-Free" Detection

As already mentioned in Section 4.2.3, the FET-based charge detection is susceptible to the charge-screening effect caused by counterions. As a result, the technique is limited to a short detectable length limit (from the gate surface), which corresponds to the thickness of the electrical double layer or the Debye length, of up to a few nanometers at most with minimized ionic strength of the surrounding environment.[32,33] This leads to an upper limit of the molecular weight for which quantitative charge detection can be feasibly performed.[34,35] For this reason, most Immuno-FET-related attempts dealing with large protein molecules whose sizes well exceed that of the Debye length remain unsatisfactory. Likewise, in the case of Gen-FETs, the detectable length of the DNA molecules (base number) is about 40. This section will summarize a unique approach of exploiting a stimuli-responsive polymer gel to carry out a FET-based, but nonetheless Debye length-free molecular detection that we have recently proposed (Fig. 4.3a).[36,37]

Stimuli-responsive polymer gels or "smart gels" are a unique class of material capable of undergoing marked changes in their physicochemical properties in response to a series of specific stimuli. They are widely studied as components forming self-regulated materials and systems in a variety of applications including biomaterials, drug delivery systems, and actuators.[38,39] As for proof of principle, a phenylboronic acid (PBA)-based glucose-responsive polymer gel, a thoroughly synthetic and well-characterized glucose-responsive material,[40–42] was covalently introduced to the FET gate surface (in this case a tantalum oxide surface) in the form of a 50-μm-thick layer, so as to obtain a glucose-sensitive FET. In this configuration, an applied chemical stimulus, that is, a change in glucose concentration, triggers an abrupt volume change of the gel, termed a "volume phase transition," which also involves other physical parameter changes such as thickness, charge density, and permittivity (Fig. 4.3a). As a key feature of the volume phase transition, the physicochemical changes commencing at the gel/outer aqueous media interface can geometrically propagate across a macroscopic thickness of the

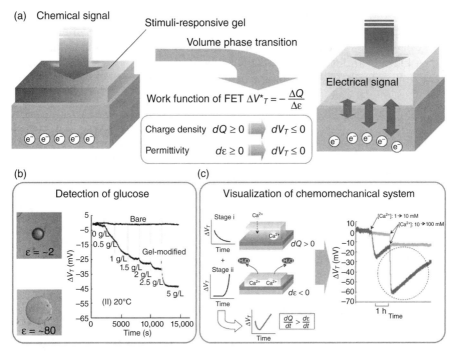

Figure 4.3 (a) Conceptual scheme for a stimulus-responsive gel-mediated signal transduction enabling "Debye length-free" FET-based molecular detection. (b) Detection of glucose by using a glucose-responsive polymer gel-modified FET.[36] (c) Kinetics of a chemomechanical system visualized by using a calcium-sensitive gel-modified FET.[37] (See color insert.)

gel layer (in the present case 50 μm)[43] and are thus able to transport the signal beyond the "barrier" of the Debye length. As a result, despite the significantly large gel thickness (a length several orders of magnitude larger than the theoretical Debye length), glucose concentrations could be measured as the change in threshold gate voltage in harmony with the glucose-responsive property of the gel (Fig. 4.3b).

In this system, a permittivity change of the gel (rather than charge density) was identified as a major source of the obtained signal. The volume change of the hydrogel herein described is practically equivalent to that of water content. A significantly high relative permittivity of water (ca. 80) compared to those typical for condensed polymeric materials (ca. 2) is responsible for this change. The permittivity change can then contribute to the altered capacitive property of the gel/gate interface, which is another determinant factor of the threshold gate voltage (V_T) aside from the charge density. Such a contribution of the apparent permittivity change to the shift of the threshold voltage (V_T) could be qualitatively explained by taking into account an operational function of the ISFET.[44]

Many other types of stimulus-responsive gels have been reported for which the present detection scheme could be applied. For example, polymer gels can be designed to perceive immunoreactions, tumor-specific biomarkers, and DNA hybridizations.[45,46] Also worthy of mention is that such a gel-transition-synchronized system is capable of detecting not only charged substances but also those electrically neutral, such as glucose. Furthermore, this gel-modified FET can exhibit "dual sensitivity," namely, to the charge density and to the permittivity. This unique property has been further exploited as a means to visualize the kinetics of multiple elemental reactions occurring in the gel-based chemomechanical systems, where changes in the two parameters could be visualized independently (Fig. 4.3c).[37] Noteworthy is that patterns of the electrical response obtained could be controlled (designed) by simply modulating the dimension of the gel. This observation implied a new principle for the design of signal communication systems in which independent sources of information (electrical, chemical, and mechanical) are connected to each other in dynamic and exchangeable manners.

4.4 NEW TARGETS OF BIO-FETs

4.4.1 Carbohydrate Chain Sialic Acid (SA) Detection Using PBA SAM-Modified FETs

Glycosylations, or the alternations of cell surface glycan structures, are dynamic and stage-specific processes during numerous normal and pathological processes including development and differentiation.[47–49] Most tumor-associated carbohydrate antigens including those clinically approved as tumor markers involve SA, an anionic monosaccharide that frequently occurs at the termini of the glycan chains. Overexpression of SA on the cell surface has been implicated in the malignant and metastatic phenotypes for many different types of cancers,[50–52] while decreased SA expression has also been identified in erythrocytes of diabetic mellitus.[53,54] Monitoring of the cell surface SA expression therefore provides rational indexes of the dynamic changes in tumor malignancy, metastatic potential, diabetic symptoms, and other SA-associated biological events.

We have recently proposed a FET-based SA detection as a new technique for label-free and live cell operative cytology (Fig. 4.4a). The principle of specific SA detection capitalizes on a reversible and covalent interaction between phenylboronic acid (PBA) and SA. PBA is a synthetic molecule capable of reversibly binding with 1,2- or 1,3-diols, hallmark structures for a majority of glycan constituent saccharides.[55–58] Our previous work had revealed that a PBA molecule with properly modulated pKa could provide a molecular basis for selective recognition of SA among other glycan constituent saccharides.[59,60] A SAM of 10-carboxy-1-decanethiol was first formed on a gold electrode followed by a condensation reaction with an amino group functionalized PBA

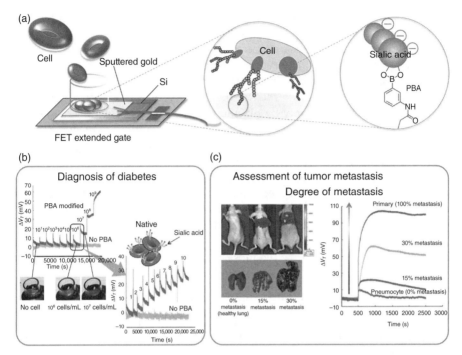

Figure 4.4 (a) Schematic representation of potentiometric SA detection using a PBA-modified gold electrode. (b) Detection of SA on the surface of rabbit erythrocytes as a relevant technique for the diagnosis of diabetes.[61] (c) Assessment of tumor metastasis based on differentiation of the (pneumocyte) surface-expressed SA.[62] (See color insert.)

(3-aminophenylboronic acid) resulting in the introduction of meta-amide-substituted PBA onto the SAM terminal. Both quartz crystal microbalance (QCM) and ellipsometric measurements had confirmed stoichiometric mono-layer formations at each step of the reaction. The apparent pKa of the surface-introduced PBA moiety, as judged from its pH-dependent changes in V_T, was found to be about 9.5 and was safely undissociated at the physiological pH (7.4), making itself SA specific under such a condition.[61] The PBA-modified gold electrode was then electrically linked to a FET gate for real-time monitoring of the charge density changes taking place on the electrode. In this configuration, anionic charges of SA (due to carboxyl groups) bound to the electrode could be detected as positive direction shifts of threshold voltage (V_T) of the FET.

The PBA-modified FET was then tested for its ability to directly capture the glycan component SA present on the cell surface. As noted earlier, under minimized ionic strength conditions, detection will only be possible within a few nanometers of the surface (i.e., the Debye length). Fortunately, the cell surface SA moieties, which generally dominate the termini of the glycan chains, should satisfy this criterion. In addition, tumor- or metastasis-associated over-expressions of SA are usually found in the form of polysialylation. Such a unit-sequential arrangement of the target SA (homopolymer of SA) present on the glycan chain termini should also help in achieving precise reflections of the altered level of the SA expressions.

As for proof of principle, erythrocytes were first investigated, for which a decline of SA content has been implicated in diabetes mellitus (Fig. 4.4b). It was demonstrated that the altered SA expressions could be directly monitored in a real-time manner simply by placing the known-count living cell suspensions onto the electrode.[61] The electrode was further applied to the assessment of the malignancy or metastasis of a tissue specimen by utilizing metastatic murine melanoma cells (for their ability to almost specifically metastasize to the healthy lungs of mice after intravenous injection) (Fig. 4.4c).[62] It was demonstrated that the PBA-modified electrode could differentiate the degree of tumor metastasis through perception of the cell membrane SA. It may be expected that these techniques could lead to a facile and quantitative adjunct to the histological evaluation of tumor malignancy and metastatic potential during intra- or postoperative diagnoses.

4.4.2 Scent Detection Using "Beetle/Chip" FETs

Lately, there are some interesting attempts at taking whole organisms or parts of an organism as the element for biorecognition events coupled with the FET, so-called beetle/chip FETs.[3,63–65] These approaches aim to make use of the specially (evolutionary) developed ability of insect species, representatively beetles, to sense smells, that is, to detect the presence of certain pheromones or plant odors, with extremely high sensitivity and selectivity. These approaches are unique in that they make use of naturally derived components to act as elements for high-performance signal transduction, taking full advantage of nature. Typically, an isolated antenna from an insect is connected on both edges to the electrolyte solution. The insect antenna consists of several segments bearing small hairs called sensilla, where the odor perception process is initiated (as they contain the olfactory receptor neurons). Upon detection of each specific odor molecule, the antenna develops electrical dipoles along the sensilla. The induced depolarization leads to modified conductance of the FET channel, giving a change in the drain–source current as the sensor signal.[63,64] Such a beetle/chip FET can achieve the detection of each specific odor molecule with concentrations on the order of ppt, in accordance with the abilities that the host biological system (insect itself) originally exhibits. Based on this concept, applications such as plant damage detection (for protection purpose), early fire detection and highly selective and sensitive chemical sensors have been proposed.

4.4.3 Aptamer-Modified Biorecognition Surfaces for a Universal Platform of bio-FETs

Many recent efforts in the area of bio-FETs have been focused on the utilization of aptamers, which are synthetic nucleic acids (DNA or RNA) that are designed to specifically bind to amino acids, proteins, carbohydrate chains, and so on, as components for specific biorecognition interactions at the gate surface of the FET.[21,22,66] Aptamers are obtained based on a technique called systematic evolution of ligands by exponential enrichment (SELEX). Aptamers exhibit significant advantages relative to protein-based receptors in terms of size, versatility in targets, synthetic accessibility, and modification while also rivaling antibodies in their strength of affinities and specificities.[67] It is also suggested that the relatively small size of aptamers (1–2 nm), as compared to typical protein receptors such as antibodies (10–15 nm), leads to a better compatibility with the FET-based detection where the size of target molecules must be within the scale of Debye length.

Such aptamer-based FETs may add a new direction to the next decade of research in the field. Many current reports of aptamer-based FETs are frequently found in a form combined with the SWNT-FET. Based on this combination (aptamers and SWNT-FETs), quantitative detection of thrombin[68] and immunoglobulin E (IgE),[69,70] both representing well-characterized classes of biomarkers, have been reported. In addition to the aforementioned advantages including its short length (thus favorable for the FET-based detection), chemical stability (reversible denaturing) and synthetic accessibility, aptamers can also cover essentially all general biological targets including amino acids, proteins, carbohydrate chains and even cells. Therefore, establishing methodologies to utilize aptamers as biorecognition components for the FET may have the potential to form the basis for a universal platform of the bio-FET.

4.5 FUTURE PERSPECTIVE

Almost 40 years have passed since the first demonstration of an ISFET by Bergveld. ISFETs and En-FETs can be categorized as the first generation of bio-FETs, some of which are already commercialized or are at the level of technical maturation. With respect to the order of appearance in history, Immuno-FETs were expected to enjoy the second fruit of the achievement in the field. However, until now, this has not been manifested to the extent of the original expectation, largely a result of the inherent technical difficulty in this approach, that is, detection of large-molecule proteins, as continuously discussed in this chapter. Meanwhile, it appears that a majority of current research interests have shifted to Gen- and Apmater-based FETs, mainly due to their better compatibility with the principle of the FET in terms of size and accessibility to targets, along with its growing relevance to clinical applications. As this trend continues to grow, development of controlled (and thus intelligent) interfaces will remain of critical importance.

Some new approaches of incorporating dynamic properties of organic materials and systems into the operation of solid-state electronics will also receive increasing attention. Hierarchically ordered processes and self-assembling features of organic (biological) substances are the important lessons provided by nature, which lend insight into the materials and systems of ultimate optimization. Such approaches, particularly when aiming to touch biological substances, become critical for the control of heterologous materials and interfaces characteristic of solid-state biosensors. Such a philosophy is already prevalent in other related research fields, for example, organic field-effect transistors (OFETs). This trend will also be true for the design of bio-FETs in the near future.

REFERENCES

1. Bergveld, P. Development of an ion-sensitive solid-state device for neurophysiological measurements. *IEEE Transactions on Biomedical Engineering* **Bm17**, 70–71 (1970).

3. Janata, J. & Moss, S.D. Chemically sensitive field-effect transistors. *Biomedical Engineering* **11**, 241–245 (1976).

3. Schoning, M.J. & Poghossian, A. Recent advances in biologically sensitive field-effect transistors (BioFETs). *Analyst* **127**, 1137–1151 (2002); references therein.

4. Yates, D.E., Levine, S., & Healy, T.W. Site-binding model of electrical double-layer at oxide-water interface. *Journal of the Chemical Society-Faraday Transactions I* **70**, 1807–1818 (1974).

5. vanHal, R.E.G., Eijkel, J.C.T., & Bergveld, P. A general model to describe the electrostatic potential at electrolyte oxide interfaces. *Advances in Colloid and Interface Science* **69**, 31–62 (1996).

6. Caras, S. & Janata, J. Field-effect transistor sensitive to penicillin. *Analytical Chemistry* **52**, 1935–1937 (1980).

7. Schasfoort, R.B.M., Kooyman, R.P.H., Bergveld, P., & Greve, J. A new approach to immunoFET operation. *Biosensors & Bioelectronics* **5**, 103–124 (1990).

8. Feng, C.L., Xu, Y.H., & Song, L.M. Study on highly sensitive potentiometric IgG immunosensor. *Sensors and Actuators. B, Chemical* **66**, 190–192 (2000).

9. Kamahori, M., Ishige, Y., & Shimoda, M. Enzyme immunoassay using a reusable extended-gate field-effect-transistor sensor with a ferrocenylalkanethiol-modified gold electrode. *Analytical Sciences* **24**, 1073–1079 (2008).

10. Kamahori, M., Ishige, Y., & Shimoda, M. A novel enzyme immunoassay based on potentiometric measurement of molecular adsorption events by an extended-gate field-effect transistor sensor. *Biosensors & Bioelectronics* **22**, 3080–3085 (2007).

11. Miyahara, Y., Sakata, T., & Matsumoto, A. Microbial genetic analysis based on field effect transistors. In: Zourob, M. et al. (eds), *Principles of Bacterial Detection: Biosensors, Recognition Receptors and Microsystems*, Vol. 14. pp. 311–337. Philadelphia, PA: Springer Science+Business Media, LLC (2008); references therein.

12. Sakata, T. & Miyahara, Y. Potentiometric detection of single nucleotide polymorphism by using a genetic field-effect transistor. *Chembiochem: a European Journal of Chemical Biology* **6**, 703–710 (2005).

13. Sakata, T. & Miyahara, Y. DNA sequencing based on intrinsic molecular charges. *Angewandte Chemie (International ed. in English)* **45**, 2225–2228 (2006).

14. Wolf, B., Brischwein, M., Baumann, W., Ehret, R., & Kraus, M. Monitoring of cellular signalling and metabolism with modular sensor-technique: the PhysioControl-Microsystem (PCM (R)). *Biosensors & Bioelectronics* **13**, 501–509 (1998).

15. Fromherz, P., Offenhausser, A., Vetter, T., & Weis, J.A. Neuron-silicon junction—a Retzius cell of the leech on an insulated-gate field-effect transistor. *Science* **252**, 1290–1293 (1991).

16. Baumann, W.H. et al. Microelectronic sensor system for microphysiological application on living cells. *Sensors and Actuators. B, Chemical* **55**, 77–89 (1999).

17. Offenhausser, A. & Knoll, W. Cell-transistor hybrid systems and their potential applications. *Trends in Biotechnology* **19**, 62–66 (2001).

18. Ingebrandt, S., Yeung, C.K., Krause, M., & Offenhausser, A. Cardiomyocyte-transistor-hybrids for sensor application. *Biosensors & Bioelectronics* **16**, 565–570 (2001).

19. Yeung, C.K., Ingebrandt, S., Krause, M., Offenhausser, A., & Knoll, W. Validation of the use of field effect transistors for extracellular signal recording in pharmacological bioassays. *Journal of Pharmacological and Toxicological Methods* **45**, 207–214 (2001).

20. Sakata, T. & Miyahara, Y. Noninvasive monitoring of transporter-substrate interaction at cell membrane. *Analytical Chemistry* **80**, 1493–1496 (2008).

21. Kim, S.N., Rusling, J.F., & Papadimitrakopoulos, F. Carbon nanotubes for electronic and electrochemical detection of biomolecules. *Advanced Materials* **19**, 3214–3228 (2007); references therein.

22. Hu, P.A. et al. Carbon nanostructure-based field-effect transistors for label-free chemical/biological sensors. *Sensors* **10**, 5133–5159 (2010).

23. Tans, S.J., Devoret, M.H., Groeneveld, R.J.A., & Dekker, C. Electron-electron correlations in carbon nanotubes. *Nature* **394**, 761–764 (1998).

24. Martel, R., Schmidt, T., Shea, H.R., Hertel, T., & Avouris, P. Single- and multi-wall carbon nanotube field-effect transistors. *Applied Physics Letters* **73**, 2447–2449 (1998).

25. Cinke, M. et al. Pore structure of raw and purified HiPco single-walled carbon nanotubes. *Chemical Physics Letters* **365**, 69–74 (2002).

26. Byon, H.R. & Choi, H.C. Network single-walled carbon nanotube-field effect transistors (SWNT-FETs) with increased Schottky contact area for highly sensitive biosensor applications. *Journal of the American Chemical Society* **128**, 2188–2189 (2006).

27. Bradley, K., Gabriel, J.C.P., Star, A., & Gruner, G. Short-channel effects in contact-passivated nanotube chemical sensors. *Applied Physics Letters* **83**, 3821–3823 (2003).

28. Star, A. et al. Label-free detection of DNA hybridization using carbon nanotube network field-effect transistors. *Proceedings of the National Academy of Sciences of the United States of America* **103**, 921–926 (2006).

29. Heller, D.A. et al. Optical detection of DNA conformational polymorphism on single-walled carbon nanotubes. *Science* **311**, 508–511 (2006).

30. Ulman, A. Formation and structure of self-assembled monolayers. *Chemical Reviews* **96**, 1533–1554 (1996).

31. Kamahori, M., Ishige, Y., & Shimoda, M. DNA detection by an extended-gate FET sensor with a high-frequency voltage superimposed onto a reference electrode. *Analytical Sciences* **23**, 75–79 (2007).

32. Bergveld, P. The future of biosensors. *Sensors and Actuators A, Physical* **56**, 65–73 (1996).

33. Schasfoort, R.B.M., Bergveld, P., Kooyman, R.P.H., & Greve, J. Possibilities and limitations of direct detection of protein charges by means of an immunological field-effect transistor. *Analytica Chimica Acta* **238**, 323–329 (1990).

34. Bergveld, P. A critical-evaluation of direct electrical protein-detection methods. *Biosensors & Bioelectronics* **6**, 55–72 (1991).

35. Stern, E. et al. Importance of the debye screening length on nanowire field effect transistor sensors. *Nano Letters* **7**, 3405–3409 (2007).

36. Matsumoto, A. et al. Chemical-to-electrical-signal transduction synchronized with smart gel volume phase transition. *Advanced Materials* **21**, 4372–4378 (2009).

37. Matsumoto, A., Endo, T., Yoshida, R., & Miyahara, Y. Electrical visualization of chemo-mechanical signal transduction using a smart gel-modified gate field effect transistor. *Chemical Communications* **37**, 5609–5611 (2009).

38. Miyata, T., Uragami, T., & Nakamae, K. Biomolecule-sensitive hydrogels. *Advanced Drug Delivery Reviews* **54**, 79–98 (2002).

39. Qiu, Y. & Park, K. Environment-sensitive hydrogels for drug delivery. *Advanced Drug Delivery Reviews* **53**, 321–339 (2001).

40. Kataoka, K., Miyazaki, H., Bunya, M., Okano, T., & Sakurai, Y. Totally synthetic polymer gels responding to external glucose concentration: their preparation and application to on-off regulation of insulin release. *Journal of the American Chemical Society* **120**, 12694–12695 (1998).

41. Matsumoto, A., Yoshida, R., & Kataoka, K. Glucose-responsive polymer gel bearing phenylborate derivative as a glucose-sensing moiety operating at the physiological pH. *Biomacromolecules* **5**, 1038–1045 (2004).

42. Matsumoto, A. et al. A totally synthetic glucose responsive gel operating in physiological aqueous conditions. *Chemical Communications* **46**, 2203–2205 (2010).

43. Matsumoto, A., Kurata, T., Shiino, D., & Kataoka, K. Swelling and shrinking kinetics of totally synthetic, glucose-responsive polymer gel bearing phenylborate derivative as a glucose-sensing moiety. *Macromolecules* **37**, 1502–1510 (2004).

44. Bergveld, P. The impact of mosfet-based sensors. *Sensors and Actuators* **8**, 109–127 (1985).

45. Miyata, T., Asami, N., & Uragami, T. A reversibly antigen-responsive hydrogel. *Nature* **399**, 766–769 (1999).

46. Miyata, T., Jige, M., Nakaminami, T., & Uragami, T. Tumor marker-responsive behavior of gels prepared by biomolecular imprinting. *Proceedings of the National Academy of Sciences of the United States of America* **103**, 1190–1193 (2006).

47. Fukuda, M. Possible roles of tumor-associated carbohydrate antigens. *Cancer Research* **56**, 2237–2244 (1996).

48. Bertozzi, C.R. & Kiessling, L.L. Chemical glycobiology. *Science* **291**, 2357–2364 (2001).

49. Raman, R., Raguram, S., Venkataraman, G., Paulson, J.C., & Sasisekharan, R. Glycomics: an integrated systems approach to structure-function relationships of glycans. *Nature Methods* **2**, 817–824 (2005).

50. Raz, A. et al. Cell-surface properties of B-16 melanoma variants with differing metastatic potential. *Cancer Research* **40**, 1645–1651 (1980).

51. Dobrossy, L., Pavelic, Z.P., & Bernacki, R.J. A Correlation between cell-surface sialyltransferase, sialic-acid, and glycosidase activities and the implantability of B-16 murine melanoma. *Cancer Research* **41**, 2262–2266 (1981).

52. Passaniti, A. & Hart, G.W. Cell-surface sialylation and tumor-metastasis—metastatic potential of B-16 melanoma variants correlates with their relative numbers of specific penultimate oligosaccharide structures. *Journal of Biological Chemistry* **263**, 7591–7603 (1988).

53. Chari, S.N. & Nath, N. Sialic acid content and sialidase activity of polymorphonuclear leucocytes in diabetes mellitus. *The American Journal of the Medical Sciences* **288**, 18–20 (1984).

54. Rogers, M.E. et al. Decrease in erythrocyte glycophorin sialic acid content is associated with increased erythrocyte aggregation in human diabetes. *Clinical science (London, England: 1979)* **82**, 309–313 (1992).

55. Boeseken, J. The use of boric acid for the determination of the configuration of carbohydrates. *Advances in Carbohydrate Chemistry* **4**, 189–210 (1949).

56. Foster, A.B. Zone electrophoresis of carbohydrates. *Advances in Carbohydrate Chemistry* **12**, 81–115 (1957).

57. Lorand, J.P. & Edwards, J.O. Polyol complexes and structure of the benzeneboronate ion. *The Journal of Organic Chemistry* **24**, 769–774 (1959).

58. Aronoff, S., Chen, T.C., & Cheveldayoff, M. Complexation of D-glucose with borate. *Carbohydrate Research* **40**, 299–309 (1975).

59. Uchimura, E., Otsuka, H., Okano, T., Sakurai, Y., & Kataoka, K. Totally synthetic polymer with lectin-like function: induction of killer cells by the copolymer of 3-acrylamidophenylboronic acid with N,N-dimethylacrylamide. *Biotechnology and Bioengineering* **72**, 307–314 (2001).

60. Otsuka, H., Uchimura, E., Koshino, H., Okano, T., & Kataoka, K. Anomalous binding profile of phenylboronic acid with N-acetylneuraminic acid (Neu5Ac) in aqueous solution with varying pH. *Journal of the American Chemical Society* **125**, 3493–3502 (2003).

61. Matsumoto, A., Sato, N., Kataoka, K., & Miyahara, Y. Noninvasive sialic acid detection at cell membrane by using phenylboronic acid modified self-assembled monolayer gold electrode. *Journal of the American Chemical Society* **131**, 12022–12023 (2009).

62. Matsumoto, A., Cabral, H., Sato, N., Kataoka, K., & Miyahara, Y. Assessment of tumor metastasis by the direct determination of cell-membrane sialic acid expression. *Angewandte Chemie (International ed. in English)* **49**, 5494–5497 (2010).

63. Schoning, M.J., Schroth, P., & Schutz, S. The use of insect chemoreceptors for the assembly of biosensors based on semiconductor field-effect transistors. *Electroanalysis* **12**, 645–652 (2000).

64. Schroth, P., Luth, H., Hummel, H.E., Schutz, S., & Schoning, M.J. Characterising an insect antenna as a receptor for a biosensor by means of impedance spectroscopy. *Electrochimica Acta* **47**, 293–297 (2001).

65. Schroth, P. et al. Extending the capabilities of an antenna/chip biosensor by employing various insect species. *Sensors and Actuators. B, Chemical* **78**, 1–5 (2001).

66. Willner, I. & Zayats, M. Electronic aptamer-based sensors. *Angewandte Chemie (International ed. in English)* **46**, 6408–6418 (2007).

67. Keefe, A.D., Pai, S., & Ellington, A. Aptamers as therapeutics. *Nature Reviews Drug Discovery* **9**, 537–550 (2010).

68. So, H.M. et al. Single-walled carbon nanotube biosensors using aptamers as molecular recognition elements. *Journal of the American Chemical Society* **127**, 11906–11907 (2005).

69. Maehashi, K. et al. Label-free protein biosensor based on aptamer-modified carbon nanotube field-effect transistors. *Analytical Chemistry* **79**, 782–787 (2007).

70. Maehashi, K., Matsumoto, K., Takamura, Y., & Tamiya, E. Aptamer-based label-free immunosensors using carbon nanotube field-effect transistors. *Electroanalysis* **21**, 1285–1290 (2009).

CHAPTER 5

Supported Lipid Bilayers: Intelligent Surfaces for Ion Channel Recordings

ANDREAS JANSHOFF and CLAUDIA STEINEM

5.1 INTRODUCTION

The structure and function of biomolecules as well as larger assemblies are intimately connected. To be able to mimic the native situation as closely as possible, while it is still possible to study individual molecules in the absence of a multicomponent environment, tailored experimental model systems are required. It is of pivotal importance to control the complexity of a system by adding or removing components to manage the investigation of their impact on the biological function. A typical example is the biological membrane, whose composition is an intricate mixture of proteins and lipids assembled in an ultrathin bimolecular sheet fulfilling a wealth of functions ranging from compartmentalization over energy conversion and mechanical sensing of the environment to tissue formation.

Model membranes that capture the essential thermomechanical, optical, and electrical features of cellular membranes encompass liposomes, black lipid membranes (BLMs), and solid-supported membranes (SSMs). These systems ensure proper function of transmembrane proteins that would otherwise denature if taken out of their native environment. In particular, the entire class of transmembrane proteins functioning as receptors, channels, and pumps loses its activity when taken out of the membranous environment.

Among the various model membranes, SSMs are the most versatile ones. By forming SSMs, in which functional membrane components have been embedded, a solid substrate is turned into a smart material. However, a solid support also holds disadvantages as it might reduce the lateral mobility of the membrane leaflet attached to the support and hinders or even prevents the observation of transport processes across the bilayer. The latter phenomenon

Intelligent Surfaces in Biotechnology: Scientific and Engineering Concepts, Enabling Technologies, and Translation to Bio-Oriented Applications, First Edition.
Edited by H. Michelle Grandin and Marcus Textor.

is particularly important if one aims at studying the barrier properties of membranes associated with channels, transporters, or pumps.

Here, we review the relevant and most recent aspects of SSM formation and characterization with special focus on ion transport across patterned and pore-spanning bilayers. We concentrate on the development of membrane structures attached to a surface to allow for the insertion and detection of transport activity of transmembrane proteins. If several requirements are fulfilled, SSMs can provide an appropriate environment for membrane proteins and, as such, can be used to investigate the proteins' response to external stimuli, thus acting as an intelligent surface. Each leaflet of the lipid bilayer should be in the fluid state and the entire membrane should be surrounded by an aqueous phase. Several different supported bilayer systems have been developed over the past 30 years including polymer-cushioned and tethered lipid bilayers, as well as systems on porous materials, which will be discussed further. A particular emphasis lies on the inevitable demand for microstructured membrane-covered surfaces pointing in the direction of chip-based array techniques. While some of the above-mentioned systems are routinely used for biophysical investigations and ligand–membrane receptor screening (see Reference 1 and references therein) to study membrane protein interactions, the main challenge remains the functional insertion of transmembrane peptides and proteins.

5.2   SUPPORTED LIPID BILAYERS

5.2.1   SSMs on Flat Interfaces

SSMs can be prepared by a variety of different methods dependent on the support (Fig. 5.1). Successful preparations have been described on hydrophilic

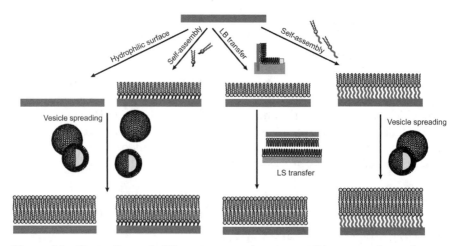

Figure 5.1   Illustrations of different ways to prepare solid-supported membranes based on vesicle spreading and Langmuir–Blodgett transfer. (See color insert.)

substrates such as mica and glass, various metal surfaces such as gold and platinum, or semiconductors such as indium tin oxide (ITO) and silicon. Bilayer deposition is generally achieved by employing the Langmuir–Blodgett (LB) method or self-assembly techniques, such as vesicle spreading[2–8] or even a combination of both. While LB films offer control over the composition and lateral pressure of both leaflets, self-assembly techniques are more versatile and the bilayers are easier to prepare. The method of choice will be dependent on its application. While anchoring of lipids via covalent or quasi-covalent bonds results in a rather stable monolayer and thus bilayer, the lateral mobility and a certain distance between solid support and the surface-facing membrane leaflet might not be sufficient to host a protein in a fully functional fashion. The solution of this apparent contradiction is one of the key challenges in the development of membrane preparation protocols.[9]

5.2.1.1 *Lipid Bilayers on Transparent Surfaces*

Brian and McConnell[10] were the first to show that adsorption and spreading of vesicles on glass supports results in planar lipid bilayers, which maintain lateral mobility of the lipids as shown by fluorescence recovery after photobleaching (FRAP).[11,12] However, the resulting lipid bilayers are in such close contact (≈1 nm) to the transparent support that incorporation of large transmembrane proteins becomes virtually impossible. To generate a distance between the bilayer and the support, a polymer, tethered to a lipid, can be used, on which unilamellar vesicles are spread. For example, 1,2-dimyristoyl-*sn*-glycero-3-phosphoethanolamine-polyethyleneglycol-triethoxysilane (DPS), with as many as 45 ethylene oxide units, was transferred to quartz or glass by the LB technique.[13,14] Similarly, Purrucker et al.[15] reported on the design of various lipopolymer tethers. By means of living cationic polymerization of 2-methyl-2-oxazolines, they were able to synthesize a series of well-defined lipopolymers, equipped with a silane coupling group on the proximal, and lipid anchors on the distal chain ends. This allowed for the functionalization of glass substrates and offered the possibility to precisely control the length of the polymer chain. Thus, the group was able to investigate the effect of the spacer length and the lateral spacer density on membrane structure and function. Another approach is to make use of polymer cushions such as polyaniline/poly(acrylic acid) multilayer films,[16] regenerated cellulose,[17] or a thermoresponsive polymer cushion.[18] Vesicles can also be spread on such functionalized surfaces forming lipid bilayers.

5.2.1.2 *Lipid Bilayers on Gold Surfaces*

To be able to perform electrochemical measurements, lipid bilayers need to be prepared on conductive surfaces serving as the working electrode. A review written by Ottova et al.[19] gives an overview of formation, characterization, patterning, and the application of so-called supported planar lipid bilayers (s-BLMs) on various metal surfaces such as platinum, gold, or silver. In particular, gold has been proven to be ideally suited for the preparation of lipid bilayers as the surface is chemically inert but still allows for functionalization via gold–sulfur-driven self-assembly processes. The electrical characteristics of membranes on gold surfaces can be investigated by impedance spectroscopy (IS), providing membrane capacitances of 0.5–1.0 $\mu F/cm^2$ and specific membrane resistances in the order of 10^5–10^7 Ω cm^2.[20,21] Membranes on gold surfaces might be classified according to their different architectures: (i) hybrid bilayers composed of a lipid monolayer on a hydrophobic support and a second leaflet atop of it, (ii) lipid bilayers on a hydrophilic or charged surface, and (iii) covalently anchored lipid bilayers on a hydrophilic surface.

(i) *Hybrid Bilayers.* For the formation of a hybrid bilayer composed of a lipid monolayer on a hydrophobic support, the gold surface is first functionalized by an alkanethiol or sulfur-bearing phospholipid derivative,[22,23] or a hydrophobic hairy-rod polymer.[24] A second monolayer can be attached by a Langmuir–Schäfer (LS) dip, where a lipid monolayer is transferred horizontally from the air–water interface to the hydrophobic solid support. Most techniques rely, however, on the physisorption/self-assembly of lipids from an organic,[25] detergent solution,[26] or from a vesicle suspension,[27,28] where only the latter one leads to solvent- and detergent-free bilayers. These supported lipid layers are well suited for the investigation of reactions at the membrane interface, that is, the binding of ligands to membrane-confined receptors. However, proper functioning of transmembrane ion channels is rarely achieved since a second aqueous compartment is missing.

(ii) *Lipid Bilayers on Hydrophilic or Charged Surfaces.* As mentioned in the previous sections, it is necessary to create an aqueous compartment between the bilayer and the support, thereby decoupling the membrane from the solid support. By using charged self-assembly molecules, oppositely charged lipid membranes can be adsorbed on the functionalized gold surface. However, this method is very susceptible to high-ionic-strength conditions, which cause detachment of the membrane from the surface.[20] Decoupling of the membranes was also pursued by creating polymer cushions in between membrane and solid support. These protocols aim at a minimized interaction of the polymer with the supported bilayer, while the hydrophilicity of the polymer is maximized. Despite strong efforts, only a small number of procedures turned out to be suited to produce modestly high surface coverage. For example, Majewski et al.[29] described the formation of lipid bilayers by fusion of 1,2-dimyristoyl-*sn*-glycero-3-phosphocholine (DMPC) vesicles on polyethyleneimine. Employing neutron reflectometry, a complex signal was obtained, which was attributed to intact vesicles coexisting with bilayers and multilayers. Based on an avidin protein cushion, we were able to show[4,30] that the formation of planar bilayers starting from biotinylated vesicles is a function of the number of biotin anchoring groups that drive their attachment and spreading on the surface. Several approaches start from a polymer, to which a lipophilic anchor has been attached in order to increase the propensity to bind spread, and fuse vesicles onto it. In a pioneer study by Spinke et al.,[31] a moderately hydrophilic methacrylic polymer with aliphatic side chains was deposited on gold, by LB transfer, and the formation of DMPC lipid bilayers by vesicle fusion was monitored by surface plasmon resonance (SPR). Several other amphiphilic polymers followed, such as polyacrylamide polymers,[32] and 1,2-distearoyl-*sn*-glycero-3-phosphoethanolamine-*N*-poly(ethyleneglycol)-2000-*N*-[3-(2-(pyridyldithio)propionate] (DSPE-PEG-PDP)[33] combined with PEG-PDP and egg–phosphatidylcholine (PC).

(iii) *Covalently Anchored Lipid Bilayers.* A third concept, first introduced by Vogel and coworkers, makes use of phospholipids[26] and cholesterol derivatives (see Reference 34 and references therein), with hydrophilic spacer groups terminated by a sulfur-bearing group, that can self-assemble as a monolayer on gold surfaces. The spacers can be based on a wide range of compounds such as oligo(ethyleneoxide)[26,35,36] or oligopeptides.[37] The resulting tethered membranes have been shown to be fluid lipid bilayers possessing an aqueous phase separating the membrane from the support. The spacer acts as an elastic buffer, decoupling the lipid layer from the solid surface and generating a water layer in between.[9,38–46] Cornell and coworkers[35,47–51] were the first to use half-membrane-spanning tether lipids with benzyl disulfide (DLP) and synthetic archaea analogue full membrane-spanning lipids (MSLs) with phytanoyl chains to stabilize the structure and polyethyleneglycol units as a hydrophilic spacer. Bilayer formation was achieved by immersion of a gold electrode in an ethanolic solution of the lipid mixture for the surface-attached leaflet, drying, and subsequent immersion in an ethanolic solution of a lipid mixture for the outer leaflet.

5.2.1.3 *Lipid Bilayers on Silicon*

Besides gold, another frequently used surface is silicon since this material is compatible with conventional photolithography and is nearly atomically flat, rendering it a superior surface if it comes to atomic force microscopy (AFM) imaging. Elender et al.[52] prepared dextran-modified silicon oxide surfaces to deposit a bilayer by a combination of the LB and LS techniques. The dextran layer exhibited a thickness of around 100 nm and was covalently bound to the thermally oxidized silicon oxide surface via epoxidation or aminosilanization. The lipid diffusion constant was 2.8 $\mu m^2/s$, which is well within the range of known diffusion coefficients for fluid lipid bilayers. Shen et al.[53] built up polymer-supported lipid bilayers on benzophenone-modified silicon dioxide substrates by a photochemical reaction, which turned out to be a versatile approach to covalently link the polymer layer to the substrate. IS on moderately and highly doped n-type silicon substrates was used to investigate 1,2-diphytanoyl-*sn*-glycero-3-phosphocholine (DPhPC) bilayers generated by an LB transfer of a mixed monolayer of 1,2-dipalmitoyl-*sn*-glycero-3-phosphoethanolamine-N-[methoxy (polyethylene glycol)-2000] and DPhPC followed by fusion of large unilamellar vesicles.[54] To generate air-stable lipid membrane systems, Saavedra and coworkers[55,56] used polymerizable lipids (1,2-bis[10-(2′,4′-hexadienoyloxy) decanoyl]-*sn*-glycero-3-phosphocholine, bis-SorbPC). The resulting membranes, after *in situ* polymerization, were not only air stable but were also resistant to organic solvents and surfactant solutions, and retained their ability to suppress nonspecific adsorption of proteins, which is characteristic for a fluid PC bilayer. Tethered lipid bilayers were also generated on silicon dioxide surfaces based on 3-di-*O*-phytanyl-*sn*-glycero-1-tetraethyleneglycol-D,L-α-lipoic acid ester lipids attached to a silane.[57]

5.2.2 SSMs on Porous/Aperture Containing Surfaces

5.2.2.1 Lipid Bilayers on Micromachined Apertures
Since the pioneering work of Müller and Rudin,[58] lipid bilayers suspended over a small aperture have become an invaluable tool to investigate ion channels. These membranes are formed by spreading a lipid solution dissolved in a nonvolatile solvent across an aperture in a thin insulating polymer foil separating two electrolyte reservoirs. The process of bilayer formation can be monitored by the changes in interference colors eventually leaving a BLM behind. This method has been extended in the following years by the Montal–Müller and the "tip-dip" techniques. In the last 10 years, planar arrangements on a solid support have been developed to be compatible with sensor technologies and automization procedures. Such micromachined supports were generated by conventional photolithography[59,60] and suspended bilayers were formed by spreading a lipid dissolved in *n*-decane on the perfluorothiol-functionalized gold surface of the aperture-containing substrate. Electrical measurements on those membranes revealed capacitances of 0.3–0.7 μF/cm^2 and resistances of around 10^7 Ω cm^2. The long-term stability, however, was not longer than 5 hours and therefore comparable to that of classical BLMs. A similar result was found by Eisenberg and coworkers.[61] The authors discussed these problems in terms of the surface energy of the oxidized silicon. An improvement in stability was achieved by attaching a polytetrafluoroethylene (PTFE) layer on the silicon dioxide layer by chemical vapor deposition, thus rendering the surface hydrophobic.[62] Fertig et al.[63–67] used apertures that were manufactured in glass substrates by the single ion track etching method with diameters between 1 and 10 μm. This invention has led to the company Nanion Technologies GmbH. Vogel and coworkers[68] developed a method to prepare a lipid bilayer, which suspends a 0.6- to 7.0-μm-large hole in silicon. To prepare the bilayer, a negatively charged giant unilamellar vesicle needs to spread on a silicon dioxide surface with a single hole and functionalized with 4-aminobutyldimethyl-methoxysilane or poly-L-lysine.

5.2.2.2 *Lipid Bilayers on Porous Materials* To combine the merits of robustness of membranes attached to a solid support with the advantage of freestanding bilayers, as discussed in Chapter 5.2.2.1, which allow for the insertion of transmembrane proteins without a capacitive coupling, substrates with pore arrays or even porous materials have been introduced as membrane supports.[69–72] Membranes spanning these holes, with diameters between 50 nm and several tens of micrometers, take advantage of the natural properties of a cell membrane, where integrated ion channels are mobile, and transport of ions from one side of the membrane to the other is not hindered by the vicinity of a substrate. To give some examples, Hemmler et al.[73] prepared membranes by spreading lipids from an organic solution onto the surfaces of laser structured pore arrays with pore diameters of 30–70 μm and track-etched polycarbonate membranes with pore diameters of 5.0 and 0.8 μm. Favero et al.[74,75] first prefunctionalized polycarbonate membranes with pore diameters of 1 μm and a pore density of 10^5–10^7 pores/cm^2 by covering the surface with gold and octadecanethiol to render it hydrophobic. Spreading of a PC solution in *n*-hexane/isobutanol results in an insulating layer, which they called mixed hybrid bilayer membranes (MHBLMs). The average lifetime of this membrane system was larger than 10 hours. Schuster et al.[76] used microfiltration membranes in combination with S-layers to support lipid membranes and hence increased the stability substantially, as compared to conventional BLMs.

We developed an artificial membrane system based on porous alumina and porous silicon substrates that can also be considered as a hybrid between an SSM and a freestanding lipid bilayer. As each of the bilayers spanning the pores of the substrate resembles a single BLM, the system was called nano-BLMs. The porous surface is first functionalized with gold and a lipid with a terminal thiol group. On this hydrophobic surface, a lipid dissolved in a non-volatile solvent, similar to the painting technique according to Müller and Rudin[58] is spread, thus resulting in highly insulating pore-suspending lipid bilayers. Impedance analysis of the membrane system revealed specific membrane capacitances that are indicative of single lipid bilayers. The membrane resistances are in the gigaohm regime allowing for single-channel measurements.[77,78] The membrane resistance remains in the gigaohm regime for several tens of hours and only slowly decreases over time, which demonstrates its high long-term stability compared to other strategies.

Solvent-free pore-spanning membranes required tailored protocols. By using the Montal–Müller technique, Mayer et al.[79] deposited lipid layers on highly ordered pore arrays in Teflon films that were microfabricated by soft lithography, leading to pores with diameters in the range of 2–800 μm. Weng et al.[80] presented the formation of fluid lipid membranes supported on nanoporous aerogel/xerogel substrates by means of vesicle spreading, resulting in solvent-free lipid membranes. Recently, we were able to produce highly insulating pore-spanning membranes on porous alumina substrates. The gold covered porous substrates were first functionalized with a thiol-bearing cholesterol derivative onto which large unilamellar vesicles were spread. Even though these pore-spanning membranes did not exhibit as high a membrane resistance as nano-BLMs, they turned out to be well suited for an integral investigation of ion channel activity by means of IS.[81]

5.2.3 Patterning of SSMs

Array fabrication with controlled and addressable composition is desirable for almost all bioanalytical applications due to higher throughput, reduced sample volume, and an increased sensitivity on a smaller sensor area when the sample volume and the analyte concentration are limited. While structuring of proteins and nucleic acids is readily achieved via soft lithography, the preparation and structuring of lipid bilayers requires continuous exposure to aqueous solutions. Moreover, methods based on microcontact printing for structuring lipid membranes are limited to a very small number of different lipid compositions since the method does not allow for individual addressability of the segments. A selection of strategies to pattern membranes on solid supports using bottom-up and top-down lithography is given in Figure 5.2. As a consequence, patterning of lipid bilayers poses particular challenges on the protocols due to the

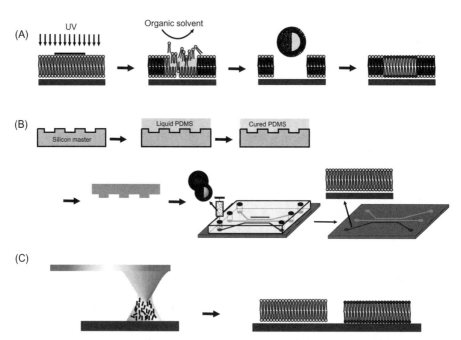

Figure 5.2 Micropatterning of solid-supported membranes. (A) Lithography based on selective polymerization of lipids and refilling of the gaps with vesicles. (B) Formation of individually addressable lipid bilayers using micromolding in capillaries. (C) Dip-pen nanolithography based on atomic force microscopy and selective deposition of lipids on the surface. (See color insert.)

nature of the bimolecular sheet, which is susceptible to air exposure. Despite these difficulties, quite a number of solutions have been found as outlined in the next chapters.

5.2.3.1 *Patterning of Hybrid SSMs*

Strategies to pattern hybrid membranes, which consist of one leaflet that is chemisorbed on the surface and the second, outer one physisorbed on top of it, are mainly based on soft lithography techniques that are frequently used to structure thiols on gold. Two or more different thiols are applied on a gold surface in a spatially defined manner using techniques such as microcontact printing or microwriting.[82,83] Either the first thiol compound is spatially delivered on the surface while the second one fills up the residual areas or micromachining and photolithography selectively remove thiols from a preformed monolayer and the resulting pattern is then filled by a second thiol species. The use of micropatterning of solid substrates with self-assembled monolayers (SAMs) has been shown to be an effective way of producing an array of bilayer patches on a surface. Jenkins et al.[84–86] introduced and characterized a hybrid system based on microcontact printing of lipophilic SAMs. The authors investigated substrates that consisted of circular hydrophilic regions functionalized with mercapto-ethanol surrounded by octadecanethiol.[84] Three geometries were studied in which the diameter of the hydrophilic portion varied between 4 and 16 µm and the center-to-center separation between 10 and 40 µm. The arrangement allowed for the study of lipid deposition on the SAMs with the same total hydrophilic surface area but with differently sized hydrophilic patches. IS revealed that for SAMs with smaller diameter hydrophilic patches, a larger lipid coverage was obtained. The results from AFM images and SPR in conjunction with IS showed that the simple picture of a bilayer spanning the hydrophilic patches is too simplistic. The real situation is considerably more complex and the hydrophobic-hydrophilic edges play an important role.

5.2.3.2 *Patterning of Nonhybrid SSMs*

Generally, structuring of fluid nonhybrid bilayers has been pioneered by Boxer and coworkers using barriers to lateral diffusion of lipids. Using blotting and stamping, Hovis and Boxer[87] managed to produce patterned fluid lipid bilayer membranes on solid supports. These methods are based on the fact that membranes undergo self-limiting lateral expansion when the bilayer material is removed from the surface or when it is deposited in a pattern on a surface. The authors describe a procedure in which the bilayer material is selectively removed from the support using a poly(dimethylsiloxane) (PDMS) stamp. Alternatively, bilayers assembled on a PDMS stamp were printed onto clean surfaces. Parikh and coworkers introduced a wet photolithography approach using light-activated, localized oxidative chemistry that directly patterns fluid phospholipid bilayers in an aqueous environment.[88,89]

Recently, Jackson and Groves applied scanning probe lithography to remove lipid membranes from prepatterned chromium arrays and then refilled these regions with new lipid components.[90] The authors also describe an aqueous aluminum lift-off process suitable for the fabrication of hybrid patterns of proteins and supported lipid membranes on silica surfaces. For this purpose, thin patterned aluminum films were employed as sacrificial protecting layers, thus defining the geometry of the protein–lipid patterns. The thin layer of aluminum is lifted off and the exposed, uncovered substrate is subsequently filled with lipids by vesicle spreading. The procedure makes it possible to obtain structures with line widths of 200 nm.[91] Along the same lines, Orth and coworkers used a polymer lift-off method to create lipid bilayer patterns down to a 1-μm resolution.[92] The patterns were formed in solution as the polymer was mechanically peeled away in one piece. Binding of antibodies and avidin on these uniform micron-scale platforms was successful.

In principle, these patterning methods are limited to a small number of different lipid compositions deposited on a single chip. Moreover, achieving individual addressability of the various segments is not feasible. To address each membrane segment individually, we and others have developed a general strategy for generating numerous selective functionalized lipid membrane compartments using micromolding in capillaries on glassy supports.[93–96] The realization of the membrane array of solid-supported lipid bilayers in the micrometer regime is based on the combination of the technique of vesicle spreading and the soft lithography microfluidic network (μFN) process. The general technique of material molding in capillaries formed by elastomers was first established by Xia and Whitesides.[82] A structured elastomer provides a network of empty channels when brought into contact with a surface. The structure in the mold is obtained by curing the two components of PDMS on a coated silicon wafer with the inverse master structure and subsequent removal of the PDMS replicate. The pretreatment of the PDMS mold in an O_2 plasma renders the surface hydrophilic, which is necessary to establish a tight seal between the mold and the glass substrate. The flow pads are individually addressed with different vesicle solutions through small holes on the top of the PDMS mold. Vesicles are injected to fill the empty channels by laminar capillary flow. Once in contact with the glass, the vesicles adhere and spread to form planar lipid bilayers. Figure 5.2B schematically illustrates the microstructuring process of SSM segments. Subsequent to the removal of the PDMS mold and rinsing of the sample with buffer, the separated lipid membrane compartments remaining on the substrate are accessible to optical techniques and high-resolution surface analysis tools.[93,94]

These individually addressable solid-supported lipid membrane segments prepared by micromolding in capillaries have been shown to be ideally suited to follow specific protein adsorption processes on small areas by AFM and fluorescence microscopy.[93] The adjacent bilayers differing in lipid composition allowed investigating the specific binding of proteins such as cholera toxin and annexins proving the selective nature of the molecular recognition in a single experiment including the proper controls.[93,97,98]

Many biosensor applications require electrically conductive substrates such as gold. We also developed a procedure that allows for the formation of individually addressable lipid bilayers, electrostatically immobilized on functionalized gold surfaces, by means of micromolding in capillaries using a chemically modified microfluidic PDMS network.[99]

Even smaller structures have been recently achieved by Lenhert et al. using dip-pen nanolithography (DPN).[100–102] DPN is a scanning probe-based fabrication technique where an atomic force microscope tip is used to transfer molecules to a surface via a solvent meniscus. DPN can be used to deposit materials on surfaces with high lateral resolution down to 100 nm. Lenhert and coworkers used parallel and multiplexed DPN of 1,2-dioleoyl-*sn*-glycero-3-phosphocholine (DOPC) mixed with phospholipids containing biotin and nitrilotriacetic acid (NTA) functional groups.[100–102] Subsequently, two different proteins were selectively bound to the lipid patterns based on biotin–streptavidin and histidine tag coupling. Recently, they succeeded in creating lipid-based lyotropic optical diffraction gratings composed of biofunctional lipid multilayers with a thickness between 5 and 100 nm using lipid DPN.[100–102] The authors showed that these lipid multilayer gratings allow for label-free and specific detection of lipid–protein interactions in solution.

Cremer and coworkers developed a method based on AFM to control the formation of SSMs down to the sub-100-nm level.[103] *Nanoshaving* employs an AFM tip to selectively remove a preexisting thin film from a substrate. The resulting uncovered regions can be subsequently filled with vesicles to create lines of planar lipid bilayers possessing widths as thin as 55 nm.

5.3   CHARACTERISTICS OF SSMs

5.3.1   Thermomechanical Properties of SSMs

SSMs are a major playground for life scientists and, in principle, they allow for the investigation of the influence of lipid composition on domain formation and protein function. However, it is pivotal to first elucidate the influence of the solid support on the physical properties of SSMs, such as their thermotropic phase behavior and their lateral organization, as it is suspected that phase transitions and lateral mobility are significantly affected by the underlying substrate. Reports on phase transitions of supported bilayers are rather controversial, ranging from those that found significantly different thermomechanical and electrical properties compared to freestanding bilayers, to others who monitored only slight differences.[104–107] Frequently, bilayer thickness as a function of temperature is used as a measure of the chain melting process during the main phase transition from the rippled gel phase or gel phase to the fluid crystalline phase.[108–113] In addition to measuring the thickness of the bilayer, thermal expansion as a response to heating or cooling of the SSM has been employed by following the closing or opening of defect areas within the bilayer.[108–116] Thermal expansion is, however, suppressed if no sufficiently large free area is provided, and only a few studies provide useful quantitative information.[113,115] We recently demonstrated that it is feasible to determine changes in membrane thickness and thermal expansion of SSMs during the main phase transition by means of temperature-controlled AFM and imaging ellipsometry utilizing microstructured bilayers prepared by micromolding in capillaries.[99] While AFM might not be ideally suited to unambiguously determine thickness changes and area expansion of the bilayer due to the naturally invasive nature of the method, imaging ellipsometry (see Methods Box 5.1 at end of chapter) is better suited to simultaneously acquiring changes in thickness and area expansion of microstructured lipid bilayers in a noninvasive manner. Parikh and coworkers demonstrated that the imaging ellipsometry of microstructured membranes allows for a quantitative determination of physicochemical properties of supported membranes such as bilayer thicknesses, molecular areas, lateral uniformity, and ligand–receptor interactions.[117] A thorough study by Faiss et al.[118] on the thermotropic behavior of individually addressable microstructured bilayers demonstrates the feasibility of the approach to obtain quantitative data on the phase behavior of SSMs. Figure 5.3A shows the impact of temperature sweeps on a membrane stripe composed of DMPC. Micropatterned bilayers have the advantage of providing the required space for lateral expansion upon heating but also allow for the comparison of the parameters with an internal standard, which might be a lipid bilayer with known thermotropic properties. Based on this setup, it became possible to systematically detect changes of the phase transition behavior as a result of the attachment of the bilayer to the solid support. Specifically, the influence of the cholesterol content and chain length on the phase behavior of supported saturated diacyl PC bilayers was investigated (Fig. 5.3A,B). Compared to results obtained with vesicles, a systematic reduction in the cooperativity of the main phase transition was observed, while the main phase transition temperatures, as well as the lateral diffusion coefficients, depend only slightly on the solid support.

Figure 5.3B shows the change in bilayer thickness and relative area expansion of DMPC, 1,2-dipentadecoyl-*sn*-glycero-3-phosphocholine (diC15PC), and 1,2-dipalmitoyl-*sn*-glycero-3-phosphocholine (DPPC) as a function of temperature. The curves show the expected dependence of the main phase transition temperature on the acyl chain length. All transition temperatures are shifted by 2°–6° to higher temperatures, while the broadness of the transition is reduced from a shorter to a longer chain length. It was found that the cooperativity of the phase transition, expressed as the cooperative unit size n, is at least a factor of 10 smaller than for multilamellar vesicles and increases with acyl chain length.

In addition to the thermotropic behavior of neat phospholipids, mixtures with cholesterol have also been investigated. Cholesterol is unique in its ability to change the phase transition behavior of lipid membranes, including the formation of a "liquid-ordered" phase at high cholesterol concentrations.[119–122] Above the main phase transition, cholesterol causes a large increase in the

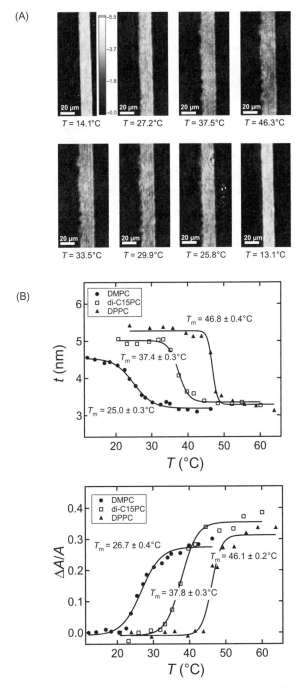

Figure 5.3 (A) Ellipsometric thickness maps of structured DMPC bilayers on Si/SiO$_2$ at various temperatures. The height scale is valid for all images. (B) Change in bilayer thickness (top) and relative area expansion (bottom) of DMPC, diC15PC, and DPPC bilayers as a function of temperature. The straight lines denote empirical sigmoidal fits to the data.

average orientational order of the lipid chains, accompanied by an increase in bilayer thickness. In the gel phase, however, this effect is small because the chains are already largely in an all-trans conformation. Therefore, one major effect of the incorporation of cholesterol into lipid bilayers is to broaden and reduce the enthalpy of the main phase transition, eventually eliminating it at 50 mol % cholesterol.[123,124] Accordingly, the cross-sectional area of the phospholipid molecule is decreased above and increased below the main phase transition temperature, thereby reducing the overall expansion of the membrane at an elevated temperature. In summary, SSMs deposited on hydrophilic surfaces most likely display the same thermotropic properties as bilayers organized in liposomes.

5.3.2 Mechanical Stability

The local mechanical properties of lipid bilayers attached to a solid support can be probed by indenting the membrane with an AFM tip (see Methods Box 5.2 at end of chapter). A typical force curve recorded on a lipid bilayer shows a repulsive component until the film eventually ruptures and the tip jumps into contact with the underlying substrate surface (Fig. 5.4). Compression of the bilayer occurs prior to rupture, thus making it possible to access the bilayer's Young modulus.[125]

Several groups[126–130] reported on material-dependent breakthrough events on different lipid bilayers with regard to imaging contrast mechanisms[126] or the activation process of the penetration of the AFM tip through the lipid bilayer,[129] respectively. A quantitative analysis of the correlation of adhesive and elastic properties and their dependence on the lipid head group, chain length, and the membrane lamellarity has been carried out by Künneke et al.[125] by employing pulsed force mode (PFM) microscopy. An automated analysis scheme for the detection of breakthrough events based on a multiparameter cluster analysis could be applied to correlate adhesion with membrane stiffness in an unequivocal fashion.

Although in principle it is possible to obtain compressional modules from force indentation curves taken on SSMs, the underlying substrate affects these measurements substantially if not dominate the elastic response entirely. Considering that the indentation depth should be below 10% of the bilayer thickness, the indentation depth to collect data in a faithful manner is rather limited.

A general solution to this problem is indentation experiments carried out on freestanding membranes such as pore-spanning lipid bilayers (Fig. 5.5). These measurements allow one to locally access the bending module of a lipid bilayer.[131–133] The elastic response of a membrane to indentation comprises contributions from bending, stretching, and lateral tension. While bending of the membrane usually influences the force indentation curves only marginally, as detailed next, stretching and lateral tension govern the elastic response of thin membranes to a large extent.

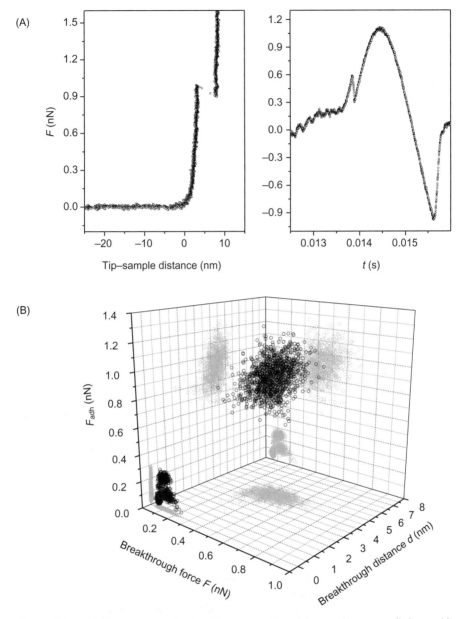

Figure 5.4 (A) Force curves obtained by conventional force microscopy (left graph) and by pulsed force mode (PFM) microscopy (right graph) on 1-palmitoyl-2-oleoyl-*sn*-glycero-3-phospho-L-serine (POPS) bilayers. Both force curves show breakthrough events in the contact regime. (B) Three-dimensional cluster analysis of breakthrough events monitored by PFM microscopy of a POPS bilayer/POPS multilayer/mica system. Orthogonal projections of the maximum adhesion force, the breakthrough force, and breakthrough distance as obtained from the same PFM periods show the cluster extensions.

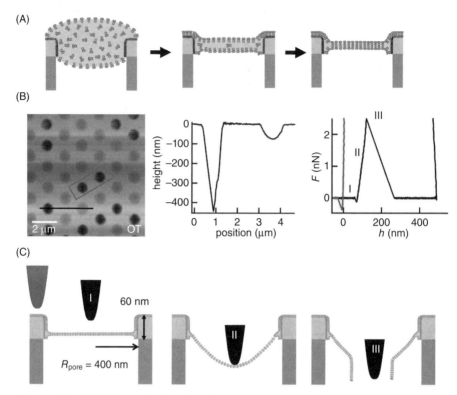

Figure 5.5 (A) Schematic drawing of the preparation of nano-BLMs on a porous matrix using the painting technique. (B) AFM image (left) and corresponding line profile (middle) of pore-spanning bilayers as well as typical force indentation curves (right) obtained from the rim (red) and the center of the pore (black). (C) Schematic illustration of the indentation event shown in the force indentation curve in (B) (I–III). (See color insert.)

Recently, we scrutinized the mechanical behavior of lipid bilayers spanning the pores of highly ordered porous silicon substrates by local indentation experiments as a function of surface functionalization, lipid composition, solvent content, indentation velocity, and pore radius.[134] Nano-BLMs as well as solvent-free pore-spanning bilayers were imaged by fluorescence microscopy and AFM prior to force curve acquisition, thus making it possible to distinguish between membrane-covered and uncovered pores. Force indentation curves on pore-spanning bilayers attached to functionalized hydrophobic porous silicon substrates reveal a predominately linear response that is mainly attributed to prestress in the membranes. This is in agreement with the observation that indentation leads to membrane rupture well below 5% area dilatation. However, membrane bending and lateral tension dominates over prestress and stretching if solvent-free supported membranes, obtained from spreading giant liposomes on hydrophilic porous silicon, are indented. In order to obtain intrinsic mechanical parameters from indentation experiments, it is inevitable to use smaller pores since the bending response increases with R^{-2}.

5.4 ION CHANNELS IN SSMs

Ion channels represent an important class of membrane-spanning protein pores that mediate the flux of ions in a variety of cell types. In particular, they are of major importance for the human physiology, and thus, they are highly attractive molecular drug targets.[135] However, investigation of ion channels and their pharmacological modulation is by no means an easy task as their function relies on a laterally mobile and highly insulating lipid bilayer. The functionality of an ion channel can best be monitored by its ion transport properties. Upon the opening of a single functional ion channel, typically 10^7–10^8 charges are transferred across the membrane per second and per channel, which gives rise to a current of around 2–20 pA that can be monitored only with high gain amplifiers. The patch clamp technique is the state-of-the-art technology for the study of ion channels,[136] but patch clamping is a laborious process requiring skilled and highly trained scientists. Owing to its ultralow throughput, conventional patch clamp is frequently applied only in the later stages of drug discovery and development. To be able to search for new drug candidates at an earlier stage of drug development, high-throughput screening assays are required. In recent years, new methods have been developed, which are a trade-off between high throughput and high information content. These so-called automated patch clamp systems[137–139] provide a platform, which allows for the investigation of ion channels from a functional perspective; that is, the electrical characteristics of ion channels and their modulation by drugs can be monitored in great detail. Automated patch clamp, however, relies on currents in the picoampere regime, which are generated by a single ion channel, and data workup of these single events is rather tedious.

Hence, integral methods such as IS (see Methods Box 5.3 at end of chapter), cyclovoltammetry, or chronoamperometry might be advantageous as these methods enable one to read out changes in ion channel activities in one single scan. Hence, it is obvious that new approaches are necessary to develop bioanalytical devices and drug screening techniques for the pharmaceutical industry, targeting ion channels in an integral manner.

A number of approaches are based on lipid membranes that are attached to a conducting solid substrate such as gold, platinum, or ITO, which were discussed in Chapter 5.2.1.2. In the following, we focus on lipid membranes on solid substrates into which ion carriers, channel-forming peptides, and proteins, as well as transporters, have been successfully incorporated.

5.4.1 Carriers

Supramolecular carriers originating either from natural or synthetic sources have attracted a lot of interest during the years as their insertion into a lipid bilayer results in a controlled and specific transport of ions across the membrane. Two different examples will be given to illustrate the applicability of ion carriers in SSMs. One of the most prominent and very well-studied examples of a natural ion carrier is the cyclic depsipeptide valinomycin from *Streptomyces fulvissimus*. It is a 12-membered ring with three identical units and facilitates the transport of alkali cations with the selectivity sequence $Rb^+ > K^+ > Cs^+ > Na^+ > Li^+$ by forming a three-dimensional complex shielding the ions from the hydrophobic membrane core. By IS, Naumann et al.[140] and we[41] were able to show that valinomycin exhibits its well-known cation selectivity in tethered bilayers on gold. An appropriate equivalent circuit had to be developed to be able to extract changes in membrane conductance from the impedance data upon adding different cation concentrations. The result was that the membrane conductance significantly decreases with increasing K^+ concentration in a linear fashion, while sodium ions have virtually no impact on the membrane conductance. Instead of using gold surfaces, Roskamp et al.[141] prepared tethered bilayer lipid membranes on aluminum oxide, thereby making use of phosphonate ether lipids, which form monolayers on aluminum oxide with a thickness of 3.7 nm and a capacitance of about 19 $\mu F/cm^2$. Such a high capacitance indicates a large number of defects in the monolayer. After vesicle fusion on the hydrophobic monolayer, a bilayer with a capacitance of 10 $\mu F/cm^2$ and a membrane resistance of 17 $M\Omega \ cm^2$ was achieved. This type of bilayer allows for the reconstitution of valinomycin, which exhibits selectivity for potassium ions as proven by impedance analysis.

Another example of the successful reconstitution of an ion carrier is monensin. Monensin is a natural antibiotic from *Streptomyces cinnamonensis*, which adopts a ringlike conformation in solution and is capable of transporting alkali cations across biological membranes. Monensin was incorporated into phospholipid/alkanethiol bilayers on gold electrodes by a paint-freeze method, in which the organic solvent was frozen out of the bilayer at −5 to −20°C. By cyclic voltammetry and potentiometry, the membrane formation was proven and the selectivity coefficient of different ion pairs (Na^+/K^+, Na^+/Rb^+, and Na^+/Ag^+) was measured.

5.4.2 Channel-Forming Peptides

One of the best investigated ion channels in SSMs is gramicidin A. The linear pentadecapeptide is synthesized by *Bacillus brevis*, forming a channel in lipid bilayers consisting of two anti-parallel-oriented monomers bound to each other by six hydrogen bonds. The resulting dimer has a length of 2.6 nm, which is sufficient to span the hydrophobic part of a membrane. Owing to the given length, a functional gramicidin channel is only formed in a single lipid bilayer, and this fact can be used to verify that single lipid bilayers have been formed on a solid substrate. The transmembrane ion channel with a van der Waals radius of 0.2 nm selectively facilitates the permeation of alkali cations. The ion selectivity following $K^+ > Na^+ > Li^+$ as well as the partial blockade with Ca^{2+} is well understood.[142,143] Thus, this peptide is widely used to investigate the integrity of novel membrane model systems with respect to transport processes.[35,144] Several different surfaces serving as support for gramicidin-doped lipid membranes have been investigated.

Nikolelis et al.[145] used gramicidin in stabilized metal-supported BLMs to develop an ammonium ion sensor. Gritsch et al.[146] and we[20,147] investigated the impact of native gramicidin D, a mixture of gramicidin A, B, C, which differ in one amino acid, in solid-supported lipid bilayers by IS on gold and ITO surfaces, respectively. Ion transport was monitored and could be modeled by equivalent circuit analysis, which allowed for the extraction of the membrane resistance. The obtained results reproduced the selectivity sequence of gramicidin toward monovalent cations and the peptide-doped membranes could be used several times without loss of selectivity and sensitivity.[147] By solving the continuum equation, it turned out that, in addition to a membrane capacitance and resistance accounting for the electrical properties of the lipid bilayer, a Warburg impedance arises, thus representing bulk diffusion of cations to the gramicidin pores. However, as the impedance spectra were obtained on gold surfaces, the Warburg impedance overlapped with the capacitance of the gold electrode, which was a drawback in unambiguously defining this element at low frequencies. Support of the Warburg element was, however, given by Wiegand,[148] who considered a one-dimensional random walk of ions in the pores as the molecular origin for linear diffusion on a macroscopic scale, and also resulted in the occurrence of the Warburg impedance. Recently, we performed impedance analysis on gramicidin D-doped lipid membranes attached to a porous alumina substrate.[81] In this configuration, there is no underlying capacitance, which overlaps with the Warburg impedance, and indeed, this impedance element could be unambiguously assigned to the low-frequency impedance response (Fig. 5.6).

Cornell and coworkers[35,47,48] engineered an elegant biosensor based on a tethered membrane attached to a gold surface composed of bola-amphiphiles derived from thermophilic archaea and their thiol-modified analogues with reconstituted gramicidin. The so-called ion channel switch detects antibody fragments (F_{ab} fragments) by effectively preventing the formation of conducting gramicidin dimers and consequently reduces the conductivity of the membrane. This could be measured by IS in the phase minimum at 10 Hz and −300 mV DC offset potential. This principal theme was varied, for example, in a competitive assay, in which a preformed complex was released by the addition of a low-molecular-weight analyte such as digoxin.[49] With this assay, a variety of molecules such as hormones, proteins, nucleic acids, and whole cells[149,150] have already been detected. A commercial version of the ion-switch biosensor for detecting multiple pathogens on an array is now available.[150]

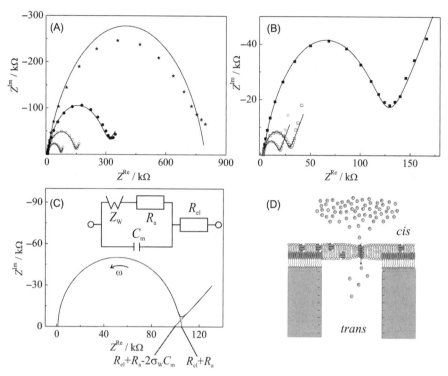

Figure 5.6 Impedance spectra of a pore-spanning membrane after incubation with DOPC vesicles containing 2 mol % gramicidin D obtained in an (A) alkali cation-free buffer ($\star$) and 1 mM ($\bullet$), 5 mM ($\square$), and 10 mM ($\circ$) LiCl-containing buffer. (B) Impedance spectra in the presence of 1 mM ($\bullet$), 5 mM ($\square$), and 10 mM ($\circ$) KCl-containing buffer. Buffer: 10 mM TRIS, 100 mM tetramethylammonium chloride (TMA), pH 8.6. (C) Simulated impedance spectrum based on the equivalent circuit shown in the inset. Electrolyte resistance $R_{el} = 100\ \Omega$, resistance $R_a = 10^5\ \Omega$, membrane capacitance $C_m = 10^{-7}$ F, Warburg impedance Z_W with $\sigma_W = 23{,}570\ \Omega/s^{0.5}$.[81] (D) Schematic representation of the diffusion of ions across a pore-spanning membrane mediated by gramicidin D.

The prerequisite for the ion transport to take place at the electrode surface is to provide a small reservoir underneath the bilayer, which is achieved by tethers at the attached lipids. Krishna et al.[51] investigated in detail the impact of this ionic reservoir on the magnitude of the overall ionic conductance. They found that the reservoir conductivity influences the overall conductivity much more than the channel conductivity itself.

Kim et al.[151] were able to realize continuously-on channels of gramicidin. Supported membranes were prepared by first depositing a partial bolalipid layer on a gold surface using a thioctic acid-modified bolalipid as an anchoring group followed by vesicle fusion of gramicidin containing 2,2'-di-O-decyl-3,3'-O-1'',20''-eicosanyl-bis-*rac*-glycero-1,1'-diphosphocholine. The membranes were inert against organic solvent such as ethanol and CH_2Cl_2, and the impedance decreased in the presence of gramicidin.

Another concept of channel-forming peptides is realized in alamethicin, a peptaibol from *Trichoderma viride*. In contrast to gramicidin, one alamethicin helix spans the entire lipid bilayer and forms voltage-gated ion channels with multiple conductance levels. This behavior can be explained by the formation of transmembrane aggregates according to the barrel stave mechanism.[152] The uptake and release of alamethicin helical monomers from a channel aggregate accounts for the observed multistate conductance levels.[153] The formation of such a helix bundle requires the lateral movement of the individual helices. Yin et al.[154] introduced a tethered lipid bilayer containing alamethicin channels. By means of impedance analysis, they were able to detect the action of amiloride-based inhibitors. If a porous substrate instead of a solid substrate is used, resulting in nano-BLMs, channel activity cannot only be monitored by integral measurements such as IS but also rather by voltage clamp experiments resolving single-channel conductance.[78] In a similar approach, Pilz and Steinem[155] managed to control the helix bundle formation of an amphipathic peptide helix in nano-BLMs. An amphipathic peptide with the sequence H_2N-(LeuSerSerLeuLeuSerLeu)$_3$CONH$_2$ was linked to a bipyridine moiety at the N-terminus, with the aim to control the conductance behavior of the peptide by complexation of the bipyridine residues with Ni.$^{2+}$ Reconstituted in nano-BLMs, the peptide activity was monitored in the current traces as characteristic rectangular steps. While in the absence of $NiCl_2$, four different opening levels were discernable with conductance levels of $G_1 = (131 \pm 19)$ pS, $G_2 = (181 \pm 20)$ pS, $G_3 = (234 \pm 20)$ pS, and $G_4 = (374 \pm 70)$ pS. In the presence of Ni^{2+}, the distribution of the conductance states was considerably different. Only the first ($G_1 = 131$ pS) and second ($G_2 = 181$ pS) conductance levels were very prominent, while the third and forth ones were greatly diminished. The relative area of the first and second conductance states amounted to 78% in the presence and only 43% in the absence of $NiCl_2$. This led to the conclusion that the complexation of bipyridine by Ni^{2+} indeed results in a considerable confinement of the observed multiple conductance states. Assuming that the lowest conductance state is a result of the formation of a six-helix bundle, helix bundles with six and seven helices are preferentially formed in the presence of Ni^{2+}, while higher-order aggregates become less likely.

Melittin, the major component of the bee venom of *Apis mellifera*, is another amphipathic α-helical peptide. However, this peptide generally does not form well-defined ion channels but rather defects in lipid membranes. However, by linking four melittin molecules together, Terrettaz et al.[156] achieved a transmembrane configuration leading to a defined pore in the bilayer. By linking a repetitive NANP sequence, which is the major B-cell epitope of the circumsporozoite protein of *Plasmodium falciparum*, the pathogen of malaria, at the C-terminus of each peptide, the system could be used as a synthetic ligand-gated ion channel (SLIC). By means of IS, the blocking of the melittin pores by an antibody against the NANP sequences was readily monitored.[157]

5.4.3 Channel-Forming Proteins

Ion channel proteins are of major importance for human physiology and, as such, great effort has been undertaken to provide reconstitution protocols for ion channels in SSMs. As a model for large ion channels, the very robust pore-forming channel hemolysin was inserted into different lipid membrane systems. Glazier et al.[158] prepared phospholipid/18-octadecyl-1-thiahexa(ethylene oxide) membranes on gold surfaces and inserted α-hemolysin. By IS, they detected a decrease in impedance, and by cyclic voltammetry, they monitored an increase in permeability of redox ions upon insertion of the large protein. Schuster and Sleytr[159] demonstrated that S-layer ultrafiltration membranes are well suited to monitoring the opening and closing of the channel even though the signals were rather noisy. Multiple insertions of α-hemolysin were monitored by Hemmler et al.[73] in membranes spanning 50 μm, laser structured, pore arrays, and 5.0- and 0.8-μm pores of track-etched membrane filters.

Gritsch et al.[146] were among the first to study the functional reconstitution of outer membrane protein F (OmpF, conducting) and outer membrane protein A (OmpA) (nonconducting, not pore forming) in solid-supported lipid bilayers electrostatically attached to ITO. The porin OmpF from *Escherichia coli* is a well-characterized protein in terms of structure[160,161] and channel activity. It is composed of 16 antiparallel aligned β-sheets (β-barrel) connected by amino acid sequences building up a water-filled pore. Three of these monomeric units with a molecular weight of 37.1 kDa and a length of 5 nm are arranged around a threefold molecular axis. One protein covers an area of roughly 80 nm^2. The authors were able to demonstrate its functionality and selectivity by measuring the membrane resistance in various electrolyte compositions. It turned out that the membrane resistance is considerably more reduced in the presence of Na^+ ions than in the presence of Cl^- ions, thus emphasizing that OmpF is a more cation-selective pore. Unexpectedly, the incorporation of the nonconducting OmpA, via vesicle fusion, also shows a reduction of membrane resistance in the presence of Cl^- ions. Stora et al.[162] reconstituted OmpF in a tethered lipid bilayer on gold surfaces. While the bilayer-forming process was monitored by SPR, IS was used to measure the electrical properties of the bilayer and the ion current through the protein pores. The association of the receptor-binding R-domain protein fragment, which is the central region of all colicins, to OmpF was identified by a reduction of the OmpF conductance by 15%, when monitored at a fixed frequency. In nano-BLMs, the porin OmpF is surrounded by just a few thousand lipids, and the question arises whether this environment disturbs the channel activity. By voltage clamp experiments, it was proven that the protein is fully functional in nano-BLMs. The insertion of the porin resulted in a three-step increase and decrease in current due to the stepwise opening and closing of each subunit pore.[163] Point histogram analysis of the current traces allowed for the determination of the three different conductance levels with $G_1 = (1700 \pm 80)$ pS, $G_2 = (3360 \pm 80)$ pS, and $G_3 = (5060 \pm 50)$ pS. In addition, it was also possible to observe the reported fast kinetics and subconductance states of the protein in nano-BLMs, thereby indicating that the close proximity of immobilized lipid bilayers on the pore rims does not influence the ion channel activity.[163] Nestorovich et al.[164] reported that the β-lactam antibiotic ampicillin is capable of blocking the OmpF channel by moving in and out of the channel. This process takes place on a rather fast timescale. It turned out that the time resolution of the nano-BLMs system is not sufficient to fully resolve every single ampicillin blockade, as was demonstrated in the work of Nestorovich et al.[164] However, blockades of ampicillin were clearly detected as downward spikes of the ion flow during the opening of one monomer.[163] Recently, we were able to show that connexin 26 can also be reconstituted in a fully functional manner in pore-suspending membranes on porous alumina substrates (Fig. 5.7). Connexin 26 (Cx26) is a member of the connexin family, the building blocks for gap junction intercellular channels. These dodecameric assemblies are involved in gap junction-mediated cell–cell communication, allowing for the passage of ions and small molecules between two neighboring cells. Mutations in Cx26 lead to the disruption of gap junction-mediated intercellular communication with consequences such as hearing loss and skin disorders. By means of single-channel recordings on pore-spanning membranes on porous alumina substrates, we were able to show that not only the wild-type Cx26 but also a mutant of Cx26, that is, Cx26 M34A, forms an active hemichannel with similar conductance values, thus indicating that, on the hemichannel level, the ion conductance of the mutant is not significantly altered.[165]

Based on a similar pore-spanning membrane system on polycarbonate filters, which is called MHBLMs, Favero et al.[71] demonstrated the insertion of the glutamate receptor. Combined with a flow-through system acting on both sides of the polycarbonate filter, the detection of glutamate was presented. A linear increase in conductance, upon the addition of glutamate, in the 10 nano-molar range was monitored.

5.5 FUTURE PERSPECTIVE: ION CHANNELS IN MICROPATTERNED MEMBRANES

Together with G protein-coupled receptors, ion channels represent around 60% of known pharmaceutical targets, which makes them a highly important class of proteins. For example, the defective function of ion channels has been linked to disorders such as cardiac arrhythmia, epilepsy, and diabetes. However, as their function relies on a membrane environment, techniques capable of screening membrane protein functions in a parallel manner are still very limited, and ion channels have recently been identified as an underrepresented drug target.[166]

Artificial lipid bilayers deposited on a solid substrate can serve as a matrix for ion channel proteins, and they can be prepared in a parallel arrangement

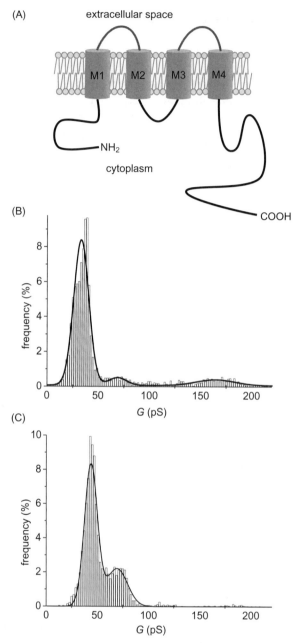

Figure 5.7 (A) Schematic drawing of a Cx26 monomer in a lipid bilayer. The mutation is located in helix M1 (B) Event histogram of the observed conductance states of Cx26 wild type obtained in nano-BLMs at +100 mV in 10 mM HEPES, 200 mM KCl, 0.02 mM EDTA, pH 7.4. The solid line is the result of fitting three Gaussian distributions to the histogram assigning three main conductance states with $G_1 = (34 \pm 8)$ pS, $G_2 = (70 \pm 8)$ pS, and $G_3 = (165 \pm 19)$ pS. (C) Event histogram analysis of the observed conductance states of Cx26 M34A in nano-BLMs obtained at +110 mV in 10 mM HEPES, 200 mM KCl, 0.02 mM EDTA, pH 7.4. The solid line is the result of fitting two Gaussian distributions to the histogram with two main conductance states at $G_1 = (44 \pm 6)$ pS and $G_2 = (69 \pm 10)$ pS.

such that high-throughput screening becomes possible. However, it is still a major challenge to individually address these membranes and to incorporate such bilayers into devices capable of measuring membrane protein function, preferentially with electrical readout systems. One approach worth following is the parallelization of membranes spanning apertures or pore arrays. Arranged in an array, these membranes would enable the investigation of the action of multiple drugs, quasi-simultaneously, on one chip. Another approach is the patterning of membranes on solid substrates with the remaining challenge to insert membrane proteins in a fully functional manner and then to design a device capable of reading out the proteins' activity. Instead of using planar patterned membranes, Heron et al.[167] have formed lipid bilayers between aqueous droplets and semisolid supports such as hydrogels. Such bilayers are exceptionally robust and allow imaging as well as single-channel recordings. This might be an alternative to patterned planar membranes, and the future will reveal which approach is the best.

METHODS BOX 5.1   ELLIPSOMETRY

Ellipsometry is a well-established method that measures the dielectric properties of thin films by monitoring the change in polarization upon reflection from the interface.[168] By this means, ellipsometry collects information about layers that are thinner than the wavelength of the probing light itself. Ellipsometry is noninvasive and gives access to fundamental physical parameters through the measurement of the complex refractive index such as thickness, morphology, chemical composition, porosity, or electrical conductivity. Single thin organic films as well as complex multilayer stacks ranging from a few nanometers to several micrometers can be measured with high accuracy.

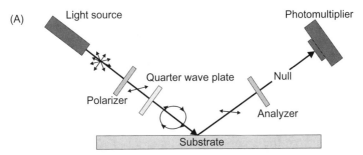

Figure Box 5.1   (A) Setup of a typical null ellipsometer in which the change in polarization upon beam reflection is assessed by rotating polarizer and analyzer, respectively. (B) Typical time traces of Δ (delta, black) and Ψ (psi, red) upon vesicle spreading (POPC:POPS in different ratios) on a silicon surface. (C) Δ-map (top) and thickness profile (bottom) of a microstructured lipid bilayer on silicon acquired using an imaging ellipsometer. (See color insert.)

(Continued)

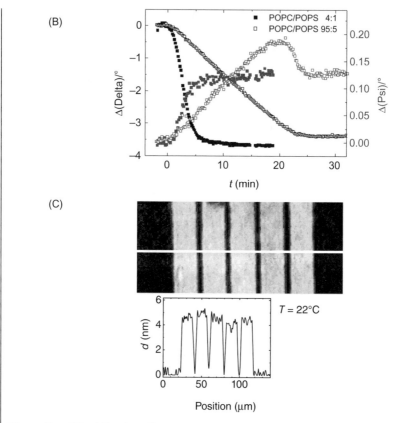

Figure Box 5.1   (*Continued*)

Technically, ellipsometry is mostly performed in a reflection setup as depicted in Figure Box 5.1.[168] Electromagnetic waves, which are emitted by a light source such as a laser diode, are linearly polarized and pass a quarter-wave plate serving as a retarder before they fall onto the sample. After reflection, the radiation passes a second polarizer (analyzer) before it falls onto the detector. Nulling of the reflected light provides the ellipsometry angles Ψ and Δ (vide infra).

In ellipsometry, the complex reflectance ratio, ρ, parameterized by the ellipsometry angles Ψ and Δ, is measured. The polarization state of the light incident upon the sample may be decomposed into an s- and a p-component (the s-component is oscillating perpendicular to the plane of incidence and parallel to the sample surface, and the p-component is oscillating parallel to the plane of incidence). The Fresnel reflection coefficients of the s- and p-components, after reflection and normalized to their initial value, are denoted by r_s and r_p, respectively:

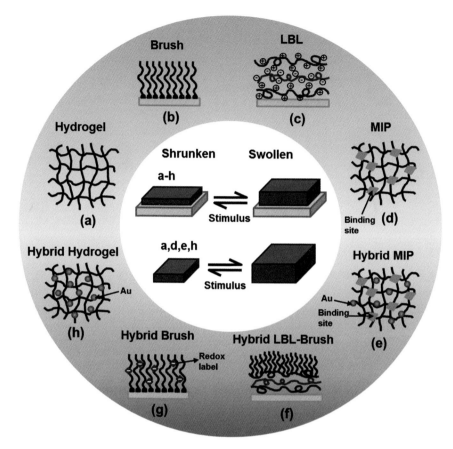

Figure 1.2 The four main architectures of stimulus-responsive polymers are (a) hydrogels, (b) polymer brushes, (c) layer-by-layer (LBL) multilayers, and (d) molecularly imprinted polymers (MIPs). Furthermore, biosensor platforms with hybrid structures that embed inorganic (AuNPs) or organic reporter molecules (redox label ferrocene) in the polymer matrix are shown (e, g, and h), and the combination of the two main structures (LBL and polymer brush) are illustrated in (f). Adapted with permission from references [8], [13], and [132].

Intelligent Surfaces in Biotechnology: Scientific and Engineering Concepts, Enabling Technologies, and Translation to Bio-Oriented Applications, First Edition.
Edited by H. Michelle Grandin and Marcus Textor.
© 2012 John Wiley & Sons, Inc. Published 2012 by John Wiley & Sons, Inc.

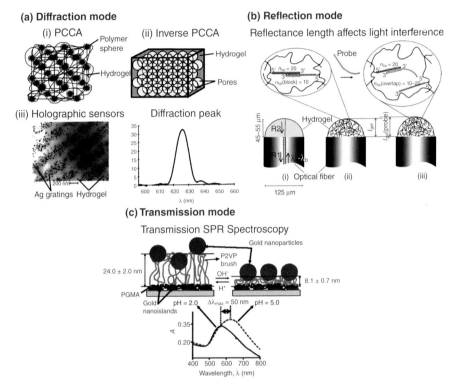

(a) Diffraction mode

(i) PCCA — Polymer sphere, Hydrogel

(ii) Inverse PCCA — Hydrogel, Pores

(iii) Holographic sensors — Ag gratings Hydrogel — 200 nm

Diffraction peak — λ (nm)

(b) Reflection mode

Reflectance length affects light interference

Probe

$n_{bp} = 20$, $n_{bp}(block) = 10$

$n_{bp} = 20$, $n_{bp}(overlap) = 10\text{–}20$

Hydrogel

(i) Optical fiber (ii) (iii)

45–55 µm, 125 µm

(c) Transmission mode

Transmission SPR Spectroscopy

Gold nanoparticles

P2VP brush — OH⁻ / H⁺

24.0 ± 2.0 nm

PGMA — Gold nanoislands

pH = 2.0, $\Delta\lambda_{max} = 50$ nm, pH = 5.0

8.1 ± 0.7 nm

A — 0.35, 0.20 — Wavelength, λ (nm) — 400 500 600 700 800

Figure 1.3 Various optical measurement modes that are exploited to transduce the response of stimulus-responsive polymer coatings. (a) In the diffraction mode, the swelling/shrinking of the polymer matrix shifts the diffraction peaks generated by (i) ordered polymer spheres, (ii) ordered porosity, or (iii) metal gratings in a hydrogel matrix. (b) In the reflection mode, the swelling and shrinking of hydrogels coated on the tip of fiber optics change the reflectivity of the coating. The volumetric response in the gel arises from the disruption in oligonucleotide junctions and changes the optical path length (top panel): (i) Hemispherical hydrogel coating at the end of the optical fiber, (ii) sensing (blue) and blocking (red) oligonucleotides in their hybridized state, and (iii) destabilization of the hybridization junctions due to the addition of probe nucleotides (green) cause the gel to swell. (c) In the transmission mode, the extension and contraction of a polymer brush due to the change in pH are coupled to the plasmon response of Au nanoislands (anchored by cross-linked thin layer of polyglycidyl methacrylate [PGMA]) and nanoparticles, which generates a shift in the absorbance peak. Adapted with permission from references [17], [29], [67], [88], and [91].

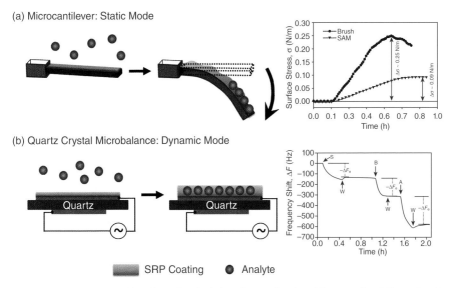

(a) Microcantilever: Static Mode

(b) Quartz Crystal Microbalance: Dynamic Mode

SRP Coating   Analyte

Figure 1.5   Two examples of mechanical signal transduction. (See text for full caption.)

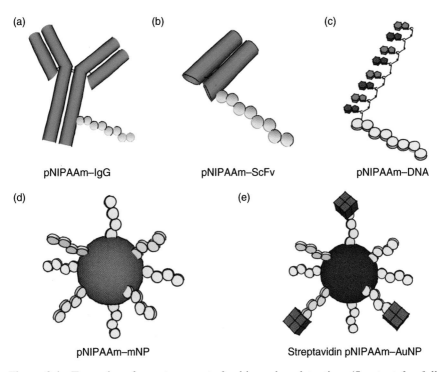

(a) pNIPAAm–IgG

(b) pNIPAAm–ScFv

(c) pNIPAAm–DNA

(d) pNIPAAm–mNP

(e) Streptavidin pNIPAAm–AuNP

Figure 2.4   Examples of smart reagents for biomarker detection. (See text for full caption.)

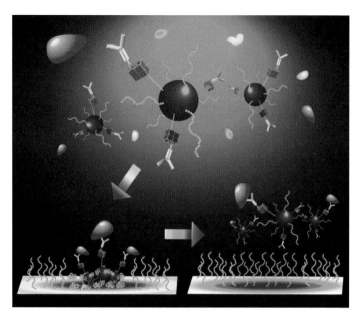

Figure 2.5 Design concept for a microfluidic system that utilizes smart nanobeads having both smart polymers and antibodies on the surface. (See text for full caption.)

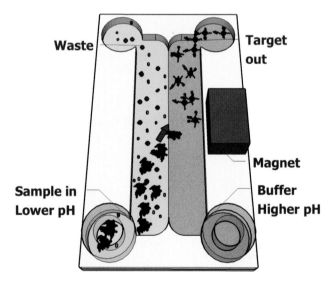

Figure 2.9 Target analyte separation in a microfluidic channel facilitated by pH-responsive magnetic nanoparticles (mNPs) under isothermal conditions. The channel contains two flow streams. The left stream (green) is the sample that has been preincubated with mNPs. mNP aggregation is triggered by the lower pH buffer in this sample flow stream. The pH of the right stream (pink) is chosen to reverse mNP aggregation. A magnet provides a sufficient field to pull the aggregates laterally into the higher pH flow stream. The conjugate aggregates move out of the sample flow stream and in to the higher pH stream, where they return to a dispersed state, carrying the bound target analyte with them. Movement of other molecules across this interface is limited by diffusion due to the laminar flow conditions. Reproduced from Lai et al.[44] by permission from the Royal Society of Chemistry.

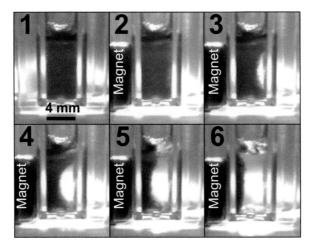

Figure 2.10 Video stills of dual AuNP/mNP coaggregation and magnetic separation. (See text for full caption.)

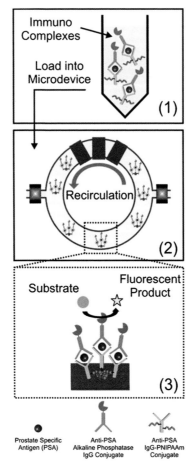

Figure 2.11 Schematic of smart immunoassay in a multilayer PDMS device. (See text for full caption.)

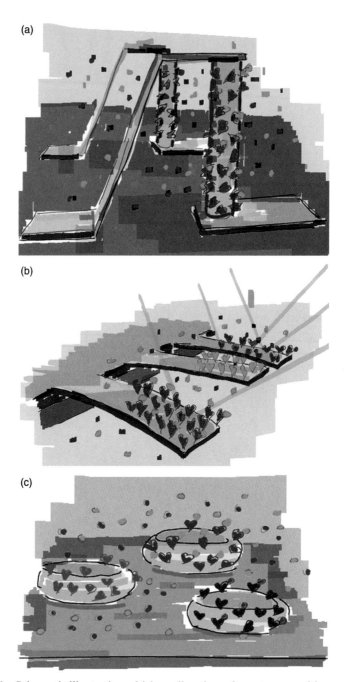

Figure 3.1 Schematic illustration of (a) small-scale surface-stress sensitive cantilevers, (b) semiconductor nanowires, and (c) nanoplasmonically active gold disks designed with immobilized probe molecules for selective detection of suspended analyte molecules. The different colors represent capture agents for different molecules immobilized on the respective sensors.

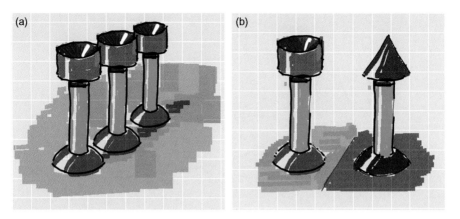

Figure 3.2 Schematic illustration of the different molecular components required to create a biosensor surface. (See text for full caption.)

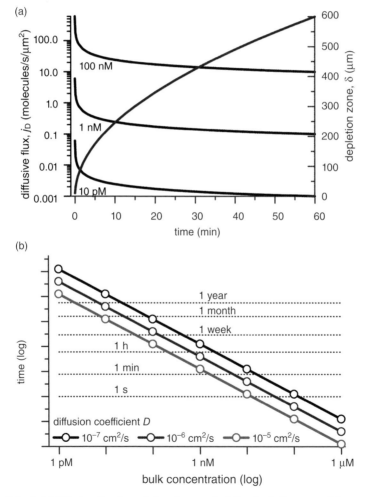

Figure 3.4 (a) Diffusive flux j_D and development of the depletion zone δ from a sensor surface over time under stagnant (i.e., no flow) conditions. $D = 10^{-6}$ cm^2/s (b), time required to reach a coverage corresponding to a detection limit of 1% of the saturated coverage (according to Eq. 3.5). Note that the absolute values given on the y-axis are not strictly correct since they have been calculated from scaling relations (Eqs. 3.2, 3.3, and 3.5) and are thus missing an unknown prefactor.

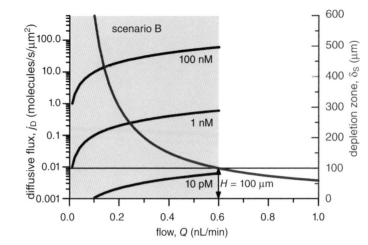

Figure 3.5 Diffusive flux j_D and size of the steady-state depletion zone δ_s for different flows Q for a channel height H of 100 µm. The channel width W is 100 µm, $D = 10^{-6}$ cm²/s. Scenario B (depletion zone expanding across the whole channel height) only occurs for flows <0.6 nL/min (gray shaded area).

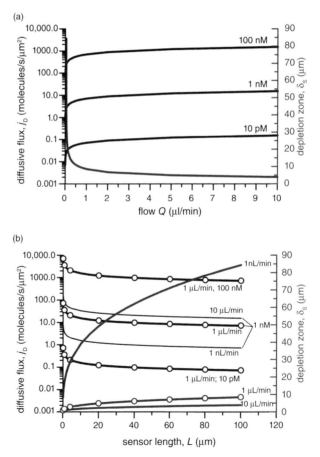

Figure 3.6 Diffusive flux j_D and size of the steady-state depletion zone δ_s in a channel with a height of 100 µm (a) for varying flows Q and different bulk concentrations for a sensor length $L = 100$ µm and (b) for varying sensor length L and different bulk concentrations and flow conditions.

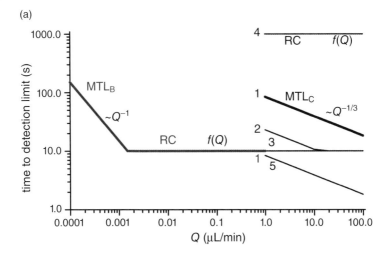

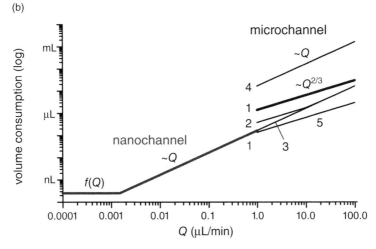

Figure 3.8 The time t_x required to reach the detection limit x (a) and the total volume consumption until the detection limit is reached (b) are plotted versus the flow Q for both a microchannel (100×100 μm², blue) and a nanochannel (100×100 nm², red). For the nanochannel, Q corresponds to the total flow through an experimentally relevant system, that is, an array of nanopores with 10 pores/μm² and a total area of 50×50 μm² (i.e., 25,000 pores in total). The average flow velocity in both the micro- and the nanochannels are of comparable magnitude. 1, "standard" conditions; 2, shorter sensor; 3, faster diffusion or lower receptor density; 4, slower binding kinetics; 5, lower detection limit. Absolute values for the parameters used in 1–5 can be found in Table 3.5. Subscript B stands for the case of full collection efficiency of target molecules (i.e., the depletion zone spans over the whole channel height and grows laterally into the channel), and subscript C stands for the case where the depletion zone is much smaller than the channel height. RC, reaction controlled regime; MTL, mass transport limited regime.

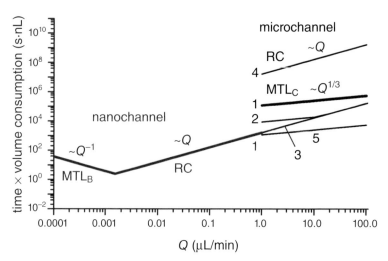

Figure 3.9 The product of the time to reach the detection limit and the sample volume consumed in that time is plotted versus the flow Q. Such a master curve can be used to assess the overall performance of a biosensor. 1, "standard" conditions; 2, shorter sensor; 3, faster diffusion or lower receptor density; 4, slower binding kinetics; 5, lower detection limit. Absolute values for the parameters used in 1–5 can be found in Table 3.5.

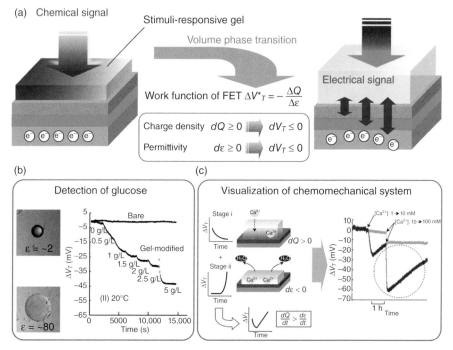

Figure 4.3 (a) Conceptual scheme for a stimulus-responsive gel-mediated signal transduction enabling "Debye length-free" FET-based molecular detection. (b) Detection of glucose by using a glucose-responsive polymer gel-modified FET.[36] (c) Kinetics of a chemomechanical system visualized by using a calcium-sensitive gel-modified FET.[37]

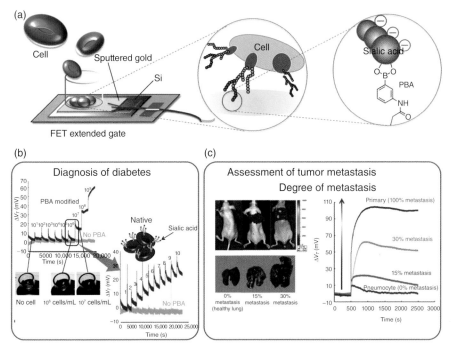

Figure 4.4 (a) Schematic representation of potentiometric SA detection using a PBA-modified gold electrode. (b) Detection of SA on the surface of rabbit erythrocytes as a relevant technique for the diagnosis of diabetes.[61] (c) Assessment of tumor metastasis based on differentiation of the (pneumocyte) surface-expressed SA.[62]

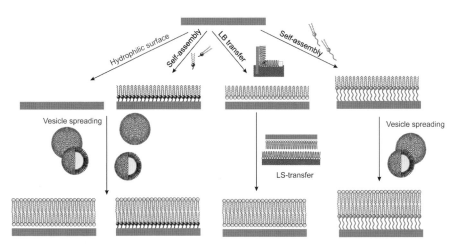

Figure 5.1 Illustrations of different ways to prepare solid-supported membranes based on vesicle spreading and Langmuir–Blodgett transfer.

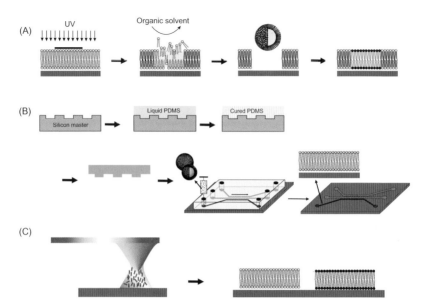

Figure 5.2 Micropatterning of solid-supported membranes. (A) Lithography based on selective polymerization of lipids and refilling of the gaps with vesicles. (B) Formation of individually addressable lipid bilayers using micromolding in capillaries. (C) Dip-pen nanolithography based on atomic force microscopy and selective deposition of lipids on the surface.

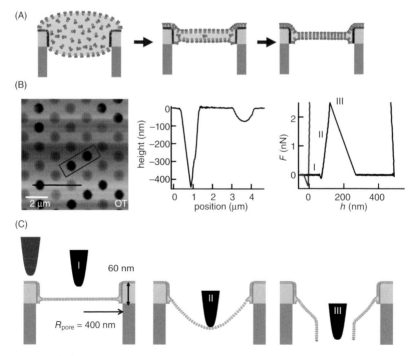

Figure 5.5 (A) Schematic drawing of the preparation of nano-BLMs on a porous matrix using the painting technique. (B) AFM image (left) and corresponding line profile (middle) of pore-spanning bilayers as well as typical force indentation curves (right) obtained from the rim (red) and the center of the pore (black). (C) Schematic illustration of the indentation event shown in the force indentation curve in (B) (I–III).

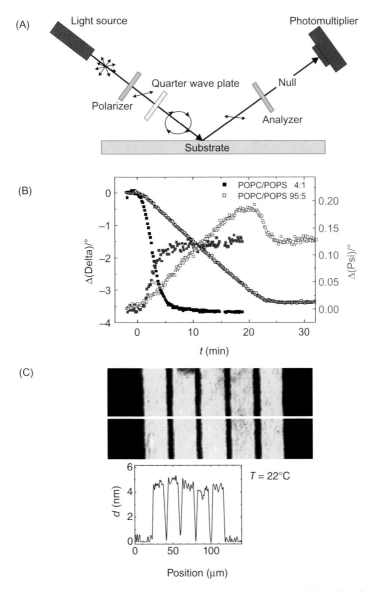

Figure Box 5.1 (A) Setup of a typical null ellipsometer in which the change in polarization upon beam reflection is assessed by rotating polarizer and analyzer, respectively. (B) Typical time traces of Δ (delta, black) and Ψ (psi, red) upon vesicle spreading (POPC:POPS in different ratios) on a silicon surface. (C) Δ-map (top) and thickness profile (bottom) of a microstructured lipid bilayer on silicon acquired using an imaging ellipsometer.

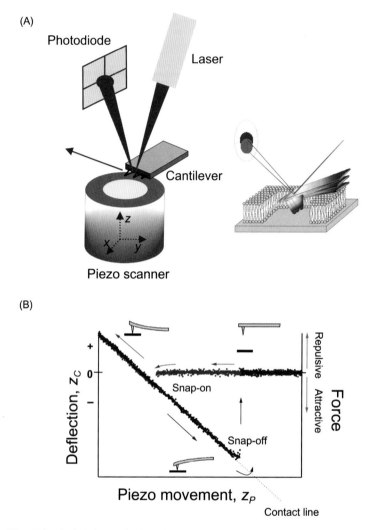

Figure Box 5.2 (A) Schematic drawing of the setup of an atomic force microscope. (B) Deflection curve of the cantilever as obtained upon approaching (red) and retracting (blue) the tip.

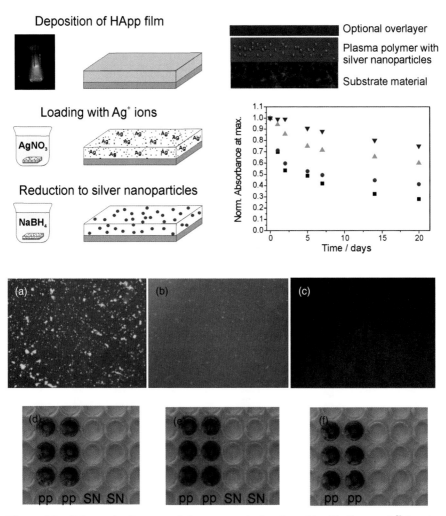

Figure 6.2 Schematic diagram of the approach developed by Vasilev et al.[50] for the loading of silver nanoparticles into amine plasma polymer coatings and the control of the release kinetics of silver ions via the adjustable thickness of an additional plasma polymer overlayer. Also shown are test results of antibacterial effectiveness against *S. epidermidis*; image (a) and rows labeled pp are samples of the control heptylamine surface (no silver), while images (b) and (c) and rows labeled SN are samples with silver-loaded coatings, with different overlayers.

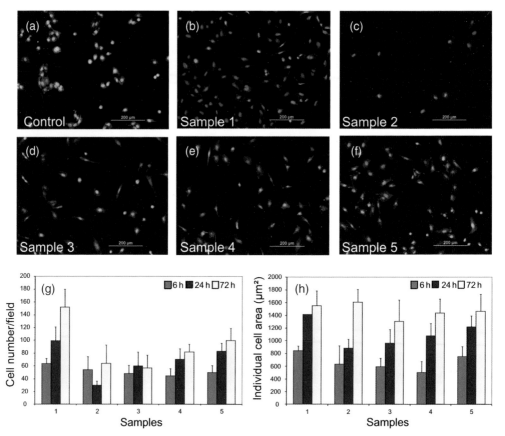

Figure 6.3 Osteoblast cell adhesion and spreading after 24 hours on (a) glass control; (b) heptylamine plasma polymer coating without silver; (c) heptylamine plasma polymer (HApp) coating loaded with silver nanoparticles without an overlayer; (d–f) same as (c) but coated with a HApp overlayer of thickness 6 nm (d), 12 nm (e), and 18 nm (f); (g) cell numbers and (h) individual cell areas after 72 hours on these samples. Adapted from Vasilev et al.[50] by permission of the American Chemical Society, © 2010.

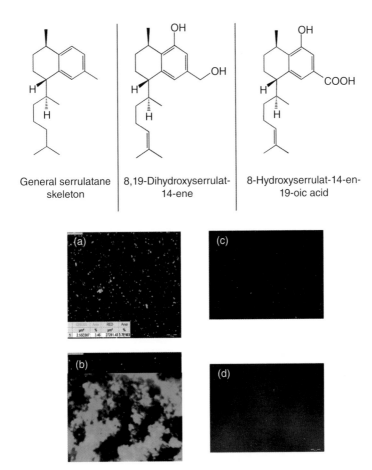

Figure 6.6 Molecular structure of serrulatanes and fluorescence microscopy images of bacterial colonization after 2 hours (top) and 6 hours (bottom) onto amine control surfaces (left) and serrulatane grafted surfaces (right). In image (b) the commencement of biofilm formation is evident. The diffuse color in (d) is due to the diffusion of dye into the polymer material, not to biofilm staining as in (b) Adapted from Ys.[81]

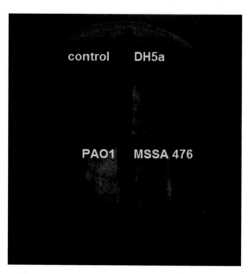

Figure 6.8 Effect of inoculating vesicle-modified fabric (a crude wound dressing material) with either HEPES buffer or nonpathogenic *E. coli* (top row) and pathogenic bacteria (bottom row).

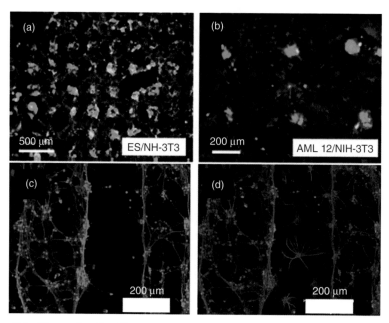

Figure 7.3 Patterning: Intelligent polymer thin films were used to achieve successful cell patterning and coculturing of multiple cell types, a significant step toward engineering of complex tissues with multiple cells. (See text for full caption.)

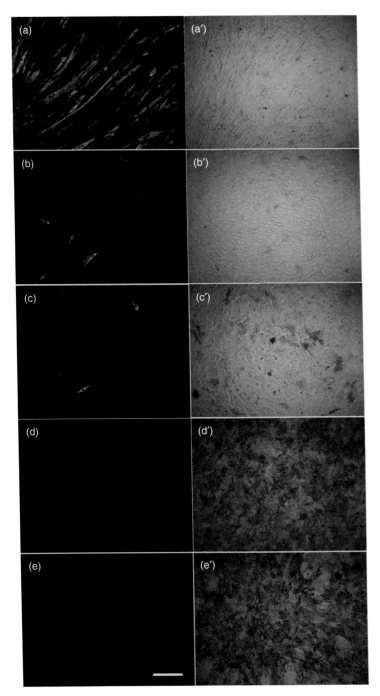

Figure 7.4 Surface-mediated delivery of growth factors: Intelligent polymer coatings are successful in presenting protein cargo, specifically growth factors, to the cultured cells. In this example, recombinant human bone morphogenic protein-2 (rhBMP-2) was incorporated into cross-linked PLL/HA multilayers and was used to induce a guided differentiation of cultured myoblasts into osteoblasts. This strategy of surface-mediated drug delivery was successful and proceeded in a dose-dependent manner (increasing concentration of rhBMP-2 from a to e), as evidenced by decreasing levels of a myogenic marker (troponin T, left column, immunochemical staining) and an accompanying increase in an osteogenic marker (alkaline phosphatase, right column, histochemical staining). Reprinted with permission from Crouzier et al.,[60] Wiley-VCH. © 2008.

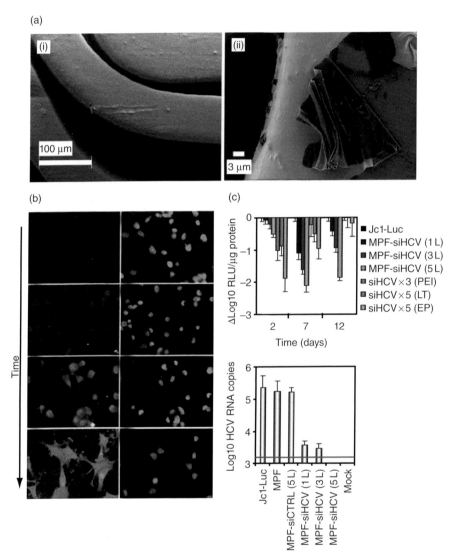

Figure 7.5 Surface-mediated delivery of nucleic acids. Multilayered polymer coatings are successful in surface-mediated drug delivery and hold promise for diverse applications, specifically localized drug delivery achieved from the surface of cardiovascular stents for the prevention of restenosis. (See text for full caption.)

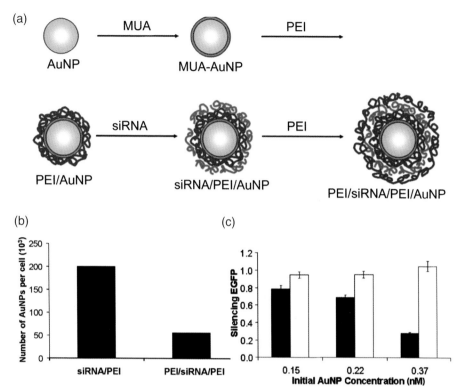

Figure 7.6 siRNA delivery using polymer-coated gold colloids: (a) 11-mercaptoundecanoic acid (MUA) was adsorbed onto ca. 15-nm gold colloids followed by the deposition of PEI, siRNA, and PEI. (b) Cellular uptake of the polymer-coated nanoparticles. The number of siRNA/PEI/AuNPs per cell was significantly higher as compared with PEI/siRNA/PEI/AuNPs. (c) Gene silencing of EGFP in CHO-K1 cells using different concentrations of PEI/siRNA/PEI/AuNPs coated with either siRNA against EGFP (black bars) or a nontargeted siRNA control (white bars). A dose-dependent specific knockdown was observed, and the cellular EGFP production was reduced to about 28% for the highest tested PEI/siRNA/PEI/AuNP concentration. Reprinted with permission from Elbakry et al.,[112] American Chemical Society. © 2009.

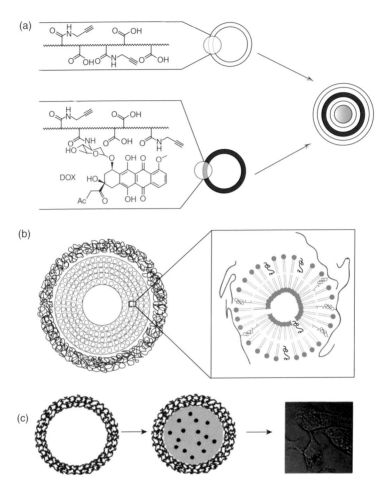

Figure 7.7 Approaches to formulate anticancer drugs using polymer capsules: (a) conjugation of the drug to a polymer, which is then used as in the capsule assembly. Reprinted with permission from Ochs et al.,[134] American Chemical Society. © 2010. (b) Incorporation of the drug into liposomes, which are then confined within polymer capsules;[40] and (c) solubilization of the lipophilic anticancer therapeutic in an oil phase and encapsulation of the emulsion droplets within the carrier capsules. Reprinted with permission from Sivakumar et al.,[138] Wiley-VCH. © 2009.

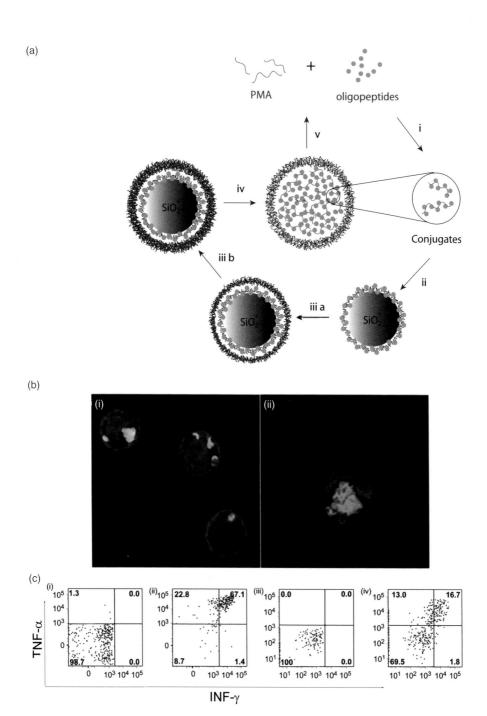

Figure 7.8 Vaccination using polymer capsules. (See text for full caption.)

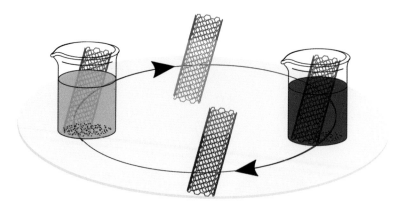

Figure Box 7.1 Schematic illustration of LBL performed via a repetitive adsorption of two interacting polymers and using a model macroscopic (planar) substrate.

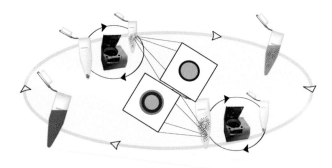

Figure Box 7.2 Schematic illustration of LBL performed via a repetitive adsorption of interacting polymers onto colloidal substrates with intermediate substrate washing achieved via multiple centrifugation-redispersion cycles.

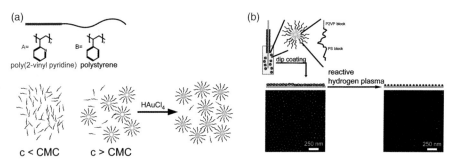

Figure 8.1 Block copolymer micelle nanolithography. (a) The diblock copolymer consists of one polystyrene and one poly(vinylpyridine) block. Below the critical micelle concentration (CMC), the polymer does not aggregate; the solution consists only of free chains. Above the CMC, micelles form, and only a constant number of molecules are in a free state. Upon the addition of $HAuCl_4$, micelles are stabilized and the thermodynamic equilibrium is shifted toward the micelles. (b) The substrate is retracted with a certain velocity from the micellar solution; micelles assemble on the surfaces in a hexagonal order. The scanning electron micrographs on the bottom show a coated substrate before (left side) and after exposure to hydrogen plasma (right side). Adapted from Aydin et al.[105] by permission of Carl Hanser Verlag, © 2011.

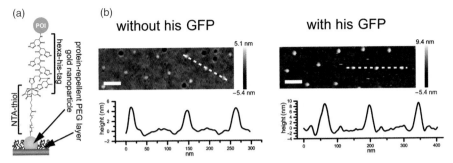

Figure 8.2 Protein immobilization. (See text for full caption.)

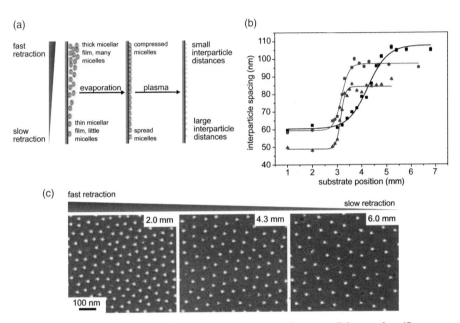

Figure 8.4 Nanoparticle spacing gradients by micellar nanolithography. (See text for full caption.)

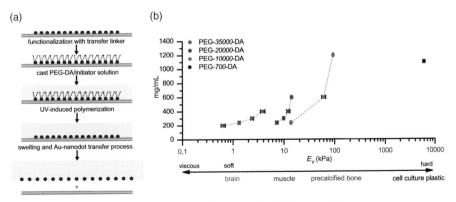

Figure 8.5 Transfer nanolithography. (See text for full caption.)

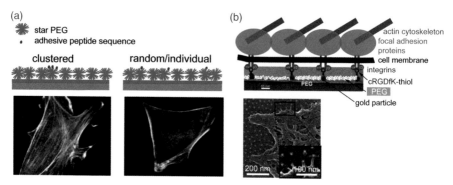

Figure 8.6 Nanoscale patterning affects cell adhesion. (See text for full caption.)

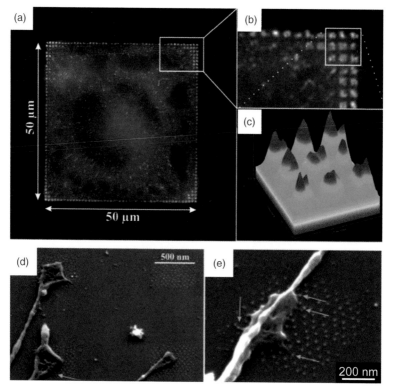

Figure 8.7 Cell adhesion to micro-nanostructured substrates with interligand distances of 58 nm. (a) Live cell fluorescence microscopy image of a REF52-yellow fluorescent protein (YFP)-paxillin cell plated for 2 hours on a 50-μm square divided into 500 × 500 nm squares, separated by 500 nm. (b) Close-up of (a) illustrating the contact site formation on squares. (c) YFP-paxillin fluorescence intensity distribution on cellular adhesion sites. (d,e) Scanning electron micrographs of filopodial structures on biofunctionalized hierarchical nanopatterns (500-nm squares separated by 1000 nm). Red arrows indicate mature contact structures, and blue arrows show ultrasmall cellular protrusions in contact with the adhesive gold nanoparticles. Reproduced from Arnold et al.[98] by permission of The Royal Society of Chemistry, © 2009.

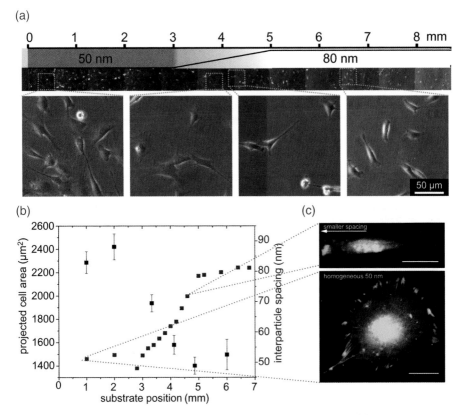

Figure 8.8 Cell adhesion to nanoscale distance gradient substrates. (a) Stitched phase-contrast micrographs showing the adhesion of MC3T3 osteoblasts to different areas of the gradient substrate. Close-up shows images at substrate areas offering 50-, 60-, 70-, and 80-nm interparticle spacing. (b) Projected cell area after 23 hours' cell culture on a substrate including a 2-mm spacing gradient from 50 to 80 nm. (c) Bottom: immunofluorescence images of MC3T3 osteoblasts after 23 hours of adhesion on a homogeneously nanopatterned area with 50 nm. Top: along the gradient on a section having a spacing of approximately 70 nm. Smaller spacings are on the left side of the image. Cells are stained for vinculin (green) and actin (red). Scale bars correspond to 20 μm. Adapted from Arnold et al.[56] and Hirschfeld-Warneken et al.[86]

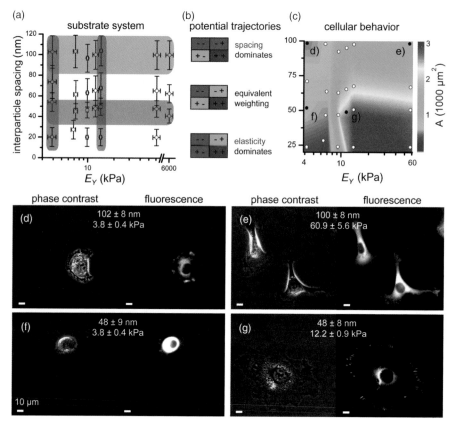

Figure 8.10 Cellular behavior within an artificial, multidimensional parameter space. (See text for full caption.)

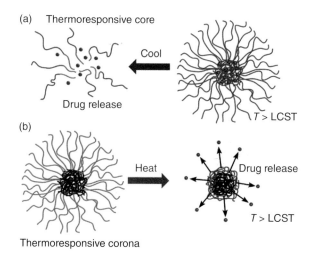

Figure 9.4 Schematic of temperature-responsive polymeric micelles either with a thermoresponsive core (a) or thermoresponsive corona (b).

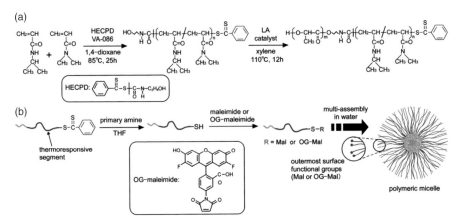

Figure 9.6 (a) Synthesis of poly(IPAAm-*co*-DMAAm)-*b*-PLA diblock copolymers. (b) Conversion of thermoresponsive polymer termini and formation of polymeric micelles. HECPD: 2-[N-(2-hydroxyethyl)-carbamoyl]prop-2-yl dithiobenzoate; THF: tetrahydrofuran; OG: Oregon Green 488; SH: sulfhydryl group.

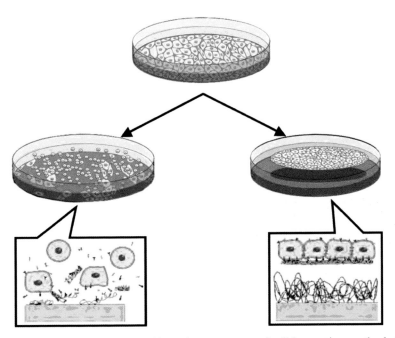

Figure 9.8 Confluent cells are subjected to two types of cell harvesting methods. The first is conventional trypsinization, in which nearly all membrane proteins, as well as deposited ECM, are digested (left). Therefore, all the cells are harvested as single cells. On the contrary, cell sheet harvesting by temperature reduction does not need proteolytic enzymes, such that all the cultured cells are harvested as a single contiguous cell sheet together with deposited ECM (right). Green materials depict deposited ECM.

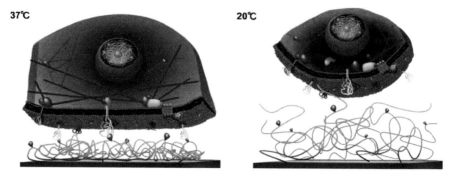

Figure 9.9 Schematic illustration of temperature-responsive affinity control between integrin receptors and RGDS ligands. At 37°C, the temperature-responsive polymer shrinks to expose RGD ligands (red beads) to the integrin receptors of cell membranes (yellow). Upon temperature reduction, the polymer swells to push cells out from the surface.

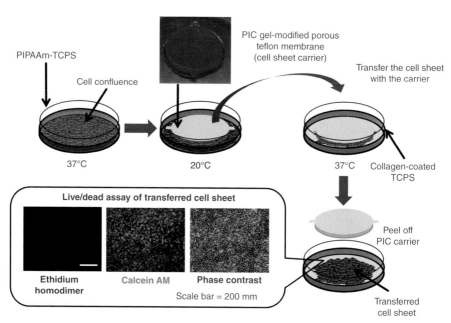

Figure 9.10 Schematic illustration of the transfer of a cell sheet using a PIC gel-modified porous Teflon membrane (cell sheet carrier). Inset shows microscopy images of a LIVE/DEAD assay of the transferred cell sheet.

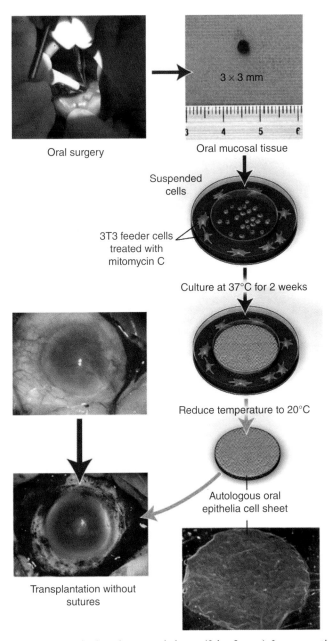

Figure 9.11 The removal of oral mucosal tissue (3 by 3 mm) from a patient's cheek. Isolated epithelial cells are seeded onto temperature-responsive cell-culture inserts. After 2 weeks at 37°C, these cells grow to form multilayered sheets of epithelial cells. The viable cell sheet is harvested, with intact cell-to-cell junctions along with the extracellular matrix, in a transplantable form simply by reducing the temperature of the culture to 20°C for 30 minutes. The cell sheet is then transplanted directly to the diseased eye without sutures.

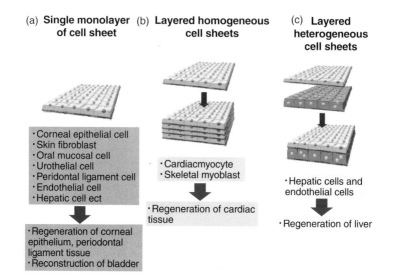

Figure 9.13 Schematic drawing of regeneration or reconstruction of tissue and organ by various cell sheet methods including (a) single-monolayer cell sheet and (b) layering of homogeneous 3-D tissue or (c) layering of heterogeneous 3-D tissue.

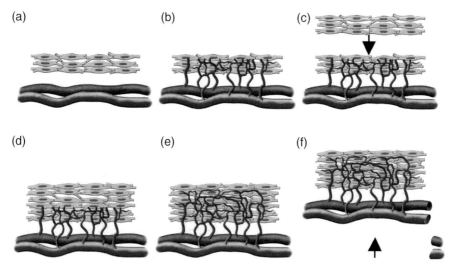

Figure 9.14 Schematic illustration of the concept used for bioengineering multilayer grafts with surgically connectable vessels. (a) First, a graft is transplanted over a surgically accessible artery and vein. (b) In this case, the graft is supplied with both new vasculature and blood directly from these existing vessels. (c,d) After sufficient vascularization has occurred, a second graft is transplanted onto the first graft. (e,f) Finally, the microvascularized construct, accompanied by graftable vessels harvested from the host, is fully perfused by host vessels and surgically resected. Ectopic transplantation of such a graft is then possible.

$$\rho = \frac{r_p}{r_s} = \tan(\Psi)\exp(i\Delta). \tag{5.1}$$

Since ρ is a complex quantity, $\tan(\Psi)$ is the amplitude ratio upon reflection and Δ is the phase shift difference. The next step comprises the conversion from Ψ and Δ into the optical constants or the thickness of the sample. Usually, an optical model is assumed, which encompasses the optical constants and thickness parameters of all individual layers in the given sequence. By means of a fitting algorithm, only the unknown optical constants and/or thickness parameters are varied, and the corresponding Ψ and Δ values are computed using the Fresnel equations. The optimization procedure provides the corresponding optical constants that best match the experimentally determined Ψ and Δ values. Since amplitude ratios are measured, ellipsometry accurately determined slight changes in the optical thickness of the sample.

In principle, one distinguishes single-wavelength ellipsometry and spectroscopic ellipsometry. While single-wavelength ellipsometry employs a monochromatic light source such as a laser (e.g., He–Ne), spectroscopic ellipsometry uses broadband light sources to cover a certain spectral range in the infrared, visible, or ultraviolet spectral region. Single-wavelength ellipsometry delivers only one pair of Ψ and Δ and is particularly well suited to monitor changes of optical thickness as a function of time for kinetic measurements, while spectroscopic ellipsometry provides the complex refractive index in the corresponding spectral region and thus allows for determining unknown optical constants.

METHODS BOX 5.2   AFM AND FORCE SPECTROSCOPY

The first atomic force microscope (AFM) was introduced by Binnig et al. in 1986.[169] It is capable of imaging the topography of a surface with atomic resolution. The microscope relies on measuring tip–sample interaction forces in the piconewton regime. A schematic setup of an AFM is shown in Figure Box 5.2. In brief, a very sharp needle with a tip diameter of only several nanometers is mounted at the end of a cantilever and probes the interaction between the tip and the sample surface. For imaging, either the cantilever or the sample is scanned in the xy-direction, while the deflection in the z-direction is monitored via reflection of a laser beam from the reflective side of the cantilever.

(Continued)

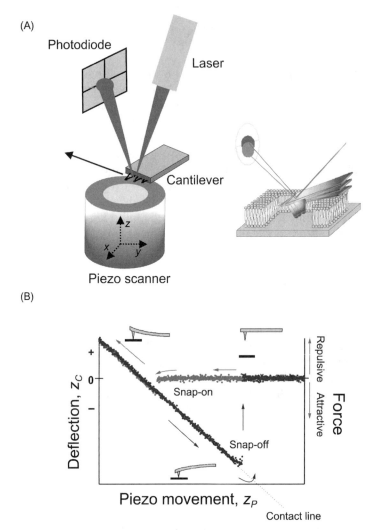

Figure Box 5.2 (A) Schematic drawing of the setup of an atomic force microscope. (B) Deflection curve of the cantilever as obtained upon approaching (red) and retracting (blue) the tip. (See color insert.)

Combining the scanning information with the deflection of the cantilever at each position provides a topographical image of the surface. While typical resolutions in the z-direction can be as low as 1 Å, the lateral resolution in the xy-direction is typically >1 nm and is usually limited by the tip size. The imaging modes are divided into static (contact mode) and dynamic modes (tapping mode, noncontact mode). Typical control parameters are deflection for static modes or oscillation amplitude for dynamic modes.

The cantilever is typically made from silicon or silicon nitride with a tip radius on the order of nanometers. Interfacial forces that are measured in AFM include viscoelastic contact forces, van der Waals and Casimir forces, capillary forces, electrostatic forces, covalent bonds, and magnetic forces. Consequently, the AFM can also be used to measure these forces rather than to provide images of surface topography.[170] Force curves, also known as force–distance curves, usually refer to the deflection of the free end of the AFM cantilever, while the fixed end is moved vertically toward and then away from the sample surface at a defined velocity. If the velocity is varied and the forces are displayed as a function of speed, the technique is called force spectroscopy.

The forces range from only a few piconewtons (rupture of hydrogen bonds) to several nanonewtons (capillary forces). The interactions are strongly dependent on the experimental conditions, such as tip and sample material, chemical modification of the surfaces, and the surrounding medium. Dependent on the medium, different interactions dominate the experimental force curves. In air, van der Waals forces, which are mostly attractive, are in general superimposed by stronger, also attractive, capillary forces caused by the condensation of water vapor in the area of the tip–sample contact. These capillary forces vanish if measurements are performed in fluids.

Force spectroscopy experiments in an aqueous solution are of major importance since they allow for the study of native biological processes and the mechanical behavior of single molecules like membranes, nucleic acids, and proteins *in situ*. Electrostatic forces are dominant in aqueous solution; they can be attractive or repulsive, dependent on the surface potential, ionic strength, and pH. In addition to electrostatic interactions, short-ranging dipole–dipole interactions, hydrogen bonding, or, in the case of ligand–receptor couples, highly specific complex combinations of different binding types, as well as covalent bonding, occur in force experiments. Forces between the tip and the sample can be investigated not only by force spectroscopy on a spatially restricted area but also by mapping the surface. The upper lateral resolution limit is given by the contact radius of the tip with the substrate, which is typically in the order of some 10 nm, while the lower limit is in the range of single molecules or atom groups.

Indentation experiments are often conducted to probe the viscoelastic nature of biological specimens. For this purpose, appropriate contact models that depend on the tip geometry and adhesion force in the contact area are applied to extract the Young modulus of the substrates. Energy dissipation due to (internal) friction might give rise to a hysteresis in the approach and retraction curves, which is often a sign of viscoelasticity.

METHODS BOX 5.3   IMPEDANCE SPECTROSCOPY

Impedance spectroscopy (IS) measures the dielectric properties of an inter-face or medium.[171] The measurement provides the complex impedance of an electrochemical system as a function of frequency. Usually, frequencies ranging from 10^3 to 10^8 Hz are applied. Figure Box 5.3 shows the general concept of impedance analysis applied to SSMs. IS provides information about a large variety of physical properties such as the dielectric function, coverage, film thickness, as well as diffusion and rate constants of electro-chemical reactions taking place at the electrode–electrolyte interface.

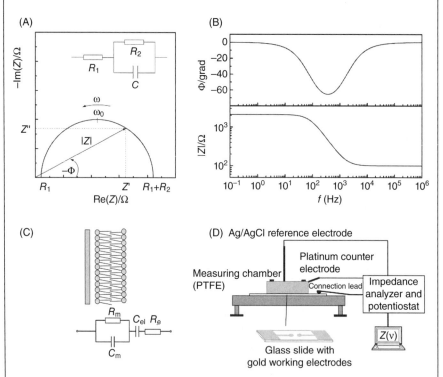

Figure Box 5.3   Principle of impedance spectroscopy applied to solid-supported membranes. (A) Nyquist plot of the electrical circuit with $R_1 = 100\ \Omega$, $R_2 = 2000\ \Omega$, and $C = 1\ \mu F$. The arrow denotes the direction in which the frequency increases. (B) Bode plot of the same circuit showing impedance magnitude $|Z|$ and the phase lag Φ. (C) Typical equivalent circuit of a solid-supported membrane. (D) Experimental setup to acquire impedance spectra of supported bilayers deposited on gold electrodes.

IS is only marginally invasive due to the small applied voltage ampli-tudes, in the 10-mV range, thus allowing the linear response theory to be applied.

In continuous-wave spectrometers, a sinusoidal voltage $\hat{U}\exp(i\omega t)$ with a discrete frequency is applied and the resulting alternating current $\hat{I}(\omega)$ $\exp(i(\omega t - \Phi(\omega)))$ is recorded. The corresponding response function, the complex impedance $Z(\omega)$, is readily obtained for each frequency:

$$Z = \frac{\hat{U}\exp(i\omega t)}{\hat{I}(\omega)\exp(i(\omega t - \Phi(\omega)))} = |Z(\omega)|\exp(i\Phi(\omega)). \tag{5.2}$$

Φ is the phase lag between voltage and current and $|Z|$ is the magnitude. Since Z is a complex quantity, it can be decomposed into a real (Z') and imaginary (Z'') part:

$$Z = |Z|\exp(i\Phi) = Z' + iZ'' \tag{5.3}$$

with the following relationships:

$$|Z|^2 = (Z')^2 + (Z'')^2, \tag{5.4a}$$

$$\Phi = \arctan\left(\frac{Z''}{Z'}\right), \tag{5.4b}$$

$$Z' = |Z|\cos(\Phi) \tag{5.4c}$$

and

$$Z'' = |Z|\sin(\Phi). \tag{5.4d}$$

Figure Box 5.3A,B illustrates these relationships by showing Nyquist and Bode plots of a simple electrical circuit consisting of an ohmic resistance in series to an element consisting of a parallel combination of a resistor and a capacitor with the complex impedance:

$$Z(\omega) = R_1 + \frac{1}{\dfrac{1}{R_2} + i\omega C}. \tag{5.5}$$

Frequently, complex quantities other than the impedance of the system are used to emphasize a particular behavior of the system. The admittance $(Y = Z^{-1})$ emphasizes relaxation processes at high frequency, while the complex dielectric function $(\varepsilon = Y/i\omega C_c)$ does it for the low-frequency regime. The real part of the complex dielectric function ε' at low frequency is often referred to as the static dielectric constant, while the imaginary part ε'' describes dissipative processes, that is, absorption of the electromagnetic waves. Other related functions are the modulus $(M = \varepsilon^{-1})$ and the complex capacitance $(C = \varepsilon C_c)$.

(Continued)

Data reduction is usually achieved by creating models that can be cast into an equivalent circuit with an explicit transfer function serving as a fitting function for the complex data. Equivalent circuits can be derived from first principles or can be of an empiric nature, depending on the complexity of the problem.

REFERENCES

1. Cooper, M.A. Advances in membrane receptor screening and analysis. *Journal of Molecular Recognition* **17**, 286–315 (2004).
2. Richter, R., Mukhopadhyay, A., & Brisson, A. Pathways of lipid vesicle deposition on solid surfaces: a combined QCM-D and AFM study. *Biophysical Journal* **85**, 3035–3047 (2003).
3. Schönherr, H., Johnson, J.M., Lenz, P., Frank, C.W., & Boxer, S.G. Vesicle adsorption and lipid bilayer formation on glass studied by atomic force microscopy. *Langmuir* **20**, 11600–11606 (2004).
4. Pignataro, B., Steinem, C., Galla, H.-J., Fuchs, H., & Janshoff, A. Specific adhesion of vesicles monitored by scanning force microscopy and quartz crystal microbalance. *Biophysical Journal* **78**, 487–498 (2000).
5. Richter, R.P. & Brisson, A.R. Following the formation of supported lipid bilayers on mica: a study combining AFM, QCM-D, and ellipsometry. *Biophysical Journal* **88**, 3422–3433 (2005).
6. Reimhult, E., Höök, F., & Kasemo, B. Intact vesicle adsorption and supported biomembrane formation from vesicles in solution: influence of surface chemistry, vesicle size, temperature, and osmotic pressure. *Langmuir* **19**, 1681–1691 (2003).
7. Dimitrievski, K., Reimhult, E., Kasemo, B., & Zhdanov, V.P. Simulations of temperature dependence of the formation of a supported lipid bilayer via vesicle adsorption. *Colloids and Surfaces B, Biointerfaces* **39**, 77–86 (2004).
8. Zhdanov, V.P. & Kasemo, B. Comments on rupture of adsorbed vesicles. *Langmuir* **17**, 3518–3521 (2001).
9. Tanaka, M. & Sackmann, E. Polymer-supported membranes as models of the cell surface. *Nature* **437**, 656–663 (2005).
10. Brian, A.A. & McConnell, H.M. Allogeneic stimulation of cytotoxic T cells by supported planar membranes. *Proceedings of the National Academy of Sciences of the United States of America* **81**, 6159–6163 (1984).
11. McConnell, H.M., Watts, T.H., Weis, R.M., & Brian, A.A. Supported planar membranes in studies of cell-cell recognition in the immune system. *Biochimica et Biophysica Acta* **864**, 95–106 (1986).
12. Tamm, L.K. & Mcconnell, H.M. Supported phospholipid-bilayers. *Biophysical Journal* **47**, 105–113 (1985).
13. Kiessling, V. & Tamm, L.K. Measuring distances in supported bilayers by fluorescence interference-contrast microscopy: polymer supports and SNARE proteins. *Biophysical Journal* **84**, 408–418 (2003).

14. Wagner, M.L. & Tamm, L.K. Tethered polymer-supported planar lipid bilayers for reconstitution of integral membrane proteins: silane-polyethyleneglycol -lipid as a cushion and covalent linker. *Biophysical Journal* **79**, 1400–1414 (2000).

15. Purrucker, O., Fortig, A., Jordan, R., & Tanaka, M. Supported membranes with well-defined polymer tethers-incorporation of cell receptors. *Chemphyschem* **5**, 327–335 (2004).

16. McBee, T.W., Wang, L.Y., Ge, C.H., Beam, B.M., Moore, A.L., Gust, D., Moore, T.A., Armstrong, N.R., & Saavedra, S.S. Characterization of proton transport across a waveguide-supported lipid bilayer. *Journal of the American Chemical Society* **128**, 2184–2185 (2006).

17. Goennenwein, S., Tanaka, M., Hu, B., Moroder, L., & Sackmann, E. Functional incorporation of integrins into solid supported membranes on ultrathin films of cellulose: impact on adhesion. *Biophysical Journal* **85**, 646–655 (2003).

18. Smith, H.L., Jablin, M.S., Vidyasagar, A., Saiz, J., Watkins, E., Toomey, R., Hurd, A.J., & Majewski, J. Model lipid membranes on a tunable polymer cushion. *Physical Review Letters* **102**, 228102 (2009).

19. Ottova, A., Tovarozek, V., & Tien, H.T. Supported Planar Lipid Bilayers (s-BLMs, sb-BLMs, etc.). In: Tien, H. & Ottova-Leitmannova, A. (eds.), *Planar Lipid Bilayers (BLMs) and Their Applications*, pp. 917–955. Amsterdam: Elsevier (2003).

20. Steinem, C., Janshoff, A., Ulrich, W.-P., Sieber, M., & Galla, H.-J. Impedance analysis of supported lipid bilayer membranes: a scrutiny of different preparation techniques. *Biochimica et Biophysica Acta* **1279**, 169–180 (1996).

21. Wiegand, G., Arribas-Layton, N., Hillebrandt, H., Erich, S., & Wagner, P. Electrical properties of supported lipid bilayer membranes. *The Journal of Physical Chemistry B, Materials, Surfaces, Interfaces & Biophysical* **106**, 4245–4254 (2002).

22. Siepmann, J.I. & Mcdonald, I.R. Simulations of self-assembled monolayers of thiols on gold. *Thin Films* **24**, 205–226 (1998).

23. Karpovich, D.S., Schessler, H.M., & Blanchard, G.J. The kinetics and thermodynamics of monolayer formation: in situ measurement of alkanethiol adsorption onto gold. *Thin Films* **24**, 43–80 (1998).

24. Sigl, H., Brink, G., Seufert, M., Schulz, M., Wegner, G., & Sackmann, E. Assembly of polymer/lipid composite films on solids based on hairy rod LB films. *European Biophysics Journal* **25**, 249–259 (1997).

25. Florin, E.L. & Gaub, H.E. Painted supported lipid membranes. *Biophysical Journal* **64**, 375–383 (1993).

26. Lang, H., Duschl, C., & Vogel, H. A new class of thiolipids for the attachment of lipid bilayers on gold surfaces. *Langmuir* **10**, 197–210 (1994).

27. Hubbard, J.B., Silin, V., & Plant, A.L. Self-assembly driven by hydrophobic interactions at alkanethiol monolayers: mechanism of formation of hybrid bilayer membranes. *Biophysical Journal* **75**, 163–176 (1998).

28. Plant, A.L., Gügütchkeri, M., & Yap, W. Supported phospholipid/alkanethiol biomimetic membranes: insulting properties. *Biophysical Journal* **67**, 1126–1133 (1994).

29. Majewski, J., Wong, J., Park, C.K., Seitz, M., Israelachvili, J.N., & Smith, G.S. Structural studies of polymer-cushioned lipid bilayers. *Biophysical Journal* **75**, 2363–2367 (1998).

30. Reiss, B., Janshoff, A., Steinem, C., Seebach, J., & Wegener, J. Adhesion kinetics of functionalized vesicles and mammalian cells: a comparative study. *Langmuir* **19**, 1816–1823 (2003).

31. Spinke, J., Yang, J., Wolf, H., Liley, M., Ringsdorf, H., & Knoll, W. Polymer-supported bilayer on a solid substrate. *Biophysical Journal* **63**, 1667–1671 (1992).

32. Théato, P. & Zentel, R. α,ω-Functionalized poly-N-isopropylacrylamides: controlling the surface activity for vesicle adsorption by temperature. *Journal of Colloid and Interface Science* **268**, 258–262 (2003).

33. Munro, J.C. & Frank, C.W. In situ formation and characterization of poly(ethylene glycol)-supported lipid bilayers on gold surfaces. *Langmuir* **20**, 10567–10575 (2004).

34. Jeuken, L.J.C., Connell, S.D., Nurnabi, M., O'Reilly, J., Henderson, P.J.F., Evans, S.D., & Bushby, R.J. Direct electrochemical interaction between a modified gold electrode and a bacterial membrane extract. *Langmuir* **21**, 1481–1488 (2005).

35. Cornell, B.A., Braach-Maksvytis, V.L.B., King, L.G., Osman, P.D.J., Wieczorek, L., Raguse, B., & Pace, R.J. A biosensor that uses ion-channel switches. *Nature* **387**, 580–583 (1997).

36. Schiller, S.M., Naumann, R., Lovejoy, K., Kunz, H., & Knoll, W. Archaea analogue thiolipids for tethered bilayer lipid membranes on ultrasmooth gold surfaces. *Angewandte Chemie (International ed. in English)* **42**, 208–211 (2003).

37. Bunjes, N., Schmidt, E.K., Jonczyk, A., Rippmann, F., Beyer, D., Ringsdorf, H., Graber, P., Knoll, W., & Naumann, R. Thiopeptide-supported lipid layers on solid substrates. *Langmuir* **13**, 6188–6194 (1997).

38. Knoll, W., Morigaki, K., Naumann, R., Sacca, B., Schiller, S., & Sinner, E.-K. Lipid membranes as biosensors. In: Mirsky, V.M. (ed.), *Ultrathin Electrochemical Chemo- and Biosensors*, pp. 239–253. Berlin Heidelberg: Springer (2004).

39. Sackmann, E. Supported membranes: scientific and practical applications. *Science* **271**, 43–48 (1996).

40. Sackmann, E. & Tanaka, M. Supported membranes on soft polymer cushions: fabrication, characterization and applications. *Trends in Biotechnology* **18**, 58–64 (2000).

41. Steinem, C., Janshoff, A., von dem Bruch, K., Reihs, K., Goossens, J., & Galla, H.-J. Valinomycin-mediated transport of alkali cations through solid supported membranes. *Bioelectrochemistry and Bioenergetics* **45**, 17–26 (1998).

42. Naumann, R., Jonczyk, A., Kopp, R., van Esch, J., Ringsdorf, H., Knoll, W., & Graeber, P. Incorporation of membrane proteins in solid-supported lipid layers. *Angewandte Chemie (International ed. in English)* **34**, 2056–2058 (1995).

43. Naumann, R., Schmidt, E.K., Jonczyk, A., Fendler, K., Kadenbach, B., Liebermann, T., Offenhäuser, A., & Knoll, W. The peptide-tethered lipid membrane as a biomimetic system to incorporate cytochrome c oxidase in a functionally active form. *Biosensors & Bioelectronics* **14**, 651–662 (1999).

44. Naumann, R., Baumgart, T., Gräber, P., Jonczyk, A., Offenhäuser, A., & Knoll, W. Proton transport through a peptide-tethered bilayer lipid membrane by the H^+-ATP synthase from chloroplasts measured by impedance spectroscopy. *Biosensors & Bioelectronics* **17**, 25–34 (2002).

45. Schmidt, E.K., Liebermann, T., Kreiter, M., Jonczyk, A., Naumann, R., Offenhäuser, A., Neumann, E., Kukol, A., Maelicke, A., & Knoll, W. Incorporation of

the acetylcholine receptor dimer from *Torpedo californica* in a peptide supported lipid membrane investigated by surface plasmon and fluorescence spectroscopy. *Biosensors & Bioelectronics* **13**, 585–591 (1998).

46. Knoll, W., Frank, C.W., Heibel, C., Naumann, R., Offenhäusser, A., Rühe, J., Schmidt, E.K., Shen, W.W., & Sinner, A. Functional tethered lipid bilayers. *Molecular Biotechnology* **74**, 137–158 (2000).

47. Woodhouse, G., King, L.G., Wieczorek, L., & Cornell, B.A. Kinetics of the competitive response of receptors which have been incorporated into a tethered lipid bilayer. *Faraday Discussions* **111**, 247–258 (1999).

48. Cornell, B.A., Krishna, G., Osman, P.D., Pace, R.D., & Wieczorek, L. Tethered-bilayer lipid membranes as a support for membrane-active peptides. *Biochemical Society Transactions* **29**, 613–617 (2001).

49. Woodhouse, G., King, L.G., Wieczorek, L., Osman, P.D., & Cornell, B.A. The ion channel switch biosensor. *Journal of Molecular Recognition* **12**, 328–334 (1999).

50. Krishna, G., Schulte, J., Cornell, B.A., Pace, R.J., Wieczorek, L., & Osman, P.D. Tethered bilayer membranes containing ionic reservoirs: the interfacial capacitance. *Langmuir* **17**, 4858–4866 (2001).

51. Krishna, G., Schulte, J., Cornell, B.A., Pace, R.J., & Osman, P.D. Tethered bilayer membranes containing ionic reservoirs: selectivity and conductance. *Langmuir* **19**, 2294–2305 (2003).

52. Elender, G., Kühner, M., & Sackmann, E. Functionalisation of Si/SiO$_2$ and glass surfaces with ultrathin dextran films and deposition of lipid bilayers. *Biosensors & Bioelectronics* **11**, 565–577 (1996).

53. Shen, W.W., Boxer, S.G., Knoll, W., & Frank, C.W. Polymer-supported lipid bilayers on benzophenone-modified substrates. *Biomacromolecules* **2**, 70–79 (2001).

54. Lin, J., Merzlyakov, M., Hristova, K., & Searson, P.C. Impedance spectroscopy of bilayer membranes on single crystal silicon. *Biointerphases* **3**, FA33–FA40 (2008).

55. Ross, E.E., Bondurant, B., Spratt, T., Conboy, J.C., O'Brien, D.F., & Saavedra, S.S. Formation of self-assembled, air-stable lipid bilayer membranes on solid supports. *Langmuir* **17**, 2305–2307 (2001).

56. Ross, E.E., Rozanski, L.J., Spratt, T., Liu, S., O'Brien, D.F., & Saavedra, S.S. Planar supported lipid bilayer polymers formed by vesicle fusion. 1. Influence of diene monomer structure and polymerization method on film properties. *Langmuir* **9**, 1752–1765 (2003).

57. Atanasov, V., Knorr, N., Duran, R.S., Ingebrandt, S., Offenhäusser, A., Knoll, W., & Koeper, I. Membrane on a chip: a functional tethered lipid bilayer membrane on silicon oxide surfaces. *Biophysical Journal* **89**, 1780–1788 (2005).

58. Müller, P. & Rudin, D.O. Action potentials induced in bimolecular lipid membranes. *Nature* **217**, 713 (1968).

59. Ogier, S.D., Bushby, R.J., Cheng, Y., Evans, S.D., Evans, S.W., Jenkings, T.A., Knowles, P.F., & Miles, R.E. Suspended planar phospholipid bilayers on micromachined supports. *Langmuir* **16**, 5696–5701 (2000).

60. Cheng, Y., Bushby, R.J., Evans, S.D., Knowles, P.F., Miles, R.E., & Ogier, S.D. Single ion channel sensitivity in suspended bilayers on micromachined supports. *Langmuir* **17**, 1240–1242 (2001).

61. Goryll, M., Wilk, S.J., Laws, G.M., Thornton, T.J., Goodnick, S.M., Saranti, M., Tang, J., & Eisenberg, R. S. Silicon-based ion channel sensor. *Superlattices and Microstructures* **34**, 451–457 (2003).

62. Wilk, S.J., Goryll, M., Laws, G.M., Goodnick, S.M., Thornton, T.J., Saranti, M., Tang, J., & Eisenberg, R.S. Teflon-coated silicon apertures for supported lipid bilayer membranes. *Applied Physics Letters* **85**, 3307–3309 (2004).

63. Fertig, N., Tilke, A., Blick, R.H., Kotthaus, J.P., Behrens, J.C., & tenBruggencate, G. Stable integration of isolated cell membrane patches in a nanomachined aperture. *Applied Physics Letters* **77**, 1218 (2000).

64. Fertig, N., Meyer, C., Blick, R.H., Trautmann, C., & Behrends, J.C. Microstructured glass chip for ion-channel electrophysiology. *Physical Review. E, Statistical Physics, Plasmas, Fluids, and Related Interdisciplinary Topics* **64**, 040901(R) (2001).

65. Fertig, N., Blick, R.H., & Behrends, J.C. Whole cell patch clamp recording performed on a planar glass chip. *Biophysical Journal* **82**, 3056–3062 (2002).

66. Fertig, N., Klau, M., George, M., Blick, R.H., & Behrends, J.C. Activity of single ion channel proteins detected with a planar microstructure. *Applied Physics Letters* **81**, 4865–4867 (2002).

67. Brueggemann, A., George, M., Klau, M., Beckler, M., Steindl, J., Behrends, J.C., & Fertig, N. Ion channel drug discovery and research: the automated nano-patch-clamp technology. *Current Drug Discovery Technologies* **1**, 91–96 (2004).

68. Schmidt, C., Mayer, M., & Vogel, H. A chip-based biosensor for the functional analysis of single ion channels. *Angewandte Chemie (International ed. in English)* **39**(17), 3137–3140 (2000).

69. Chien, M.-C., Wang, G.-J., & Yu, W.C. Modeling ion diffusion current in nanochannel using infinitesimal distribution resistor-capacitor circuits. *Japanese Journal of Applied Physics* **46**, 7436–7440 (2007).

70. Danelon, C., Suenaga, A., Winterhalter, M. & Yamato, I. Molecular origin of the cation selectivity in OmpF porin: single channel conductances vs. free energy calculation. *Biophysical Chemistry* **104**, 591–603 ((2003).).

71. Favero, G., Campanella, L., Cavallo, S., D'Annibale, A., Perrella, M., Mattei, E., & Ferri, T. Glutamate receptor incorporated in a mixed hybrid bilayer lipid membrane array, as a sensing element of a biosensor working under flowing conditions. *Journal of the American Chemical Society* **127**, 8103–8111 (2005).

72. Reimhult, E. & Kumar, K. Membrane biosensor platforms using nano- and microporous supports. *Trends in Biotechnology* **26**, 82–89 (2007).

73. Hemmler, R., Böse, G., Wagner, R., & Peters, R. Nanopore unitary permeability measure by electrochemical and optical single transporter recording. *Biophysical Journal* **88**, 4000–4007 (2005).

74. Favero, G., D'Annibale, A., Capanella, L., Santucci, R., & Ferri, T. Membrane supported bilayer lipid membrane array: preparation, stability and ion-channel insertion. *Analytica Chimica Acta* **460**, 23–34 (2002).

75. Favero, G., Capanella, L., D'Annibale, A., Santucci, R., & Ferri, T. Mixed hybrid bilayer lipid membrane incorporating valinomycin: improvements in preparation and function. *Microchemical Journal* **74**, 141–148 (2003).

76. Schuster, B., Pum, D., Sára, M., Braha, O., Bayley, H., & Sleytr, U.B. S-layer ultrafiltration membranes: a new support for stabilizing functionalized membranes. *Langmuir* **17**, 499–503 (2001).

77. Römer, W., Lam, Y.H., Fischer, D., Watts, A., Fischer, W.B., Göring, P., Wehrspohn, R.B., Gösele, U., & Steinem, C. Channel activity of a viral transmembrane peptide

in micro-BLMs: Vpu1-32 from HIV-1. *Journal of the American Chemical Society* **126**, 16267–16274 (2004).

78. Römer, W. & Steinem, C. Impedance analysis and single-channel recordings on nano-black lipid membranes based on porous alumina. *Biophysical Journal* **86**, 955–965 (2004).

79. Mayer, M., Kriebel, J.K., Tosteson, M.T., & Whitesides, G.M. Microfabricated Teflon membranes for low-noise recordings of ion channels in planar lipid bilayers. *Biophysical Journal* **85**, 2684–2695 (2003).

80. Weng, K.C., Stalgren, J.R., Duval, D.J., Risbud, S.H., & Frank, C.W. Fluid biomembranes supported on nanoporous aerogel/xerogel substrates. *Langmuir* **20**, 7232–7239 (2004).

81. Schmitt, E.K., Weichbrodt, C., & Steinem, C. Impedance analysis of gramicidin D in pore-suspending membranes. *Soft Matter* **5**, 2247–2253 (2009).

82. Xia, Y.N. & Whitesides, G.M. Soft lithography. *Annual Review of Materials Science* **28**, 153–184 (1998).

83. Qin, D., Xia, Y.N., & Whitesides, G.M. Soft lithography for micro- and nanoscale patterning. *Nature Protocols* **5**, 491–502 (2010).

84. Jenkins, A.T.A., Bushby, R.J., Evans, S.D., Knoll, W., & Offenhaeusser, A. Lipid vesicle fusion on μCP patterned self-assembled monolayers: effect of pattern geometry on bilayer formation. *Langmuir* **18**, 3176–3180 (2002).

85. Jenkins, A.T.A., Boden, N., Bushby, R.J., Evans, S.D., Knowles, P.F., Miles, R.E., Ogier, S.D., Schönherr, H., & Vancso, G.J. Microcontact printing of lipophilic self-assembled monolayers for the attachment of biomimetic lipid bilayers to surfaces. *Journal of the American Chemical Society* **121**, 5274–5280 (1999).

86. Jenkins, A.T.A., Bushby, R.J., Boden, N., Evans, S.D., Knowles, P.F., Liu, Q., Miles, R.E., & Ogier, S.D. Ion-selective lipid bilayers tethered to microcontact printed self-assembled monolayers containing cholesterol derivatives. *Langmuir* **14**, 4675–4678 (1998).

87. Hovis, J.S. & Boxer, S.G. Patterning barriers to lateral diffusion in supported lipid bilayer membranes by blotting and stamping. *Langmuir* **16**, 894–897 (2000).

88. Yee, C.K., Amweg, M.L., & Parikh, A.N. Membrane photolithography: direct micropatterning and manipulation of fluid phospholipid membranes in the aqueous phase using deep-UV light. *Advanced Materials* **16**, 1184–1189 (2004).

89. Yee, C.K., Amweg, M.L., & Parikh, A.N. Membrane photolithography: UV light-directed micro-patterning and manipulation of fluid phospholipid membranes in aqueous phases. *Biophysical Journal* **86**, 196a–197a (2004).

90. Jackson, B.L. & Groves, J.T. Scanning probe lithography on fluid lipid membranes. *Journal of the American Chemical Society* **126**, 13878–13879 (2004).

91. Jackson, B.L. & Groves, J.T. Hybrid protein-lipid patterns from aluminum templates. *Langmuir* **23**, 2052–2057 (2007).

92. Orth, R.N., Kameoka, J., Zipfel, W.R., Ilic, B., Webb, W.W., Clark, T.G., & Craighead, H.G. Creating biological membranes on the micron scale: forming patterned lipid bilayers using a polymer lift-off technique. *Biophysical Journal* **85**, 3066–3073 (2003).

93. Künneke, S. & Janshoff, A. Visualization of molecular recognition events on microstructured lipid-membrane compartments by in situ scanning force microscopy. *Angewandte Chemie (International ed. in English)* **41**, 314–317 (2002).

94. Janshoff, A. & Künneke, S. Individually addressable solid supported lipid membranes formed by micromolding in capillaries. *European Biophysics Journal* **29**, 549–554 (2000).

95. Yang, T., Jung, S., Mao, H., & Cremer, P.S. Fabrication of phospholipid bilayer-coated microchannels for on-chip immunoassays. *Analytical Chemistry* **73**, 165–169 (2001).

96. Holden, M., Jung, S.-Y., Yang, T., Castellana, E.T., & Cremer, P.S. Creating fluid and air-stable solid supported lipid bilayers. *Journal of the American Chemical Society* **126**, 6512–6513 (2004).

97. Kastl, K., Menke, M., Luthgens, E., Faiss, S., Gerke, V., Janshoff, A., & Steinem, C. Partially reversible adsorption of annexin A1 on POPC/POPS bilayers investigated by QCM measurements, SFM, and DMC simulations. *Chembiochem* **7**, 106–115 (2006).

98. Faiss, S., Kastl, K., Janshoff, A., & Steinem, C. Formation of irreversibly bound annexin Al protein domains on POPC/POPS solid supported membranes. *BBA. Biomembranes* **1778**, 1601–1610 (2008).

99. Schuy, S. & Janshoff, A. Microstructuring of phospholipid bilayers on gold surfaces by micromolding in capillaries. *Journal of Colloid and Interface Science* **295**, 93–99 (2006).

100. Lenhert, S., Mirkin, C.A., & Fuchs, H. In situ lipid dip-pen nanolithography under water. *Scanning* **32**, 15–23 (2010).

101. Lenhert, S., Sun, P., Wang, Y.H., Fuchs, H., & Mirkin, C.A. Massively parallel dip-pen nanolithography of heterogeneous supported phospholipid multilayer patterns. *Small* **3**, 71–75 (2007).

102. Sekula, S., Fuchs, J., Weg-Remers, S., Nagel, P., Schuppler, S., Fragala, J., Theilacker, N., Franzreb, M., Wingren, C., Ellmark, P., Borrebaeck, C.A., Mirkin, C.A., Fuchs, H., & Lenhert, S. Multiplexed lipid dip-pen nanolithography on subcellular scales for the templating of functional proteins and cell culture. *Small* **4**, 1785–1793 (2008).

103. Shi, J.J., Chen, J.X., & Cremer, P.S. Sub-100 nm patterning of supported bilayers by nanoshaving lithography. *Journal of the American Chemical Society* **130**, 2718–2719 (2008).

104. Heimburg, T. Mechanical aspects of membrane thermodynamics. Estimation of the mechanical properties of lipid membranes close to the chain melting transition from calorimetry. *Biochimica et Biophysica Acta* **1415**, 147–162 (1998).

105. Lee, C.-H., Lin, W.-C., & Wang, J. Using differential confocal microscopy to detect the phase transition of lipid vesicle membranes. *Optical Engineering* **40**, 2077–2083 (2001).

106. Raudino, A., Zuccarello, F., La Rosa, C., & Buemi, G. Thermal expansion and compressibility coefficients of phospholipid vesicles: experimental determination and theoretical modeling. *The Journal of Physical Chemistry* **94**, 4217–4223 (1990).

107. White, S.H. & King, G.I. Molecular packing and area compressibility of lipid bilayers. *Proceedings of the National Academy of Sciences of the United States of America* **82**, 6532–6536 (1985).

108. Charrier, A. & Thibaudau, F. Main phase transitions in supported lipid single-bilayer. *Biophysical Journal* **89**, 1094–1101 (2005).

REFERENCES **179**

109. Enders, O., Ngezahayo, A., Wiechmann, M., Leisten, F., & Kolb, H.A. Structural calorimetry of main transition of supported DMPC bilayers by temperature-controlled AFM. *Biophysical Journal* **87**, 2522–2531 (2004).

110. Feng, Z.V., Spurlin, T.A., & Gewirth, A.A. Direct visualization of asymmetric behavior in supported lipid bilayers at the gel-fluid phase transition. *Biophysical Journal* **88**, 2154–2164 (2005).

111. Keller, D., Larsen, N.B., Moeller, I.M., & Mouritsen, O.G. Decoupled phase transitions and grain-boundary melting in supported phospholipid bilayers. *Physical Review Letters* **94**, 025701/025701–025701/025704 (2005).

112. Tokumasu, F., Jin, A.J., & Dvorak, J.A. Lipid membrane phase behaviour elucidated in real time by controlled environment atomic force microscopy. *Journal of Electron Microscopy* **51**, 1–9 (2002).

113. Xie, A.F., Yamada, R., Gewirth, A.A., & Granick, S. Materials science of the gel to fluid phase transition in a supported phospholipid bilayer. *Physical Review Letters* **89**, 246103/246101–246103/246104 (2002).

114. Kaasgaard, T., Leidy, C., Crowe, J.H., Mouritsen, O.G., & Jorgensen, K. Temperature-controlled structure and kinetics of ripple phases in one- and two-component supported lipid bilayers. *Biophysical Journal* **85**, 350–360 (2003).

115. Leonenko, Z.V., Finot, E., Ma, H., Dahms, T.E.S., & Cramb, D.T. Investigation of temperature-induced phase transitions in DOPC and DPPC phospholipid bilayers using temperature-controlled scanning force microscopy. *Biophysical Journal* **86**, 3783–3793 (2004).

116. Yarrow, F., Vlugt, T.J.H., van der Eerden, J.P.J.M., & Snel, M.M.E. Melting of a DPPC lipid bilayer observed with atomic force microscopy and computer simulation. *Journal of Crystal Growth* **275**, e1417–e1421 (2005).

117. Howland, M.C., Szmodis, A.W., Sanii, B., & Parikh, A.N. Characterization of physical properties of supported phospholipid membranes using imaging ellipsometry at optical wavelengths. *Biophysical Journal* **92**, 1306–1317 (2007).

118. Faiss, S., Schuy, S., Weiskopf, D., Steinem, C., & Janshoff, A. Phase transition of individually addressable microstructured membranes visualized by imaging ellipsometry. *The Journal of Physical Chemistry. B, Materials, Surfaces, Interfaces & Biophysical* **111**, 13979–13986 (2007).

119. Mouritsen, O.G. & Zuckermann, M.J. What's so special about cholesterol? *Lipids* **39**, 1101–1113 (2004).

120. Ohvo-Rekilä, H., Ramstedt, B., Leppimäki, P., & Slotte, J.P. Cholesterol interactions with phospholipids in membranes. *Progress in Lipid Research* **41**, 66–97 (2002).

121. Ipsen, J.H., Karlström, G., Mouritsen, O.G., Wennerström, H., & Zuckermann, M.J. Phase equilibria in the phosphatidylcholine-cholesterol system. *Biochimica et Biophysica Acta* **908**, 162–172 (1987).

122. Vist, M.R. & Davis, J.H. Phase equilibria of cholesterol/dipalmitoylphosphatidylcholine mixtures: ^2H Nuclear magnetic resonance and differential scanning calorimetry. *Biochemistry* **29**, 451–464 (1990).

123. McMullen, T.P.W., Lewis, R.N.A.H., & McElhaney, R.N. Cholesterol-phospholipid interactions, the liquid-ordered phase and lipid rafts in model and biological membranes. *Current Opinion in Colloid & Interface Science* **8**, 459–468 (2004).

124. Mabrey, S., Mateo, P.L., & Sturtevant, J.M. High-sensitivity scanning calorimetric study of mixtures of cholesterol with dimyristoyl- and dipalmitoylphosphatidyl-cholines. *Biochemistry* **17**, 2464–2468 (1978).

125. Kunneke, S., Kruger, D., & Janshoff, A. Scrutiny of the failure of lipid membranes as a function of headgroups, chain length, and lamellarity measured by scanning force microscopy. *Biophysical Journal* **86**, 1545–1553 (2004).

126. Schneider, J., Dufrene, Y.F., Barger, W.R., & Lee, G.U. Atomic force microscope image contrast mechanisms on supported lipid bilayers. *Biophysical Journal* **79**, 1107–1118 (2000).

127. Butt, H.J. & Franz, V. Rupture of molecular thin films observed in atomic force microscopy. I. Theory. *Physical Review. E, Statistical Physics, Plasmas, Fluids, and Related Interdisciplinary Topics* **66**, 031601 (2002).

128. Loi, S., Sun, G., Franz, V., & Butt, H.J. Rupture of molecular thin films observed in atomic force microscopy. II. Experiment. *Physical Review. E, Statistical Physics, Plasmas, Fluids, and Related Interdisciplinary Topics* **66**, 031601 (2002).

129. Franz, V., Loi, S., Muller, H., Bamberg, E., & Butt, H.H. Tip penetration through lipid bilayers in atomic force microscopy. *Colloid Surface B* **23**, 191–200 (2002).

130. Dufrene, Y.F., Barger, W.R., Green, J.B.D., & Lee, G.U. Nanometer-scale surface properties of mixed phospholipid monolayers and bilayers. *Langmuir* **13**, 4779–4784 (1997).

131. Fine, T., Mey, I., Rommel, C., Wegener, J., Steinem, C., & Janshoff, A. Elasticity mapping of apical cell membranes. *Soft Matter* **5**, 3262–3265 (2009).

132. Lorenz, B., Mey, I., Steltenkamp, S., Fine, T., Rommel, C., Muller, M.M., Maiwald, A., Wegener, J., Steinem, C., & Janshoff, A. Elasticity mapping of pore-suspending native cell membranes. *Small* **5**, 832–838 (2009).

133. Steltenkamp, S., Muller, M.M., Deserno, M., Hennesthal, C., Steinem, C., & Janshoff, A. Mechanical properties of pore-spanning lipid bilayers probed by atomic force microscopy. *Biophysical Journal* **91**, 217–226 (2006).

134. Mey, I., Stephan, M., Schmitt, E.K., Muller, M.M., Ben Amar, M., Steinem, C., & Janshoff, A. Local membrane mechanics of pore-spanning bilayers. *Journal of the American Chemical Society* **131**, 7031–7039 (2009).

135. Ashcroft, F.M. *Ion Channels and Disease.* San Diego: Academic Press (2000).

136. Neher, E. & Sakmann, B. Single channel currents recorded from membrane of denervated frog muscle fibers. *Nature* **260**, 799–802 (1976).

137. Farre, C., Geroge, M., Brüggemann, A., & Fertig, N. Ion channel screening—automated patch clamp on the rise. *Drug Discovery Today: Technologies* **5**, e23–e28 (2008).

138. Suzuki, H., Tabata, K.V., Noji, H., & Takeuchi, S. Electrophysiological recordings of single ion channels in planar lipid bilayers using a polymethyl methacrylate microfluidic chip. *Biosensors & Bioelectronics* **22**, 1111–1115 (2007).

139. Zagnoni, M., Sandison, M.E., Marius, P., Lee, A.G., & Morgan, H. Controlled delivery of proteins into bilayer lipid membranes on chip. *Lab on a Chip* **7**, 1176–1183 (2007).

140. Naumann, R., Walz, D., Schiller, S.M., & Knoll, W. Kinetics of valinomycin-mediated K^+ ion transport through tethered bilayer lipid membranes. *Journal of Electroanalytical Chemistry* **550–551**, 241–252 (2003).

141. Roskamp, R.F., Vockenroth, I.K., Eisenmenger, N., Braunagel, J., & Koper, I. Functional tethered bilayer lipid membranes on aluminum oxide. *Chemphyschem* **9**, 1920–1924 (2008).

142. Bamberg, E. & Läugner, P. Blocking of gramicidin channel by divalent cations. *The Journal of Membrane Biology* **35**, 351–375 (1977).

143. Finkelstein, A. & Andersen, O.S. The gramicidin A channel: a review of its permeability characteristics with special reference to the single-file aspect of transport. *The Journal of Membrane Biology* **59**, 155–171 (1981).

144. Purrucker, O., Hillebrandt, H., Adlkofer, K., & Tanaka, M. Deposition of highly resistive lipid biayer on silicon-silicon dioxide electrode and incorporation of gramicidin studied by ac impedance spectroscopy. *Electrochimica Acta* **47**, 791–798 (2001).

145. Nikolelis, D.P., Siontorou, C.G., Krull, U.J., & Katrivanos, P.L. Ammonium ion minisensors from self-assembled bilayer lipid membranes using gramicidin as an ionophore. Modulation of ammonium selectivity by platelet-activating factor. *Analytical Chemistry* **68**, 1735–1741 (1996).

146. Gritsch, S., Nollert, P., Jähnig, F., & Sackmann, E. Impedance spectroscopy of porin and gramicidin pores reconstituted into supported lipid bilayers on indium-tin-oxide electrodes. *Langmuir* **14**, 3118–3125 (1998).

147. Steinem, C., Janshoff, A., Galla, H.-J., & Manfred, S. Impedance analysis of ion transport through gramicidin channels incorporated in solid supported lipid bilayers. *Bioelectrochemistry and Bioenergetics* **42**, 213–220 (1997).

148. Wiegand, G. *Fundamental Principles of the Electric Properties of Supported Lipid Membranes Investigated by Advanced Methods of Impedance Spectroscopy.* Aachen: Shaker Verlag (2000).

149. Lucas, S.W. & Harding, M.M. Detection of DNA via an ion channel switch biosensor. *Analytical Biochemistry* **282**, 70–79 (2000).

150. Lee, S.-K., Cascão-Pereira, L.G., Sala, R.F., Holmes, S.P., Ryan, K.J., & Becker, T. Ion channel switch array. *Industrial Biotechnology* **1**, 26–31 (2005).

151. Kim, J.-M., Patwardhan, A., Bott, A., & Thompson, D.H. Preparation and electrochemical behavior of gramicidin-bipolar monolayer membranes supported on gold electrodes. *Biochimica et Biophysica Acta* **1671**, 0–21 (2003).

152. Milov, A.D., Samiloiva, R.I., Tsvetkov, Y.D., Formaggio, F., Toniolo, C., & Raap, J. Self-aggregation of spin-labeled alamethicin in ePC vesicles studied by pulsed electron-electron double resonance. *Journal of the American Chemical Society* **129**, 9260–9261 (2007).

153. Cafiso, D.S. Alamethicin: a peptide model for voltage gating and protein-membrane interactions. *Annual Review of Biophysics and Biomolecular Structure* **23**, 141–165 (1994).

154. Yin, P., Burnsa, C.J., Osmana, P.D.J., & Cornell, B.A. A tethered bilayer sensor containing alamethicin channels and its detection of amiloride based inhibitors. *Biosensors & Bioelectronics* **18**, 389–397 (2003).

155. Pilz, C. & Steinem, C. Modulation of the conductance of a 2,2-bipyridine-functionalized peptide ion channel by Ni^{2+}. *European Biophysical Journal* **37**, 1065–1071 (2008).

156. Terrettaz, S., Ulrich, W.-P., Guerrini, R., Verdini, A., & Vogel, H. Immunosensing by a synthetic ligand-gated ion channel. *Angewandte Chemie (International ed. in English)* **40**, 1740–1743 (2001).

157. Terrettaz, S., Mayer, M., & Vogel, H. Highly electrically insulating tethered lipid bilayers for probing the function of ion channel proteins. *Langmuir* **19**, 5567–5569 (2003).

158. Glazier, S.A., Vanderah, D.J., Plant, A.L., Bayley, H., Valincius, G., & Kasianowicz, J.J. Reconstitution of the pore-forming toxin a-hemolysin in phospholipid/18-octadecyl-1-thiahexa(ethylene oxide) and phospholipid/n-octadecanethiol supported bilayer membranes. *Langmuir* **16**, 10428–10435 (2000).

159. Schuster, B. & Sleytr, U.B. Single channel recordings of a-hemolysin reconstituted in S-layer-supported lipid bilayers. *Bioelectrochemistry* **55**, 5–7 (2002).

160. Buehler, L.K., Kusumoto, S., Zhang, H., & Rosenbusch, J.P. Plasticity of *Escherichia coli* porin channels. Dependence of their conductance on strain and lipid environment. *The Journal of Biological Chemistry* **266**, 24446–24450 (1991).

161. Cowan, S.W., Schirmer, T., Rummel, G., Steiert, M., Ghosh, R., Pauptit, R.A., Jansonius, J.N., & Rosenbusch, J.P. Crystal structures explain functional properties of two *E. coli* porins. *Nature* **358**, 727–733 (1992).

162. Stora, T., Lakey, J.H., & Vogel, H. Ion-channel gating in transmembrane receptor proteins: functional activity in tethered lipid membranes. *Angewandte Chemie (International ed. in English)* **38**, 389–391 (1999).

163. Schmitt, E.K. & Steinem, C. Channel activity of OmpF monitored in nano-BLMs. *Biophysical Journal* **91**, 2163–2171 (2006).

164. Nestorovich, E.M., Danelon, C., Winterhalter, M., & Bezrukov, S.M. Designed to penetrate: time-resolved interaction of single antibiotic molecules with bacterial pores. *Proceedings of the National Academy of Sciences of the United States of America* **99**, 9789–9794 (2002).

165. Gassmann, O., Kreir, M., Ambrosi, C., Pranskevich, J., Oshima, A., Roling, C., Sosinsky, G., Fertig, N., & Steinem, C. The M34A mutant of connexin 26 reveals active conductance states in pore-suspending membranes. *Journal of Structural Biology* **168**, 168–176 (2009).

166. Dunlop, J., Bowlby, M., Peri, R., Vasilyev, D., & Arias, R. High-throughput electrophysiology: an emerging paradigm for ion-channel screening and physiology. *Nature Reviews Drug Discovery* **7**, 358–368 (2008).

167. Heron, A.J., Thompson, J.R., Mason, A.E., & Wallace, M.I. Direct detection of membrane channels from gels using water-in-oil droplet bilayers. *Journal of the American Chemical Society* **129**, 16042–16047 (2007).

168. Tompkins, H. *A Users's Guide to Ellipsometry*. London: Academic Press (1993).

169. Binnig, G., Quate, C.F., & Gerber, C. Atomic force microscope. *Physical Review Letters* **56**, 930–933 (1986).

170. Janshoff, A., Neitzert, M., Oberdorfer, Y., & Fuchs, H. Force spectroscopy of molecular systems—single molecule spectroscopy of polymers and biomolecules. *Angewandte Chemie (International ed. in English)* **39**, 3213–3237 (2000).

171. Barsoukov, E. & Macdonald, J. *Impedance Spectroscopy: Theory, Experiment, and Applications*. Hoboken: Wiley-Interscience (2005).

CHAPTER 6

Antimicrobial and Anti-Inflammatory Intelligent Surfaces

HANS J. GRIESSER, HEIKE HALL, TOBY A. JENKINS, STEFANI S. GRIESSER, and KRASIMIR VASILEV

6.1 INTRODUCTION

In many applications of biomedical devices, bacterial infections can arise and can seriously interfere with the intended function of the device. Yet, the literature on bacterial colonization and biofilm formation on biomaterials is far less extensive than the literature on the attachment and spreading of mammalian cells on biomaterials. The fundamental understanding of bacterial attachment mechanisms is also less well developed than the mechanistic understanding of mammalian cell attachment. Some approaches have been developed and commercialized; probably the best known of these are based on coatings that release silver ions to combat bacteria.[1] However, in terms of design sophistication, reported antibacterial coatings are not built on the same advanced biointerfacial molecular concepts as cell-supporting or cell-repellent coatings are. There is much scope for improving the sophistication of the design of antibacterial coatings by utilizing specific bioactive molecules that target a specific biomolecular function in bacteria but do not interfere in any way with mammalian cell functions. Such "intelligent" molecules can either be delivered by controlled release systems or by performing long-term protective function via covalent grafting onto biomaterial surfaces.

Thus, we will focus our discussion on such systems that are designed for controlled specific activity or for release in a manner more controlled than with many reported systems to date. Accordingly, while some mention needs to be made of existing strategies such as those utilizing quaternary ammonium cationic molecules or transition metal ions, the fact that such approaches usually cause as much damage to mammalian cells as to bacterial cells seems to make them less suitable for inclusion within intelligent approaches.

Intelligent Surfaces in Biotechnology: Scientific and Engineering Concepts, Enabling Technologies, and Translation to Bio-Oriented Applications, First Edition.
Edited by H. Michelle Grandin and Marcus Textor.
© 2012 John Wiley & Sons, Inc. Published 2012 by John Wiley & Sons, Inc.

This chapter also discusses anti-inflammatory surfaces and coatings. While this may at first glance appear to be topically disparate, it is recognized that bacterial infection may affect the inflammatory response to the presence of a biomaterial. Given this interplay, it may, in fact, be advantageous to design surfaces that exercise both antibacterial and anti-inflammatory activities (while also allowing good integration with tissue or blood).

Yet, one needs to recognize that in wound healing, the inflammatory response arises from the act of tissue damage, causes a systemic inflammatory response, and is necessary for the repair of injured tissue.[2] Thus, it may not be optimal if a biomaterial surface completely suppresses the inflammatory response; it may be much more advantageous if an intelligent biomaterial surface can be designed such that it can modulate the inflammatory response to stay within desirable limits. As bacteria affect the inflammatory response, causing additional inflammatory activity, ultimately, an intelligent surface to be utilized in wound-healing situations might be designed such as to recognize and mediate the extents of inflammation and bacterial invasion.

In this chapter, we will therefore discuss the design and development of surfaces and coatings intended to address the specific problems of bacterial infection of biomedical devices and implants and of inflammatory responses, with a focus on intelligent surfaces/coatings that are distinguished by biological hypotheses and/or predictable, specific biomolecular activity rather than indiscriminate responses, but necessarily also including some studies with less well-defined rationales. We will not endeavor to produce a comprehensive literature survey; for the sake of conciseness as well as given the volume of literature on antibacterial coatings and unavoidable duplications and close similarities in the literature, we prefer to use selected examples. We apologize for the omission of many other deserving literature reports.

6.2 ANTIBACTERIAL STRATEGIES

6.2.1 The Infection Problem

Biomedical devices have contributed greatly to saving lives and restoring the quality of life of large numbers of patients. Many devices and biomaterials have been used successfully, although their design may not be optimal from a fundamental biomolecular perspective. Yet, problems remain in the usage of biomedical devices, and a key problem is that of bacterial infection, with the formation of bacterial biofilm colonies that can be difficult to treat.

So-called device-related infections (DRIs) arise when bacteria attach and proliferate on surfaces of biomedical devices and implants. DRIs cause considerable problems in implant surgery and also with short-term biomedical devices such as catheters.[3–5] DRIs can pose a marked health risk to patients, often requiring reoperation and replacement of the infected device, and cause large costs to the healthcare system. While infections on contact lenses and catheters become manifest soon after infection, in the case of implants, DRIs often are not detected at an early stage. The severity of DRIs varies greatly among devices[5] and patients but can be very serious and even fatal at times. While contact lens-related infections rarely cause serious problems because eye soreness alerts the user to its onset, there are no early warning signs for bacterial infections of many implants and devices; the onset of an infection is masked by the ongoing soreness of the tissue after surgery or insertion of a catheter, for example. DRI diagnosis on orthopedic implants usually occurs when a full-blown infection has already caused damage to the adjacent tissue and the entire host organism (patient), which then weakens the healing process and may result in suboptimal results in terms of the utility of the device. Reoperation of infected implants has, at times, led to the death of elderly patients weakened by the previous operation or by underlying disease conditions such as diabetes mellitus.

Polymeric surface treatments and coatings have been used extensively in biomaterials research and applications, for example, in commercial products such as oxidative surface treatments for polystyrene (PS) tissue culture ware,[6] as coatings for extended-wear contact lenses,[7] and as adhesive interlayers for the subsequent covalent immobilization of bioactive molecules. Much of that work has aimed to achieve either better tissue integration or resistance to the adhesion of biological molecules, cells, and tissue. The avoidance of cellular adhesion by fouling-resistant layers can, of course, also serve to reduce the adhesion of bacteria, as discussed further. However, antiadhesive strategies also prevent the attachment of human cells and tissue, which may be a disadvantage for wound healing and implant integration. Accordingly, our focus is not on "passive" anti-adhesive strategies but on the design and development of technologies that lead to "active" surfaces that deter the adhesion of bacteria and the consequent development of biofilms and implant infection via a molecule with biological action, while enabling integration with mammalian cells and tissue. Systems seek to minimize the risk of infection on short-term biomedical devices by prophylactic measures. For instance, catheters are replaced at frequent intervals. Such preventative replacement schedules impose, however, considerable costs to healthcare systems. For implants, the problem is more complex. Improved procedures in sterilization and operating theaters have reduced significantly the frequency of early-stage infections of implants, but delayed infections, occurring many weeks or months after surgery, have barely decreased and continue to pose a serious problem. It is believed that such late-stage infections are not caused by the act of surgery but by planktonic bacteria circulating in the vascular system and eventually landing at an incompletely healed wound site where they may attach onto the implant surface, multiply, and form a biofilm that leads to infection.

Bacteria can colonize surfaces of synthetic materials in versatile ways using their own synthesized adhesion molecules or via adsorbed layers of biomolecules, particularly cell-adhesive proteins (while some bacteria can attach and proliferate on synthetic surfaces without adsorbed protein layers, in general, adsorbed protein layers appear to enhance bacterial colonization). Attached and growing bacterial colonies soon produce an exocellular polysaccharide matrix, which protects them against antibiotics and the host body's innate defense system.[4,8] Thus, bacterial biofilms on biomedical device surfaces are much more difficult to eradicate by antibiotics than planktonic/circulating bacteria, hence, the need for surgical removal of a substantial proportion of infected implants and surrounding tissue. Accordingly, a promising strategy for reducing the occurrence of DRIs is to attempt to prevent the initial attachment of bacteria to implant and device surfaces. This aim has spurred research efforts on the development of thin coatings that can be applied onto biomedical devices to combat bacterial colonization. Antibacterial coatings should deter DRIs while not affecting other properties such as the visual clarity of contact lenses or the flexibility of vascular grafts nor should, of course, such coatings adversely affect human cells or fluids (e.g., blood and tear fluid).

However, the development of antibacterial surfaces for biomedical devices needs to take into account that with the wide variety of devices and implants, as well as causative bacteria, a single approach may not be universally successful. Antibacterial strategies may need to be tailored to specific product needs. For some products, such as contact lenses, resistance to the attachment of bacteria is required along with biofouling resistance, whereas for hip and knee implants, one wishes to deter bacteria while encouraging close apposition of host cells for strong interfacial integration of the implant with human tissue. Such device-specific requirements have to be tackled using different designs of antibacterial biointerfaces.

Antibacterial strategies are, of course, also applicable to other products where problems arise from bacterial biofilm formation, for example, in water filtration and purification systems. There is a substantial body of literature on the reduction of biofouling for various applications, but the most sophisticated strategies are found in the biomaterials literature, as the consequences of infection arising at implant or device surfaces are much more serious in human health care, and the biomedical devices/implants market is much less price sensitive.

6.2.2 Approaches to Antibacterial Device Surfaces

Polymeric materials offer great flexibility for the design of biomedical devices. However, most polymers are readily colonized by bacteria. A few polymers are known to kill bacteria[9–12] or to prevent bacteria from attaching,[13–16] but those polymers are often not suitable as bulk materials for the fabrication of devices due to other considerations such as strength, flexibility, or processability. Thus, emphasis has been on using bactericidal or attachment-resistant polymers as surface coatings applied onto existing devices.

Both synthetic and natural polymers offer promise for use as antibacterial coatings. Polymer coatings can be placed onto device surfaces via various techniques such as dip coating, spin coating, layer by layer, plasma polymerization, Langmuir–Blodgett, and extrusion. For example, a coated layer of poly(dimethylaminomethyl styrene) has been deposited onto nylon fabrics.[12] This provides enormous flexibility for applying various polymers onto surfaces of biomedical devices (exploiting the reactivity of amine groups in this case) and implants for achieving antibacterial action.

Most synthetic polymers that have been reported to be bactericidal[9–12] as well as the natural polymer chitosan[17,18] are cationic. It appears reasonable to assume that their mode of action is membrane lysis, analogous to the better-known, older approaches of using cationic peptides and quaternary amine compounds (discussed further). The main issue with such cationic polymers is that they cause adverse effects on human cells and thus may find limited use as biomedical coatings. However, Salick et al.[19] reported a hydrogel scaffold, made from a self-assembling peptide and intended for tissue regeneration applications, whose surface exhibited a broad-spectrum antibacterial activity against gram-positive and gram-negative bacteria while being nonlytic for human erythrocytes, which maintained a healthy morphology when in contact with the scaffold surface.

In contrast to the relatively small number of inherently antibacterial polymers, a considerable number of low-molecular-weight molecules and some inorganic ions are known to possess antibacterial effectiveness in solution. However, it is challenging to use such antibiotics to protect implant surfaces because, unlike bactericidal polymers, they cannot be applied directly by themselves, for example, by solvent coating, onto device surfaces as they may adhere too weakly and thus may be rapidly displaced and dispersed in biological fluids. Low-molecular-weight antibiotics can be used in two ways to combat DRIs. Figure 6.1 displays schematically four major strategies for the prevention of DRIs on biomaterial surfaces.

One approach is to use a controlled release approach, in which the antibiotic is released from the biomedical device and intercepts bacteria in the vicinity. This has been studied with some organic compounds, but by far, the most common antiseptic used thus is silver; many silver-based approaches have been reported. The extensive literature on the development of devices releasing biocides and antibiotics has been the subject of several reviews.[20–22] Various antimicrobial compounds have been loaded into polymers or polymer composite films, including organic antibiotics,[23–25] silver,[26–28] and nitric oxide $(NO)^{29}$ for various intended biomedical applications. Other metal ions have also been tested, but adverse effects on human tissue present a concern. The disadvantage of the release approach is that the duration and effectiveness of antibacterial action is limited by loading and release kinetics. While polymeric carrier materials have been used most often for the delivery of antibiotics, other approaches have been reported, such as the delivery of silver sulfadiazine to wounds via liposomal encapsulation.[30]

The second approach consists of the application of a molecular surface layer of covalently immobilized ("grafted") antibiotic molecules that can prevent bacterial attachment to material surfaces. In addition to potentially much

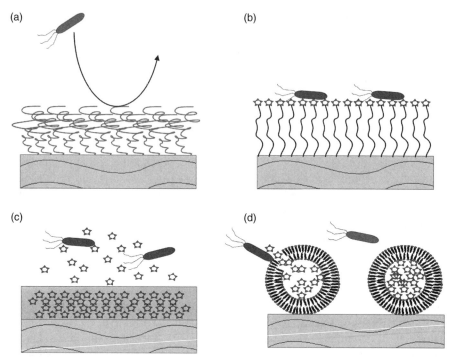

Figure 6.1 Schematic depiction of strategies for the generation of antibacterial coatings: (a) surfaces that prevent bacterial adhesion, (b) coatings that kill on contact, (c) coatings that release antimicrobial agents, and (d) smart coatings that release upon the presence of bacteria.

longer—perhaps indefinite—effectiveness, this approach is also favorable when seeking regulatory approval for new devices; if it can be ascertained that the antibiotics are durably grafted such as to remain on the device surface, one can eliminate concerns about possible adverse effects due to accumulation of antibiotic molecules or ions in body tissues such as the brain, liver, and spleen.

Polymers that by themselves are not resistant to bacterial colonization are used as vehicles for the controlled outdiffusion of dispersed antibiotics or for the covalent grafting of antibacterial small molecules. In some cases, antibiotics may be delivered from "bulk" polymers used for device manufacture, but in many cases, this may be incompatible with manufacturing processes, such as extrusion, which would destroy imbibed antibiotics. Often, it may be advantageous to first manufacture a device and then to apply a polymeric coating that can deliver or surface graft an antibiotic. Polymeric coatings are particularly useful as carriers for antibiotics on metallic and ceramic devices, such as hip and knee implants, into which antibiotic molecules usually can be neither imbibed nor grafted directly onto the inorganic surface. Exceptions exist, such as the use of carbonated hydroxyapatite coatings precipitated onto titanium implants in a manner suitable for incorporation of antibiotics containing carboxylic groups, such as cephalothin, carbenicillin, and cefamandol,[31] and hydroxyapatite loaded with gentamycin for cementless joint prostheses[24] and posttraumatic osteomyelitis.[32] In most cases, however, a thin polymeric coating serves as an essential vehicle.

A number of studies have reported the attachment of antibacterial moieties onto polymer chains (thus producing derivatized polymer chains, as opposed to surface-derivatized solid polymer materials discussed in a later section). For instance, biocidal N-halamines were incorporated into copolymers containing N-halamine siloxane and quaternary ammonium salt siloxane units, and were applied as water-based coatings.[33] Polyurethanes (PUs) with soft blocks containing end-fluorinated (-$CH_2OCH_2CF_3$) and 5,5-dimethylhydantoin pendant groups were studied as biocidal polymeric surface modifiers.[34] Polysiloxanes with pendant biocidal N,N'-dialkylimidazolium salt groups were synthesized and compared with polysiloxanes bearing conventional biocidal quaternary ammonium salt groups; the former polymers were found to have high antibacterial potency against all bacteria studied, similar to the latter polymers but with better thermal stability.[35] Such derivatized polymers can then be used either as materials per se for device fabrication or, more commonly, as coatings on existing devices.

However, when coating thin polymeric layers onto bulk biomaterials, the question needs to be considered whether the coating is stable in the biological environment. While the antibacterial polymeric coating may not spontaneously desorb in water to a significant extent, the many surface-active molecules present in biological fluids may be able to displace surface-adsorbed polymers. A safer strategy may be to attach antibacterial coatings via covalent bonding to the substrate biomaterial. Unfortunately, few studies exist that address the question of longer-term stability and performance of solvent-coated protective antibacterial polymer layers. Instructive is a study by Kingshott et al., which showed that physisorbed poly(ethylene oxide) (PEO) polymers did not provide lasting reduction in bacterial adhesion, whereas PEO chains covalently attached to a bulk material showed stable effectiveness.[15] A likely explanation is that bacteria can act as megasurfactants with high interfacial affinity for the material surface, displacing physisorbed polymer chains from the bulk material surface, whereas covalently attached (surface-grafted) polymer chains resist such displacement. It would therefore seem advisable to use the pathway of *covalent* attachment of antibacterial polymer coatings onto devices in order to prevent possible loss in biological milieus. For low-molecular-weight antibacterial compounds, discussed in a later section, covalent attachment is essential for long-term performance anyway, as they are more readily detached from a surface than polymeric coatings, but the main point to note here is that even polymeric coatings may not remain on the device surface when in contact with biological fluids, in which many surface-active proteins and cellular entities may have sufficient affinity for the surface of biomedical devices to displace physisorbed coatings.

6.2.3 Release of Antimicrobial Compounds from Polymers and Polymeric Coatings

The release of antiseptics and antimicrobial compounds from biomedical devices has attracted considerable attention. Compared to systemic drug delivery, a key advantage of local delivery of antibiotics at a specific site is that high local doses can be administered without exceeding the systemic toxicity level of a drug and risking, for example, renal and liver complications. Thus, increased doses could be applied at the site of a medical implant. An important issue concerning releasing devices is the kinetics of release of the antimicrobial compound. Fast release provides relatively high doses but short-term action. Slow release may not reach the required therapeutic level and might also lead to bacterial resistance at the release site due to survival of strains that adapt. The released antibacterial molecules must act before a protective exocellular matrix layer protects the bacterial colony. Bacteria protected by a biofilm can require 1000 times the antibiotic dose necessary to combat bacteria in suspension. An ideal release coating should provide fast initial release in the first 6 hours after intervention to protect the site while the immune system is weakened, followed by continuous "prophylactic" slow release over a period of days or weeks.

In this section, some representative strategies will be discussed for the release of antibiotic molecules or ions by diffusion or matrix degradation. Active "on-demand" release will be discussed in Section 6.4.

Many polymers suitable for biomedical devices, such as silicones, can be blended or loaded by in-diffusion, with antimicrobial compounds that are then released when in contact with a fluid environment. For example, Gaonkar et al.[36] impregnated silicone catheters with various antibiotic and antiseptic compounds and investigated their ability to prolong the onset of urinary tract infection. Catheters loaded with both chlorhexidine and triclosan showed the best performance, delaying infections for up to 31 days. A similar approach was used by Park et al.,[37] who incorporated norfloxacin into polymer coatings that were applied onto catheters. While in these cases the release of the antibiotic occurs by diffusion of the low-molecular-weight compound out of the polymer or polymer coating, an alternative approach is the use of a polymer matrix that degrades in the body environment and thereby provides delivery of the antibiotic by a combination of diffusion and polymer matrix erosion. The release of gentamicin from poly(hydroxybutyric-co-hydroxyvalerate) was studied by Rossi et al.,[38] who were able to control its release by varying the content of hydroxyvalerate in their formulations. Analogously, biodegradable polymeric nanofibers of poly(lactide-co-glycolide) (PLAGA) and nanofibers of PLAGA fabricated by electrospinning were used for the delivery of cefazolin.[39] Biodegradable poly(L-lactic acid) and poly(D,L-lactic-co-glycolic acid) films containing gentamicin suitable for application on the surface of metallic or polymeric fracture fixation devices have been reported,[40] and the release of amikacin and gentamycin from biodegradable polymeric scaffolds was studied in Reference 41.

Other systems have been reported in which specific combinations offer advantages. For example, Blanchemain et al.[42] developed an antibacterial delivery system by coating Dacron (poly(ethylene terephthalate) [PET]) vascular grafts with cyclodextrins and subsequently loading this with vancomycin. Linear release of vancomycin was observed over 50 days.

The release of NO as an antibacterial agent has been the subject of several studies. NO-releasing sol-gel polymer coatings for orthopedic devices showed a significant reduction of bacterial adhesion.[43] Polymers incorporating NO-releasing/generating moieties were shown not only to be effective against bacterial adhesion but also to improve biocompatibility of blood-contacting medical devices.[44]

6.2.4 Silver-Releasing Coatings

The release of silver (ions) from various carrier vehicles deserves a section of its own due to its prominence in the literature; reports on antibacterial action of silver-loaded materials far outweigh those on any other antibacterial biomaterial approach. Silver, silver compounds, and silver nanoparticles have enjoyed a great deal of attention in recent years and such research has recently been reviewed in considerable detail.[45,46] A number of commercial products including wound dressings,[1] bandages for burns and chronic wounds, silver and silver nanoparticle-coated catheters, and other medical devices have emerged. The efficiency of some of the coatings has, however, been subject to controversy. A number of factors associated with both the coating and the environment come into play in determining the efficiency of silver-based coating. It was found that coatings based on metallic silver are the least efficient. This is because silver needs to be in its oxidized form (Ag^+) in order to exhibit antibacterial action. However, Ag^+ ions can be complexed by chloride ions to produce insoluble silver chlorides, and this is detrimental for antibacterial efficiency. Another important problem is that in many cases, most of the loaded silver is released very quickly from the coating, thus limiting the time of protection.

There have been substantial research efforts toward engineering thin polymer films loaded with silver and silver nanoparticles in order to achieve a more prolonged and/or more controllable release. Many studies show effectiveness *in vitro*, but these newer approaches need yet to be verified *in vivo*. While some studies have applied contiguous silver film coatings onto substrates such as fibers,[47] most studies focus on silver (nano)particles incorporated within polymeric matrices. For biomedical devices, it may be advantageous to use thin polymer films containing silver nanoparticles fully encapsulated within the polymer matrix, as opposed to the situation where larger silver particles partly protrude from the polymer film layer. Ho et al.[48] presented an interesting approach, first forming silver nanoparticles within a thin film of polyethyleneimine, followed by copolymerization with 2-hydroxyethyl acrylate, which allowed further surface grafting of poly(ethylene glycol) (PEG). In this manner, bifunctional coatings were generated, with the PEG layer preventing bacterial adhesion and the silver ions releasing from the coating producing activity against *Staphylococcus aureus* bacteria present in the vicinity. Silver nanoparticles were loaded into these hydrogel coatings via *in situ* reduction of silver nitrate using sodium borohydride as a reducing agent. Analogously, Lee et al.[49] generated multilayer films, by layer-by-layer assembly, comprising catechol, which was used to ligate and reduce silver ions to metallic silver when immersed in an aqueous silver salt solution. This resulted in the generation of silver nanoparticles within the films.

In most reported studies, however, neither the amount of silver nor the release rate can readily be tailored to specific requirements. For a technology to be applicable to a range of biomedical devices, a smarter approach is needed, which enables control over those parameters with minor process variation when using one basic technology. In particular, it is desirable to adjust the release rate of silver ions to comply with the different requirements of different biomedical devices so that effective therapeutic dosage can be delivered over time periods as short as a few days or as long as a month or more. Moreover, in most systems, the loading and the release kinetics cannot be tailored independently. The design and implementation of a system that enables independent control over both loaded amounts and delivery kinetics has been reported recently.[50] An ultrathin barrier overlayer of adjustable thickness was used to control the rate of outdiffusion of silver ions. The silver loading could be controlled independently, leading to an approach with considerable flexibility and a wide range of controllable properties. Plasma polymerization of n-heptylamine or allylamine was used to create amine-rich uniform polymeric coatings into which silver ions were in-diffused by placing samples in a solution of $AgNO_3$; the time of immersion can be used to control the loaded amount. Silver ions were then reduced to silver using a reducing agent, and the silver atoms coalesced spontaneously into nanoparticles (Fig. 6.2), detected by a characteristic plasmon band in the UV–vis absorption spectrum. When placing such samples into an aqueous solution, oxidation causes the release of silver ions. The rate of release was shown to be adjustable by the application of a second plasma polymer layer (not containing silver ions and applied after loading the first coated layer with silver nanoparticles), with the thickness of this overlayer providing a convenient means of tailoring the release rate (Fig. 6.2). In this way, the loading and the release kinetics were adjustable independently over a considerable range. Even when slowing the rate of release such as to achieve sustained release over several weeks, antibacterial effectiveness was obtained *in vitro* (Fig. 6.2).

An antibacterial coating can also be produced by the plasma polymerization of a phosphine-stabilized silver maleimide complex.[51] This method is attractive in terms of comprising a single step but requires synthesis of

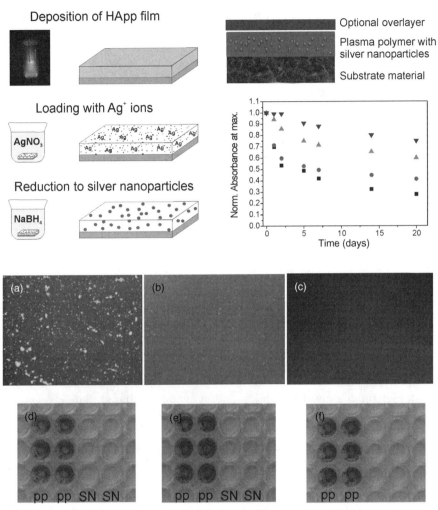

Figure 6.2 Schematic diagram of the approach developed by Vasilev et al.[50] for the loading of silver nanoparticles into amine plasma polymer coatings and the control of the release kinetics of silver ions via the adjustable thickness of an additional plasma polymer overlayer. Also shown are test results of antibacterial effectiveness against *S. epidermidis*; image (a) and rows labeled pp are samples of the control heptylamine surface (no silver), while images (b) and (c) and rows labeled SN are samples with silver-loaded coatings, with different overlayers. (See color insert.).

the precursor molecule used for the plasma deposition of the antibacterial coating.

Silver appears to be the broadest spectrum antibiotic available, and it generally does not appear to induce resistance. While contradictions exist in the literature (reviewed recently in Reference 52), it appears to tend toward the view that metallic silver has little activity (despite reference to contact activation) and that it is silver ions, released from silver metal coatings or polymer materials or coatings doped with silver nanoparticles, that exert biological functions. These ions may interact with bacterial cell walls, complex with proteins and DNA, and affect their biological functions. Different scenarios have been proposed for the mode of action of silver against bacteria; one is that silver ions bind to the bacterial cell membrane and damage it by interfering with membrane receptors and bacterial electron transport (impeding the production of adenosine triphosphate, the cell's energy source). Another scenario is that silver ions bind to bacterial DNA and thus damage their replication, and cause intracellular formation of insoluble compounds with nucleotides and proteins; particularly, the amino acids histidine and cysteine will readily complexate with Ag^+ ions. Gordon et al.[53] have reported the binding of silver ions to sulfhydryl groups and the consequent inactivation of respiratory chain enzymes, hydroxyl radical formation, and ensuing DNA damage.

Given the similarity of many structural elements that constitute human and bacterial cells, the question arises whether silver ions also interfere analogously with human cell and tissue functions. Indeed, Schrand et al.[54] reported induction of reactive oxygen species (ROS), degradation of mitochondrial membrane integrity, disruption of the actin cytoskeleton, and reduction in proliferation upon stimulation with nerve growth factor upon exposing neuroblastoma cells to silver nanoparticles. It has also been shown that a thin coating of an antimicrobial composite of poly(4-vinylpyridine)-co-poly(vinyl-N-hexylpyridinium bromide) and AgBr nanoparticles on Tygon elastomer tubes caused disruption and activation of blood platelets, making this coating unsuitable for blood-contacting devices applications.[55] It was, however, not clear whether it is the cationic copolymer or the Ag^+ ions, or both, that caused the adverse effects. In addition, another study found that the extent of adverse effects from silver ions differed for different cell lines,[56] which may help explain the inconsistencies in the literature where studies using only one cell line each, and different lines in different studies, have reported conflicting findings. The system developed by Vasilev et al.,[50] described earlier (Fig. 6.2), for obtaining control over loading and rate of release may allow obtaining antibacterial effectiveness while reducing damage to mammalian cells and tissue, as suggested by data (Fig. 6.3) showing that osteoblast cells were able to attach and spread on multilayer coatings of the type shown in Figure 6.2 despite silver ion release. Animal model studies are currently in progress to assess the extent of possible effects on tissue *in vivo* from silver ion release.

Despite concerns regarding toxicity to human cells and tissue and the absence of effectiveness in some *in vivo* studies,[57,58] a range of companies are building their business on silver-releasing coatings or nanosilver-containing products, and research continues on variations of the theme. Perhaps more thought needs to be given where and when such coatings may be suitable or unsuitable; for example, does it matter if a layer of cells next to an implant is

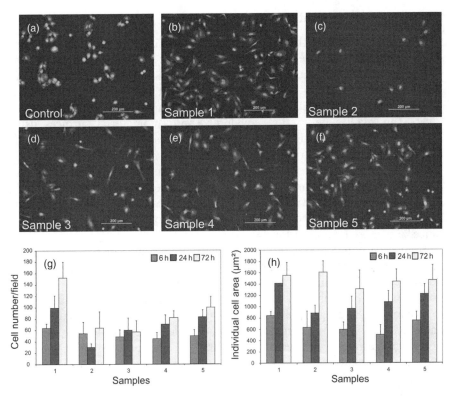

Figure 6.3 Osteoblast cell adhesion and spreading after 24 hours on (a) glass control; (b) heptylamine plasma polymer coating without silver; (c) heptylamine plasma polymer (HApp) coating loaded with silver nanoparticles without an overlayer; (d–f) same as (c) but coated with a HApp overlayer of thickness 6 nm (d), 12 nm (e), and 18 nm (f); (g) cell numbers and (h) individual cell areas after 72 hours on these samples. Adapted from Vasilev et al.[50] by permission of the American Chemical Society, © 2010. (See color insert.)

killed by antibacterial silver? For some devices, it may, whereas for others, it may not matter. The amounts and rates of release may also be important but often have not been adequately characterized. Finally, in cases such as antibacterial skin wound dressings, the short-term uptake of silver ions and the possible death of some human cells may be acceptable when balanced with the need to keep skin wounds free of infections.

In summary, silver ions are clearly effective against various bacteria *in vitro*. However, their clinical effectiveness and their potential for damage to human cells are subject to continuing controversy and concern. The same is likely to apply to other, less well-studied transition metal ions such as copper and selenium. An interesting approach is the use of gallium to interfere with iron uptake by bacteria,[59] but the consequences on human metabolism appear not to be established.

6.2.5 Nonfouling Coatings

It would appear likely that surfaces that can resist protein adsorption and mammalian cell attachment might also be able to resist bacterial colonization. There exists an enormous body of literature on nonfouling surfaces. Permanent attachment-resistant surfaces can be obtained by the grafting of hydrogel polymer layers, with PEG by far the most prominent. Thin PEG hydrogel layers can readily be grafted covalently onto biomaterial surfaces using aqueous solution conditions (e.g., see References 60–63), though marginal salvation conditions are required to obtain a high graft density and complete resistance to protein adsorption.[60] Other nonfouling coatings have been produced by "grafting-to" or surface-initiated polymerization ("grafting-from") of various hydrogel polymers. Several hydrogel coatings, for example, from PEG,[64] polyacrylamide,[16] and polylysine–PEG copolymers[14] have shown resistance to bacterial colonization.

It must be noted, however, that *in vivo* fouling is more complex than what *in vitro* models can mimic at present,[63] and *in vitro* tests of protein and cell resistance may not directly translate to resistance to bacterial attachment *in vivo*. It is also of interest to note that there is a need for *covalent* attachment of nonfouling hydrogel polymers onto the biomaterial surface in order to achieve long-lasting resistance to bacterial settlement.[15] While that study did not speculate on possible reasons, one likely explanation would be that bacteria are capable of displacing adsorbed macromolecules from solid material surfaces due to interfacial energy considerations.

6.2.6 Surface-Grafted Antibacterial Molecules

The covalent grafting of antibacterial compounds onto polymer surfaces has been the subject of considerable research in the search for antibacterial surfaces with longer-lasting effectiveness than is possible via diffusive release approaches. The polymer surfaces onto which grafting was performed were either bulk materials or coatings themselves; in the latter approach, the polymeric coating serves as an adhesive interlayer providing chemical surface groups for covalent grafting, which are not available on the underlying bulk material/device. Antimicrobial agents containing chemically reactive groups such as hydroxyl, carboxyl, and amino can be covalently linked to a wide variety of polymer surfaces using well-established conjugation reactions. While typically covalent grafting is preferred for the reason of, in principle, better adhesive stability, noncovalent attachment modes can also provide useful coatings in some circumstances. For example, Statz et al.[65] synthesized antimicrobial peptoid oligomers with an adhesive peptide moiety that enabled anchoring onto TiO_2 substrata.

Many different compounds have been grafted covalently onto biomaterial surfaces with the aim of producing antibacterial surfaces. Examples of the covalent grafting of bioactive compounds will be presented in Section 6.3; here, we will review briefly the use of compounds that do not possess specific and selective bioactivity; quaternary ammonium compounds (QACs) are the prime example for this class of strategies.

Surfaces modified with QAC layers have attracted considerable interest since the pioneering work of Tiller et al.[66] QACs are antiseptics that act against both gram-positive and gram-negative bacteria. Various reactions have been used to immobilize them onto various biomaterials. Many studies have demonstrated antimicrobial effectiveness of QAC-grafted surfaces, yet the mechanism of antibacterial action of QACs is still not fully resolved; however, two hypotheses appear to be lead contenders. The first and most cited hypothesis is that sufficiently long cationic polymer chains penetrate cell membranes.[66,67] The second hypothesis, proposed by Kugler et al.,[68] suggests that a highly charged surface can induce ion exchange between the positive charges on the surface and structurally essential mobile cations within the bacterial membrane. Being in close contact with a cationic surface, vital divalent cations cannot perform their normal role in charge neutralization of the head groups of membrane lipids, which results in a loss of membrane function, fluidity, and finally integrity. Murata et al.[69] attempted to weigh these hypotheses by varying the chain length containing the QA group and the surface density of QA groups in a gradient manner. It was concluded that the density of surface QA groups, and thus the density of cationic surface charges, is a key parameter; however, the authors did not exclude that membrane insertion of alkyl chains may also be a possible mechanism of action. The relative contributions of these modes may well differ with the molecular nature of the QAC.

As for silver, there is no doubt that QAC coatings can be strongly antibacterial *in vitro*, but the same concern of cytotoxicity applies. It stands to reason that membrane disruption by QACs by insertion or an ion disruption mechanism (or both) would equally apply to human cell membranes. Again, however, in some clinical implant applications, the disruption and death of a layer of cells may be tolerable, whereas, for example, for contact lenses, the irritation caused by QACs affecting cell membranes on the eye and the eyelid would likely not be tolerable.

Other cationic molecules have also been investigated, but as for QACs, the issue of membrane damage to human cells needs to be considered. A number of cationic peptides are known to have antibacterial activity; a well-known example is the bee sting venom melittin.[70] An example of the covalent immobilization of antibacterial peptides is a study in which a polymer surface containing epoxide groups[71] was used to achieve covalent binding, and such peptide-grafted surfaces prevented biofilm formation.[72] Another example reports the use of the peptide magainin, which is found in the skin of a frog, for the creation of an antibacterial coating.[73] However, the formation of pores in eukaryotic cell membranes by such peptides may restrict their use for human clinical applications. It is thus highly desirable to find and surface immobilize compounds with analogous strong activity but less deleterious consequences for cell membranes. A number of studies have immobilized the natural cationic biopolymer chitosan onto material surfaces (e.g., see References 74–76), as chitosan may be better tolerated by the human host body than many other cationic compounds. However, chitosan-coated surfaces appear to be substantially less effective than some other approaches.

6.3   BIOACTIVE ANTIBACTERIAL SURFACES

Antiseptics such as silver (ions) and QACs are nonspecific and nonselective in their action, affecting bacterial cells as well as mammalian cells. A more desirable strategy would seem to be the utilization of bioactive compounds that can exercise a specific action via a known biochemical mechanism. Thus, this section will discuss the use of antibacterial compounds that act via a known, specific pathway or are currently under investigation and may (or may not) act via a biochemically selective pathway for their activity.

The covalent attachment of bioactive antibacterial compounds onto medical device surfaces may provide long-term protection against biofilm formation if the compounds are resistant to degradation by the human body's healing reaction after the surgical procedure. There are, however, a number of other issues that also need to be addressed in the design and development of such coatings. First, covalent grafting may cause side reactions that may convert the molecules to a different molecular structure; for example, β-lactams and furanones readily undergo ring opening in alkaline and acid media. Thus, grafting must be performed in close to neutral pH conditions. Second, covalently grafted molecules may have a geometrically restricted ability to perform their function, such as integrin docking or interaction with the cell membrane. Third, some antibiotics are thought to have an intracellular action, such as the gyrase inhibition of novobiocin and the lux gene deactivation by furanones. Can such compounds be active at all when covalently attached onto a medical implant and thus unable to diffuse into bacterial cells?

6.3.1   Established, Commercially Available Antibiotics

An obvious strategy is the covalent immobilization of known antibiotic compounds onto material surfaces. An example of such surface modification of a bulk polymer is attaching penicillin to poly(tetrafluoroethylene) via a PEG glycol spacer.[77] Wach et al. used an analogous approach to immobilize vancomycin, also via a PEG graft interlayer.[78] Earlier work, also on titanium substrate, suggests that the PEG linker is not necessary for antibacterial activity of vancomycin[79] but is advantageous in reducing surface adhesion of dead bacteria.[78] Vancomycin and polymyxin-B were covalently attached onto hyperbranched poly(N-isopropyl-acrylamide) polymer[80]; in both cases, the conjugated antibiotic did not have bactericidal activity but bound bacteria.

An illustrative example, because of the mechanistic questions it raises, is the work by Ys[81] in which novobiocin was grafted onto a hydrophilic amine

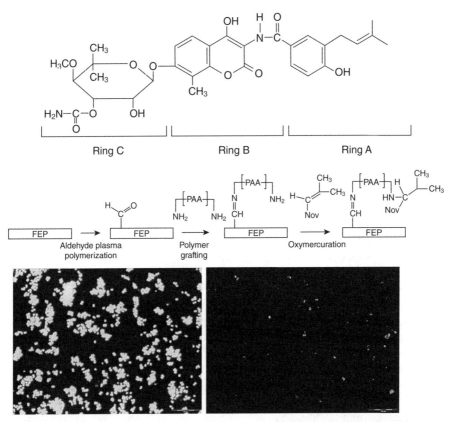

Figure 6.4 Molecular structure of novobiocin, grafting scheme for novobiocin, and bacterial colonization after 4 hours on surfaces of polyallylamine "control" (left) and novobiocin grafted onto polyallylamine (right). Adapted from Ys.[81]

surface coating (polyallylamine grafted onto an aldehyde polymer surface) via a Michael-type addition reaction of the distal C=C bond on novobiocin (structure in Fig. 6.4) via oxymercuration catalysis (Fig. 6.4), onto several material surfaces, including silicon wafers (for spectroscopic analyses) to fluorinated ethylene-propylene copolymer (FEP) sheet material as a model for catheters. Incubation of samples with broth containing *Staphylococcus epidermidis* showed a marked reduction in bacterial attachment (Fig. 6.4). It is thought that the residual few spots of bacterial attachment were at least in part due to coating defects that were unavoidable under the conditions used. With the coating steps not performed under clean room conditions, dust particles were temporarily or permanently adhered to the surface at various steps, as observed in optical microscopy, and this can cause such small coating defects. Nevertheless, a substantial reduction in bacterial attachment is clearly evident. Moreover, whereas on the control surface the bacteria formed clumps and multiplied, on the novobiocin-grafted surface, the few attached bacteria appeared to be static, neither multiplying nor assembling to colonies. Thus, the difference between the novobiocin surface and the control amine surface became more pronounced over time. The absence of formation of bacterial colonies and biofilm on the novobiocin-coated surface is promising, but preclinical (animal model) testing has not been performed yet.

These results raise an interesting question regarding the mechanism of action. Novobiocin is thought to be active intracellularly. The amino-coumarin structure of ring B is considered to be important to the activity of novobiocin as a DNA gyrase-inhibiting agent.[82] It inhibits competitively DNA gyrase (also known as bacterial topoisomerase II) through the blocking of ATP binding. It will then hinder DNA replication and thus bacterial reproduction. Novobiocin is much more effective in inhibiting prokaryote than eukaryote topoisomerase II.[83] However, how can surface-bound novobiocin, presumably unable to enter bacterial cells, act on DNA gyrase? Does it act via a transmembrane switch or is it able to insert into the bacterial membrane such that ring B is exposed to the cytoplasm? It is not understood at present why surface-grafted novobiocin is effective even when covalently linked to solid surfaces and thus presumably unable to enter bacterial cells. Molecular microbiology studies are essential for addressing these questions. The advantage of a novobiocin-grafted surface over the biochemically nonselective approaches discussed in earlier sections derives from the stronger activity of novobiocin against bacterial topoisomerase II compared with the eukaryotic analogues, which may offer an avenue toward a coating that, unlike QACs and several other compounds, causes less damage to human cells and, with a suitably adjusted surface density, may have potential for clinical applications.

Lysozyme is a cationic protein that is well-known for its antibacterial activity; it catalyzes the hydrolysis of 1,4-glycosidic linkages between N-acetymuramic acid and N-acetylglucosamine, which are components of the cell wall peptidoglycans of bacteria. Accordingly, lysozyme is an efficient antibacterial (bacteriolytic) agent against gram-positive bacteria. In contrast to QACs and other cationic polymers, however, it does not affect human ocular epithelial cell membranes. Lysozyme has been grafted onto solid material surfaces in a number of studies, including cografting with PEG,[84] which led to nonfouling surfaces resistant to protein adsorption and bacterial adhesion.

It is, however, not clear whether lysozyme immobilized on a biomedical device surface would be able to survive the proteolytic activity associated with the acute inflammation caused by surgical trauma. Human endogenous host–defense peptides derived from larger proteins, such as CNY21 (CNYITELRRQHARASHLGLAR), a peptide derived from the C-terminal part of complement factor C3a, are effective against bacteria yet are hydrolytically relatively stable and possess low cell toxicity; a recent review discusses interactions between cell wall membranes and such proteins and mutants thereof.[85] It also points out that differences in lipid compositions of prokaryotic and eukaryotic cells lead to differences in the membrane affinity of such peptides.

6.3.2 Experimental Antibiotics

Host–defense peptides typically adopt an amphiphilic conformation, which is hypothesized to be part of their mechanism of antibacterial activity. An interesting approach involves the preparation of synthetic analogues of host–defense peptides from β-peptides,[86] with the intention of mimicking the biological activity of amphiphilic, cationic α-helical antimicrobial peptides found in nature. Antibiotic activity resulted, yet a 17-residue β-peptide also showed very low hemolytic activity against human red blood cells, which indicates selectivity for bacterial cells over mammalian cells. Some of the factors important for activity in this class of peptides were examined.[86] An amphiphilic helix was necessary, and the ratio of cationic to hydrophobic residues was also important. It was suggested that the mode of action involves disruption of microbial membranes. This class of β-peptides is not degraded by proteases, which offers advantages for some biological applications. The same group later found that nylon-3 copolymers, which are much less expensive to produce, likewise can mimic amphiphilic antibacterial host–defense proteins,[87] and structure–activity relationships were elucidated.[88] Particularly encouraging is that surfaces coated with nylon-3 copolymers allowed attachment and spreading of 3T3 fibroblast cells.[89] Biomedical device surfaces carrying such intelligently designed bioactive molecules appear to offer considerable promise for the selective achievement of antibacterial effectiveness with low side effects on human cells and tissue.

β-Lactams form a well-known class of antibiotics, including penicillins. An experimental β-lactam with structural similarity to furanones was covalently attached onto contact lens surfaces and was used in an *in vitro* and *in vivo* study by Zhu et al.[90] Extended-wear silicone hydrogel contact lenses were first equipped with a layer of covalently grafted poly(allylamine), which offered high hydrophilicity. The surface amine groups were then reacted with acrylate groups on the β-lactam (Fig. 6.5). Contact lenses coated thus were studied in both guinea pigs, with the lenses inserted for 1 month, and human volunteers during a 22-hour wear. Reduction in microbial adhesion of up to 92% was observed when comparing coated lenses with control lenses (Fig. 6.5). While these results are promising, cytotoxicity and mutagenic properties of this compound have not been documented, and other antibacterial compounds have shown even greater antibacterial activity.

Many existing antibiotics are derived from leads provided by compounds extracted from natural sources, and plants and marine organisms continue to provide interesting lead compounds. Antibiotics extracted from natural sources form the basis of many novel therapeutic agents as their chemical diversity provides many opportunities for new drug leads. Defense mechanisms against microbial colonization, commonly through the biosynthesis of antimicrobial

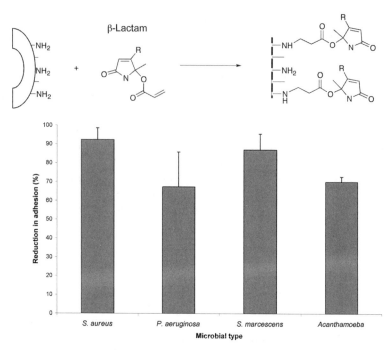

Figure 6.5 Covalent immobilization of an experimental β-lactam onto a contact lens surface and ensuing reductions in microbial adhesion. Adapted from Zhu et al.[90]

compounds, are observed in a variety of organisms, from microorganisms to marine life and terrestrial plants. In fact, many established antibiotics are derived from such leads, for example, penicillin, vancomycin, and erythromycin. Here, two classes of experimental compounds derived from natural sources will serve to illustrate the potential and the challenges when desiring to use them as surface-grafted protective antibacterial coatings.

Halogenated furanones extracted from the Australian marine algae *Delisea pulchra* and synthetic analogues were found to have antibacterial activity against a number of bacteria including the biomedically important *S. epidermidis*.[91] The antibacterial nature of furanones is attributed to their ability to interfere, by structural similarity with homoserine lactone signaling molecules, with bacterial cell communication[92]; quorum sensing is an essential step in the phenotype transformation of surface-adhered bacteria progressing to biofilm formation. Resistance is unlikely to arise since the bacteria are not killed by the furanone. Al-Bataineh et al.[93–96] employed a nitrene-based method for the covalent immobilization of furanones onto surfaces of model biomedical device materials via PEG or poly(acrylic acid) interlayers to achieve hydrophilicity. Coated surfaces were analyzed by X-ray photoelectron spectroscopy[93,94] and time-of-flight secondary ion mass spectrometry[95] to probe for molecules attached to the surface and to check that the functional groups important for antibacterial activity (the lactone ring and the bromines) were still present. It was found that nitrene-grafted furanones showed considerable antibacterial activity, with a 90% reduction in biofilm formation by S. aureus,[96] and thus a sufficient percentage of the molecules must have been attached in ways that did not interfere with their biological function. It was shown later, however, that surface-immobilized furanones did not act on quorum sensing[97]; the activity obtained by Al-Bataineh et al. may have been the result of membranolytic action arising from alkyl side chains. This conjecture is also supported by the fact that Kuehl et al.[97] found the furanone compound used in their study to be toxic to fibroblasts when used in solution. The use of surface-immobilized furanones for biomedical device coatings thus may be limited by the same issue of potential adverse effects on human cells and tissue as for other antimicrobials discussed earlier. Of particular relevance to the present review, however, is that a specific mechanism of activity that pertains in solution may no longer be feasible when a compound is covalently grafted onto surfaces, for example, interference with bacterial adhesion, proliferation, and/ or quorum sensing.

Another example of novel experimental compounds are serrulatanes, which comprise a class of diterpenes found in the Australian plant genus *Eremophila*, some members of which were extensively used in traditional Australian aboriginal medicine in ways that suggest antibacterial activity. Structural elucidation of antimicrobially active compounds isolated from several *Eremophila* plant species has led to the identification of more than 10 diterpene compounds of the serrulatane class that possess activity in solution against gram-positive bacteria associated with biomedical device infections, including methicillin-resistant S. aureus.[98,99] Figure 6.6 shows the general serrulatane skeleton and the structures of representative serrulatanes with antibacterial activity. Active serrulatanes possess hydrophilic substituents such as –COOH, –OH, –OMe, or –OAc in one or both rings, with acetylation or methylation reducing activity.

The compound 8-hydroxyserrulat-14-en-19-oic acid was immobilized covalently onto polymer surfaces carrying amine groups in two ways and orientations: either via carbodiimide formation involving its carboxyl group or via reaction between the pendant alkene bond and surface amine groups catalyzed by mercury salt.[81] The former approach resulted in coatings that showed >99% reduction in bacterial attachment (Fig. 6.6) and biofilm formation *in vitro*. As for novobiocin-grafted surfaces (above), a few isolated attached bacteria did not progress to colony formation and biofilm formation during observation for up to 48 hours. The latter approach was much less effective, indicating a role of the nonpolar "tail," perhaps for membrane insertion. These *in vitro* results suggest potential of these compounds as molecularly grafted antibacterial coating layers, but *in vivo* studies have not been performed yet. Nor is the mechanism elucidated; the phenolic hydroxyl group appears to play a key role; hence, a redox reaction may be involved.

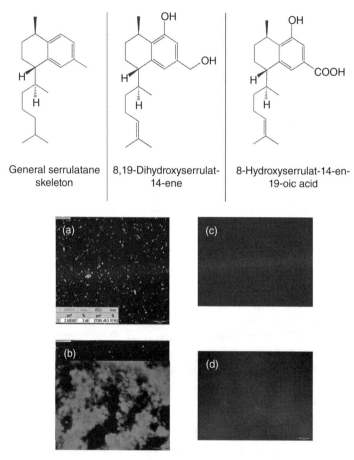

| General serrulatane skeleton | 8,19-Dihydroxyserrulat-14-ene | 8-Hydroxyserrulat-14-en-19-oic acid |

Figure 6.6 Molecular structure of serrulatanes and fluorescence microscopy images of bacterial colonization after 2 hours (top) and 6 hours (bottom) onto amine control surfaces (left) and serrulatane grafted surfaces (right). In image (b) the commencement of biofilm formation is evident. The diffuse color in (d) is due to the diffusion of dye into the polymer material, not to biofilm staining as in (b). Adapted from Ys.[81] (See color insert.)

6.4 STIMULUS-RESPONSIVE ANTIBACTERIAL COATINGS FOR WOUND DRESSINGS

The antimicrobial systems discussed thus far are all essentially passive: They either slowly elute their antimicrobial moiety over time, providing a high concentration zone of, for example, silver, close to the surface, prevent attachment of bacteria, or attempt to kill bacteria on contact as in the case of QACs. These are all valid strategies and are often highly effective, but there are some specific situations where continually eluting an antimicrobial into its local environment may cause problems. It may be much preferable in some applications to utilize a stimulus-responsive system that can sense the onset of an infection and initiate mitigating action. This can, however, be quite challenging, and little has been published on this with regard to antimicrobial action, although in the general biomaterials literature, there has been a substantial increase in interest in materials that respond to various stimuli.[100] A recent review by Gupta surveyed what were termed "smart" wound dressings: dressings that positively assisted the wound to heal and/or fight infection.[101]

Wounds are highly susceptible to infection when skin, the primary defense against infection, becomes compromised. Most wounds are accidental, but the insertion of central venous catheters and other fluid lines into patients effectively creates a wound that can be highly susceptible to infection. As a result of line sepsis, patients have an on average 5 days longer stay in intensive care units and 9 days longer in hospital.[102] Based on a conservative estimate, the total extra costs due to line sepsis are almost $1 billion annually in the United States alone.[103] One of the other big infection problems in clinical settings is that of burn infection. Burns are very common and are also very susceptible to bacterial infection. It is estimated that infection is responsible for greater than 50% of all burn-related fatalities. Children under 5 years old are a subgroup particularly susceptible to scald burns; in the United Kingdom, they comprise 7% of the population yet receive 53% of all scald injuries. Although not always so serious in older children and adults, young children can be severely burnt, with full and partial thickness burns just from a cup of tea. Babies under 2 years old, with relatively underdeveloped immune systems, can fall victim to toxic shock syndrome (TSS), caused by toxic shock toxin expressed by *Streptococcus pyogenes* and some *Staphylococcus* species.[104] TSS causes a massive immune system overresponse, with massive cytokine activation often leading (if untreated) rapidly to death.

A case study illustrates the problem of infection in children:[105] 2-year-old Amy was camping with her parents in South West England when she pulled a cup of tea over herself. She suffered 15% body surface area partial thickness burns from the scalding water. She was treated at Frenchay Hospital using a non-antimicrobial coated dressing, which promotes rapid healing. This dressing, once applied, needs to be left *in situ* without being changed, for up to 2 weeks, to allow skin re-epithelialization without scarring. Unfortunately, Amy developed a bacterial infection under the dressing a few days after injury. This could only be treated by the removal of the dressing and by thorough cleaning of the wound under anesthesia, nursing in critical care, an extended hospital stay (with associated cost), and tragically, permanent, life-long scarring. If the dressing had the ability to treat or prevent biofilm development allowing the wound-healing properties of the dressing to fully realize their effect, Amy's outcome may well have been different with complete wound healing.

A number of antimicrobial wound dressings do exist, including Acticoat™ made by Smith & Nephew and Melgisorb Ag made by Mölnlycke. They work very effectively in many clinical situations by releasing silver ions into the wound environment, preventing infection from taking hold. However, there is some cause for concern regarding silver for three principal reasons:

(1) Virtually all antimicrobials are somewhat cytotoxic, and silver is no exception. The goal is to use an antimicrobial at concentrations below its cytotoxic level but above its antimicrobial minimum inhibition concentration (MIC). A study published in 2004 showed evidence of *in vitro* toxicity of Acticoat against keratinocytes.[106]

(2) Continually exposing a bacterial population to an antimicrobial, especially at subcritical concentrations required to kill all the population, is a highly effective method to accelerate the evolution of resistant species.[107]

(3) Many silver-based dressings contain nanocrystaline silver. Shape-mediated toxicity, particularly from nanoparticles, is still poorly understood, but there is a risk both of generalized toxicity and/or removal of regulatory approval for such dressings. A study by Asharani et al. in 2008 considered silver nanoparticle toxicity in developing zebra fish and found evidence of both systemic and developmental toxicity.[108]

All these factors are not necessarily a reason not to use silver as an antimicrobial, but suggest that having silver ions continually present in a wound may not always be desirable. One simple alternative to using antimicrobial-enabled dressings on burns, for example, is not to use them from the time of initial treatment but only if infection takes hold. The difficulty with this approach, particularly with children, is that the clinical symptoms of infection can be virtually indistinguishable from clinical shock and nonspecific sickness. Moreover, the removal of dressings to apply antimicrobial therapy can delay healing, leading to scar formation.

Accordingly, there is increasing interest in creating responsive wound dressing systems, but most are based on monitoring changes in wound pH, which may indicate the state of wound healing and the presence of infection.[109] For example, Garbern et al. have developed a polymer gel drug delivery system designed to respond to pH and temperature around wound and/or tumor sites.[110]

The concept being developed by a team at the University of Bath in the United Kingdom toward developing antimicrobial dressings is to engineer a responsive dressing: that is to say, a dressing that detects infection in a wound/burn, and *only* if bacteria are present above a threshold population, responds by releasing a previously encapsulated antimicrobial substance, such as silver nitrate, while also signaling colorimetrically that infection has taken hold.[111] The trigger for response in this system is not, however, based on pH, but instead utilizes the lytic toxins secreted by key pathogenic bacteria such as *S. aureus* and *Pseudomonas aeruginosa* as infection takes hold. Such bacteria secrete toxins to break down host tissue, providing nutrients and assisting the bacteria in colonizing the host wound environment. Many *S. aureus* strains,

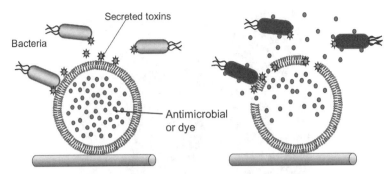

Figure 6.7   Virulence factors (toxins and enzymes) released from pathogenic bacteria break down vesicles in a wound dressing, inducing release of the vesicle contents, which could be an antimicrobial and/or a dye.

for example, secrete hemolysins and leukocidins, which create pores in healthy cells, thus causing their death, while *P. aeruginosa* expresses phospholipases (among other toxins and enzymes), which catalytically hydrolyze cell phospholipids.

The technology in the putative Bath dressing utilizes these secreted virulence factors against their hosts by using them to lyse lipid vesicles (liposomes) containing an antimicrobial or a dye, as illustrated in Figure 6.7.[112]

Data published in Reference 112 show that only pathogenic *S. aureus* and *P. aeruginosa* induce vesicle lysis, with a nonpathogenic strain of *Escherichia coli* not affecting vesicle integrity. Recent work has investigated methods to stabilize the vesicles out of water yet retain their toxin susceptibility. A number of methods are currently being studied, but promising early results have utilized an approach originally pioneered by Ringsdorf in 1971 and developed by Kolusheva[113] using photopolymerizable fatty acids to "strengthen" the lipid bilayer membrane. Results are shown in Figure 6.8, where nonwoven fabric has been treated with stabilized lipid vesicles containing self-quenched carboxyfluorescein. This molecule forms a dimer at concentrations above ~10 mmol/dm³, quenching its own fluorescence, but upon dilution, it "switches on" its fluorescence. Figure 6.8 shows the effect of inoculating the vesicle-containing fabric with pathogenic *S. aureus* and *P. aeruginosa*, and nonpathogenic *E. coli*, after drying the fabric for 2 days before rewetting. The pathogenic bacteria appear to induce fluorescence "switch on."

Recent work has looked at evaluating the optimum antimicrobial for encapsulation. The antimicrobial must not permeate the lipid membrane and should therefore be water soluble. Good results with sodium azide, silver nitrate, and gentamicin sulfate have all been recorded so far, with selective killing of only pathogenic but not nonpathogenic bacteria. This project, funded by the European Commission, is in its infancy in early 2011, but it is hoped to have manufacturable prototype dressings being tested in preclinical trials by 2014. The concept has been patented (EPO, Munich, March 2010).

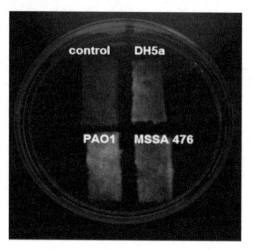

Figure 6.8   Effect of inoculating vesicle-modified fabric (a crude wound dressing material) with either HEPES buffer or nonpathogenic *E. coli* (top row) and pathogenic bacteria (bottom row). (See color insert.)

6.5   ANTI-INFLAMMATORY SURFACES

6.5.1   The Inflammatory Response

The inflammatory response is one of the first reactions of the human body to infection, irritation, or other injuries, such as insertion of a foreign material, a medical device, or implant, and is recognized as one type of nonspecific immune response. The macroscopic features are redness, warmth, swelling, and often pain. The inflammatory response directs the immune system components to the site of injury or infection and is manifested by increased blood supply and vascular permeability, which allows chemotactic peptides, neutrophils, and mononuclear cells to leave the blood vessels and enter the inflamed tissue area. Microorganisms, dirt particles, or degradable implant materials are engulfed by phagocytic cells (such as neutrophils and macrophages) in an attempt to restrict the infection/tissue damage to a small area. In the natural situation, the inflammatory response precedes healing and ends with the removal of the infected or damaged tissue by phagocytosis.

In the case of an inflammatory response after implantation of a medical device, the material characteristics, as well as the production of degradation products, affect the inflammatory response. Moreover, the size, shape, and physical/chemical properties of the implanted devices contribute to variations in the intensity and duration of the inflammatory response and subsequent wound-healing process.[114,115] One distinguishes between acute and chronic inflammatory responses. The acute inflammatory response starts immediately after medical device implantation as fluids, plasma proteins, and inflammatory cells migrate to the implantation site.[115,116] The acute inflammatory response lasts for the first 24–48 hours and is characterized by the presence of blood-derived neutrophils, which are later replaced by monocytes differentiating into macrophages. The anti-inflammatory sequence ends with the departure of macrophages through the lymphatics.

The switch to an at least intermediate chronic inflammatory phase is manifested by the occurrence of lymphocytes, plasma cells, and mononuclear cells. The chronic inflammatory response to biomaterials is usually of short duration (less than 2 weeks) and is restricted to the implant site.[115,116] The inflammatory response must be actively terminated when no longer needed to prevent unnecessary further tissue damage. Failure to stop inflammation results in chronic inflammation, cellular destruction, and attempts to heal the inflamed tissue. One intrinsic mechanism employed to terminate inflammation is the short half-life of inflammatory mediators *in vivo*. They have a limited time frame to affect their targets before breaking down into nonfunctional components; therefore, constant inflammatory stimulation is needed to propagate their effects. Active mechanisms that serve to terminate inflammation include transforming growth factor (TGF)-β secretion by macrophages, anti-inflammatory lipoxins, and inhibition of proinflammatory molecules, such as leukotrienes. Lipoxins are short-lived endogenously produced nonclassic eiconosaids whose appearance signals the end of inflammation. At present, two lipoxins have been identified; lipoxin A_4 (LXA_4) and lipoxin B_4 (LXB_4). Leukotrienes are naturally produced eicosanoid lipid mediators of the immune system that contribute to inflammation, for example, in asthma and bronchitis. Leukotriene antagonists are used to treat asthma and bronchitis.

6.5.2 Contact Activation of the Complement System

During the implantation process, the medical device or biomaterial will have direct contact with human blood. Therefore, in addition to the inflammatory response, a part of the nonspecific immune system will be activated; namely, the complement system, which consists of ca. 30 plasma- and membrane-bound proteins that are activated in a cascade manner. The complement system is able to discriminate between "self" and "nonself." The complement cascade can be activated by three different pathways; one of them is triggered by direct contact of blood with biomaterial surfaces. This pathway is referred to as the alternative pathway (for a review, see Reference 117). The complement system tries to destroy and remove substances either by direct lysis or by mediating leukocyte functions in inflammatory responses and nonspecific (innate) immunity. The main event in the activation of the complement cascade is the enzymatic generation of anaphylatoxic peptides, C3a and C5a, which induce damage through their effects on monocytes/macrophages, polymorphonuclear leukocytes (PMNs), and mast cells. Cleavage of C3 into C3b and C3a is achieved by two enzyme complexes, the C3 convertases(C4b,2a and C3b,Bb, respectively), which can be assembled by three different activation pathways, one of which is the alternative pathway taking place directly on the surface of an implanted biomaterial (Fig. 6.9).

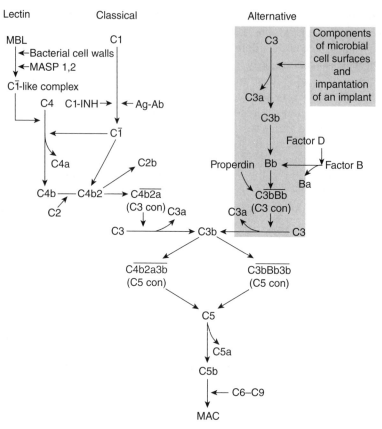

Figure 6.9 The classical, lectin, and alternative pathways converge into a final common pathway when C3 convertase (C3 con) cleaves C3 into C3a and C3b. Ab, antibody; Ag, antigen; C1-INH, C1 inhibitor; MAC, membrane attack complex; MASP, mannose-binding lectin-associated serine protease; MBL, mannose-binding lectin; P, properdin, overbar indicates activation. Adapted from http://www.merckmanuals.com/professional/immunology_allergic_disorders/biology_of_the_immune_system/complement_system.html[238].

Different biomaterial surfaces activate the complement differently. Hydrophobicity and hydrophilicity affect the activation, with hydrophobic surfaces being more potent activators than hydrophilic ones. Biomaterial surfaces with free OH and NH_2 groups are generally regarded as more prone to activate the complement than others since these groups are essential for the covalent binding of C3b.[118,119] It was shown that the very small amount of C3 adsorbed with serum and blood proteins in the first minutes after the implantation of a biomaterial is sufficient to assemble C3 convertase complexes.[120,121] *In vitro*, the activation of the C3 convertase complex was demonstrated after C3 adsorption on human albumin and immunoglobulins but not on fibrinogen.[118,120] Once C3b is generated and covalently bound to the protein coat on the biomaterial surface, the alternative pathway amplification loop can be triggered. This amplification loop then generates the majority of C3b molecules adsorbed to the material surface. C3a and C3b are ligands for receptors on leukocytes (PMNs, monocytes, and mast cells) that then trigger inflammation and release proinflammatory cytokines such as IL-1β, TNF-α, IL-6, and chemokine IL-8. Another effect of complement activation is the upregulation of receptors on leukocytes (e.g., CD11b/CD 18 and CD35), which, together with downregulation of L-selectin, makes the cells very adhesive and prone to interact with platelets and endothelial cells of adjacent blood vessels.[122,123] Therefore, the complement system is a major inflammatory system that acts upstream to induce a number of secondary inflammatory mediators, and generating biomaterials that are complement compatible is therefore of great importance.

6.5.3   Foreign Body Reaction

Depending on the size and chemical composition of the implanted biomaterial, macrophages are able to phagocytose and remove objects (smaller than 5 μm); the classical foreign body reaction is induced when the objects are larger than ~10 μm. The foreign body reaction follows a series of processes that are induced by the implantation of a medical device, a biomaterial, or an implant.[115] The initial steps that occur already during implantation will be direct contact with human blood and injured tissue, leading to adsorption of serum proteins onto the surface of the implant. Initially, the most abundant and relatively small serum protein albumin (42 mg/mL) will cover the surface that will then, depending on the surface chemistry and charge, be replaced by less abundant but larger glycoproteins such as fibrinogen (3 mg/mL), immunoglobulins (11 mg/mL), and less by vitronectin, plasma fibronectin, von Willebrand factor, and members of the complement system such as C3 and C3 convertases. This replacement will take place during the first few minutes to hours after implantation; it is commonly referred to as the Vroman effect.[124,125]

In parallel, tissue healing is initiated with the recruitment and infiltration of inflammatory cells: PMNs, monocytes, and lymphocytes. In the initial acute inflammatory phase, mast cells and PMNs secrete interleukin-4 (IL-4) and interleukin-13 (IL-13), which might lead to a transient chronic inflammatory phase, thereby stimulating T-helper cells and monocyte-to-macrophage differentiation on the biomaterial surface. In later stages of the healing response around the biomaterial, granulation tissue is formed. It contains a variety of cell types including fibroblasts that are responsible for the secretion and production of the provisional wound-healing matrix initially consisting of fibrin, later containing mostly collagen type I. Within the granulation tissue, many new blood vessels are formed that allow tissue perfusion with oxygen and nutrition.

On biomaterial surfaces, blood-bound monocytes adhere and differentiate, induced by IL-4 and IL-13, into adherent macrophages that upregulate the expression of mannose receptors on their surfaces. Mannose receptors are accumulated at contact areas between adjacent macrophages and facilitate macrophage fusion to foreign body giant cells.[115,126,127] The foreign body giant cells cover the biomaterial/medical implant and recruit fibroblasts that then start producing the fibrous capsule. Once the fibrous capsule is formed, direct contact between the implant (surface) and the tissue is inhibited.

6.5.4 Anti-inflammatory Medication

Certain types of surgeries such as cardiac surgery and cardiopulmonary bypass (CPB) produce a systemic whole-body inflammatory response induced by the contact with foreign material surfaces.[128] This is followed by the activation of the complement system producing a massive acute inflammatory response.[129] During and after implanting a CPB, more than 70 hormones, cytokines, chemokines, vasoactive substances, cytotoxins, ROS, and proteases of the coagulation and fibrinolytic systems induce mild to huge interstitial fluid shifts, generate a host of microemboli of less than 500 microns, and result in a temporary dysfunction of nearly every organ.[128–132] In such cases, systemic treatment of inflammation is needed as the inflammatory response spreads over the entire patient's body, and a local reduction of the inflammatory response by an intelligent surface coating on an implanted device would not be sufficient. Current treatments against inflammation involve glucocorticosteroids (GCs), non-steroidal anti-inflammatory drugs (NSAIDs), and therapeutic proteins.

GCs bind to glucocorticoid receptors and reduce swelling and inflammation. Corticosteroid treatment may reduce the inflammatory response in humans by several distinct mechanisms. GCs act by binding to a cytosolic glucocorticosteroid receptor (GR), which are subsequently activated by a conformational change and are able to translocate to the nucleus.[133] Once in the nucleus, the GR either binds to DNA and switches on the expression of anti-inflammatory genes or acts indirectly to repress the activity of a number of distinct signaling pathways such as nuclear factor (NF)-kB and activator protein (AP)-1, cAMP response element-binding protein (CREB), interferon regulatory factor 3 (IRF3), nuclear factor of activated T cells (NFAT), signal transducer and activator of transcription (STAT), T-box expressed in T cells (T-Bet), and GATA-3.[134,135] Typical target genes regulate a vast number of inflammatory proteins such as IL-1α, IL-2, IL-4, IL-5, IL-6, IL-8, IL-12, IL-18, cyclooxygenase (COX)-2, E-selectin, inducible nitric oxide synthase (iNOS), interferon (IFN)-α, TNF-α, and intercellular adhesion molecule (ICAM), monocyte chemoattractant protein 1 (MCP-1) chemokine (C-C motif), and ligand 2 vascular cell adhesion molecule (VCAM). Because of their variety in functions, GCs are used clinically to treat inflammatory, autoimmune, and allergic disorders; to attenuate organ rejection after transplantation, to treat brain edema, shock, and various blood cancers; and to balance out adrenal cortex insufficiencies.

A number of synthetic analogues of the natural human glucocorticoid cortisol have been developed by the pharmaceutical industry and include, among others, dexamethasone (DEX), betamethasone, triamcinolone, prednisone, prednisolone, and methylprednisolone.[136] Methylprednisolone, for example, lowers post-CPB concentrations of the proinflammatory cytokines TNF-α, IL-6, and IL-8, and increases concentrations of the anti-inflammatory cytokines IL-10 and IL-1ra, but not IL-4.[137–139] Corticosteroids also attenuate post-CPB leukocyte activation, neutrophil adhesion molecule upregulation, and pulmonary neutrophil sequestration.[137,138]

NSAIDs act by blocking the activity of COXs and by inhibition of blood clot formation. The body produces several different forms of COX, including COX-1, which is involved in pain, clotting, and protecting the gastrointestinal tract, and COX-2, which is involved in the pain produced by inflammation. Most of the NSAIDs (such as aspirin) inhibit both; however, some newer drugs, the so-called COX-2 inhibitors, are much more active against COX-2 than against COX-1. COX-2 inhibitors are effective against inflammation and seem to avoid damage to the gastrointestinal tract, but unfortunately, they increase the risk of blood clot formation.

Other possibilities consist of application of high doses of free radical scavengers and antioxidants such as high doses of vitamin C (250 mg/day) and E (300 mg/day) or N-acetylcysteine.[140] Generation of ROS, such as hydrogen peroxide and the superoxide and hydroxyl radicals, occurs upon contact with implant materials and usually retards the healing process. Free radical scavengers decrease cell membrane lipid peroxidation, reducing the neutrophil oxidative burst response and elastase activity,[141] thus reducing the inflammatory response. Moreover, vitamin E inhibits platelet aggregation *in vitro*,[142,143] thus potentially rendering biomaterial surfaces less thrombogenic.

Lipoproteins such as HDL at physiological concentrations protect against inflammatory responses by inhibiting the interaction of monocytes with endothelial cells and smooth muscle cells as well as the adhesion of monocytes to endothelial cells.[144,145] Recent studies have shown that cytokine-induced expression of VCAM-1, ICAM-1, and E-selectin is inhibited by HDL.[146,147] Moreover, transforming growth factor-β2 (TGF-β2) expression was specifically increased, mediating HDLs anti-inflammatory actions.[145]

Several therapeutic proteins have been recombinantly produced and used to reduce the inflammatory response. Aprotinin, also called Trasylol, is the best known and most studied therapeutic protein. Aprotinin is a monomeric (single-chain) globular polypeptide derived from bovine lung; it has a molecular weight of 6512 Da.[148,149] Aprotinin is a nonspecific serine protease inhibitor and has multiple actions that may suppress the inflammatory response, particularly at higher doses. Anti-inflammatory effects include attenuation of platelet activation, maintenance of platelet function, reduced complement activation, inhibition of kallikrein production, decreased release of TNF-α, IL-6, and IL-8, inhibition of endogenous cytokine-induced NO synthase induction, decreased CPB-induced leukocyte activation, and inhibition of the upregulation of monocyte and granulocyte adhesion molecules. Aprotinin was used to reduce bleeding during complex surgery, such as heart and liver surgery, where its main effect was to slow down the breakdown of blood clots. However, aprotinin was temporarily withdrawn from clinical use worldwide in 2007 after studies suggested that its use increased the risk of complications or death.[150] These findings were confirmed by follow-up studies and aprotinin/Trasylol was permanently withdrawn from the market in May 2008.

An alternative therapy has been described as antiselectin therapy: It is supposed to prevent the adhesion of leukocytes. L-selectin plays an important role in the complex process of leukocyte recruitment in the initial stages of inflammation.[123] By functioning as both adhesion and signaling molecule, L-selectin contributes to both the early adhesive events as well as the later stages of chemotaxis and cell migration. L-selectin ligand expression at sites of inflammation results in L-selectin playing an important role in the development of autoimmune and chronic inflammatory diseases. Only one selectin-directed therapy has so far demonstrated clinical success: the pan-selectin antagonist bimosiamose. Bimosiamose is a low-molecular-weight nonoligosaccharide selectin inhibitor and has been reported to prevent P-, E-, and L-selectin-mediated adhesion *in vitro*.[151,152] However, further studies *in vivo* have indicated that bimosiamose functions primarily by blocking E-selectin-mediated adhesion.[153] Clinical trials using bimosiamose have shown some promise.

To reduce the activation of the immune system upon direct contact with the surface of a medical implant, targeting of the complement cascade may be a useful strategy to limit the inflammatory response. Therapies that utilize endogenous soluble complement inhibitors may be suitable for reducing contact activation and thereby controlling the inflammatory response. A recent two-stage randomized clinical trial of a monoclonal antibody specific for human C5 demonstrated efficacy and safety in patients undergoing CPB.[154] The generation of activated complement mediators and leukocyte adhesion molecule formation was inhibited in a dose-dependent manner. These data suggest that C5 inhibition may represent a promising therapeutic modality for preventing complement-mediated inflammation. Other promising strategies might include monoclonal antibodies against C3 and C5a and strategies that attenuate complement receptor-3-mediated adhesion of inflammatory cells to the surface of a medical implant. Other therapeutic proteins include an IL-1 antagonist that binds and inactivates the IL-1 receptor[155]; a soluble version of the TNF-α receptor can be used to competitively bind TNF-α, thus preventing it from carrying out its many inflammatory actions.[156,157] Infliximab (trade name Remicade®) is a monoclonal antibody that binds to TNF-α, thus competitively inhibiting TNF-α.[158,159]

6.5.5 Local Prevention of the Inflammatory Reaction on Medical Device/Implant Surfaces

Many efficient systemic anti-inflammatory drugs such as corticosteroids or protein C have serious side effects in that they increase the risk of infection. The bacterial burden needs to be as low as possible especially after the implantation of a biomaterial or medical device. Therefore, systemic treatment with anti-inflammatory drugs might be avoided when surfaces of biomaterials and medical devices display an anti-inflammatory character. Several approaches have been performed, which will be discussed next:

(1) prevention of contact activation of the complement system;
(2) prevention of the foreign body reaction by preventing macrophage adhesion and fusion;
(3) prevention of inflammation on material surfaces by the production and release of nitrous oxide (NO), which inhibits platelet adhesion and activation; and
(4) reduction of the inflammatory response by increasing hemocompatibility.

6.5.5.1 *Prevention of Contact Activation of the Complement System*
Compstatin represents a potent inhibitor of the complement system. Compstatin is a cyclic peptide that binds to C3 and inhibits cleavage to C3a and C3b and has been shown to prevent binding of C3/C3 fragments to a polyvinylchloride (PVC) surface.[122] The study was carried out by surface plamon resonance, where 300 µg/cm^2 of C3b was coupled by amine bonds to CM5 chips and binding constants of Compstatin to different C3b forms were determined. Moreover, soluble C3a and C3b complexes were detected by ELISA after circulating EDTA-anticoagulated human whole blood in two models for extracorporeal circulation involving PVC tubings.

Downstream reactions of adhesion and activation of PMNs were significantly reduced. Compstatin was developed from a clone of a phage-displayed random peptide library that was screened for binding to C3b. Compstatin consists of 13 amino acids (ICVVQDWGHHRCT-NH2) that form a cyclic structure by the formation of a disulfide bond. Further studies with analogues and the solution structure of the peptide have indicated that a type-1 β-turn of the peptide is critical for the preservation of its conformational stability and probably forms the C3 binding site.[160,161] The mechanism of action seems to be that cleavage of native C3 was completely inhibited when C3 was added to surface-bound C3 convertase complexes in the presence of Compstatin, thus not preventing adsorption and assembly of the C3 convertase complex on a polymer surface but inhibiting the amplification loop.[122] In an *in vitro* tubing loop model, a 40× excess compared to C3 was necessary to inhibit the amplification loop. Importantly, leukocyte and erythrocyte counts were not affected, which suggests that Compstatin is not toxic to blood cells.[122] Therefore, surface-attached Compstatin might be a good option for the prevention of biomaterial-induced complement activation. However, it needs to be investigated if Compstatin is equally efficient when immobilized on a biomaterial surface.

6.5.5.2 *Prevention of the Foreign Body Reaction by Preventing Macrophage Adhesion and Fusion*

The foreign body reaction on the surface of an implant might be reduced or inhibited if macrophage adhesion and fusion can be inhibited (Fig. 6.10). Macrophages are the key cells that induce the foreign body reaction by the recruitment of leucocytes as well as by the upregulation of proteolytic enzymes (e.g., matrix metalloproteinase MMP-9) and their inhibitors TIMP-1 and TIMP-2. Macrophage migration toward the implant surface might be inhibited by several strategies as human macrophages were shown to exhibit both amoeboid and mesenchymal migration.[162] In the native situation, these migratory mechanisms should allow macrophages to migrate through all the anatomical boundaries found in the body and reach the site of injury and inflammation. Macrophages adapt their migration mode according to the matrix architecture. Pharmacological targeting of

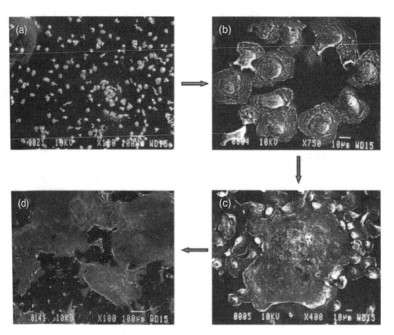

Figure 6.10 Scanning electron microscopy images of Elasthane 80A polyurethane samples from an *in vivo* case study showing the morphological progression of the foreign body reaction. The sequence of events at the polyurethane surface includes (a) monocyte adhesion (0 days), (b) monocyte-to-macrophage development (3 days), (c) ongoing macrophage–macrophage fusion (7 days), and (d) foreign body giant cells (14 days). Adapted from Anderson et al.[115] with permission from Elsevier, © 2008.

macrophage migration-related molecules for the development of new anti-inflammatory drugs, for example, directed against MMP-9 or macrophage surface integrins, might be a promising approach to inhibit macrophage attachment on a biomaterial surface.

Moreover, biomaterial surfaces that prevent adhesion of vitronectin[163] or plasma fibronectin[164] might be able to reduce macrophage adhesion and fusion. The extracellular matrix (ECM) protein fibronectin is recognized by macrophages and is frequently used on biomaterial surfaces to enhance cellular adhesion and tissue integration. Macrophage interaction with fibronectin on a biomaterial surface has been shown to induce a variety of inflammatory responses including secretion of IL-1.[165] Plasma fibronectin was found to significantly increase macrophage IL-1β mRNA expression and protein secretion after plasma fibronectin complexation with α5β1 integrin on the macrophage surface. When fibronectin was adsorbed on clinically relevant polymer surfaces such as PU, poly(dimethylsiloxane) (PDMS), polyethylene (PE), expanded polytetrafluoroethylene (ePTFE), Dacron, and PS, it was found that the physicochemical characteristics of the materials affected macrophage responses. Macrophage IL-1β secretion was decreased on polymer surfaces preadsorbed with fibronectin, IgG, or fibrinogen in comparison with surfaces without adsorbed proteins.[166] In contrast, the concentration of IL-1β increased on Dacron preadsorbed with fibronectin and was undetectable on PE. IL-1β concentrations varied among the different polymers preadsorbed with fibronectin and appeared to be related to the water contact angle of the surface. Increases in IL-1β concentration correlated with a decrease in surface water contact angle.[167,168] Further research compared PDMS and low-density polyethylene (LDPE) versus PS control surfaces. Without preadsorption of fibronectin, the IL-1β concentration was lower on PDMS as compared to PS. Following preadsorption of fibronectin, the IL-1β concentration decreased on both PDMS and PS surfaces, although the IL-1β concentration remained higher on PS controls as compared with PDMS.[166]

Generally, the chemical composition, biophysics, and topography of a biomaterial surface affect serum protein adsorption, which in turn affects the nature and amount of macrophage adhesion and fusion. It seems that each biomaterial needs to be assessed in terms of its individual capabilities in inducing an inflammatory response.

Future approaches might also include surface immobilization of antibodies against IL-4 and IL-13 as they were shown to induce the upregulation of the mannose receptors on fusing macrophages.[126,127,169] Last but not least, apoptosis of adherent macrophages might be induced by the release of TNF-α, which has been shown to induce apoptosis of biomaterial-adhered macrophages.[170]

6.5.5.3 *Prevention of Inflammation on Material Surfaces by the Release of NO* NO is a well-known inhibitor of platelet activation and adhesion and thereby reduces the inflammatory response. Polymers that release or generate NO at their surfaces have been shown to exhibit enhanced thromboresistance

in vivo when in contact with flowing blood, as well as to reduce inflammatory responses when placed subcutaneously. Locally elevated NO levels at the surface of implanted devices can be achieved by using polymers that incorporate NO donor species that can decompose and release NO spontaneously when in contact with physiological fluids, or NO-generating polymers that possess an immobilized catalyst that decomposes endogenous *S*-nitrosothiols (RSNOs) to generate NO *in situ*.

NO exerts its antiplatelet function by binding to the heme iron of soluble guanylate cyclase and subsequently increasing the production and intracellular concentrations of cyclic guanosine monophosphate (cGMP).[171] The endogenous concentration of NO as dissolved gas is very low ($\sim$3 nM).[172] Under physiological conditions, oxidized NO (in the form of NO^+ or N_2O_3) reacts with thiol groups in cysteine or cysteine-containing peptides and proteins (e.g., glutathione, albumin, and hemoglobin) to yield RSNOs.[172,173] RSNOs act as carriers of NO in the body and are thought to be responsible for the storage and bioavailability of NO.[172,174] Physiologically, NO is synthesized in endothelial cells from L-arginine and oxygen by enzymes known as nitric oxide synthases (NOSs)[175] and diffuses, for example, into circulating platelets, especially when they approach the surface of the endothelium. Platelet activation is Ca^{2+} dependent and is thus inhibited by NO.[176,177] The lifetime of NO in whole blood is very short (<1 second) due to its reaction with heme-containing compounds such as oxyhemoglobin of red blood cells.[178] Therefore, the antiplatelet effect occurs only locally when platelets are in close proximity, as the presence of red blood cells would block the NO transfer. It has been estimated that the endothelium-generated NO flux is in the range of 0.5×10^{-10} to 4.0×10^{-10} mol/cm^2/min.[179] Therefore, if the surface of a medical implant can release or generate NO at or above this range of flux, released NO will be effective only locally at the blood/biomaterial interface. Three general procedures have been used in the preparation of diazeniumdiolate-based NO-releasing polymers (Fig. 6.11): (i) dispersion of small amine-based diazeniumdiolate molecules into polymer matrices (e.g., DBHD/N_2O_2) (Batchelor et al.[180]); (ii) diazeniumdiolation of covalently linked amine sites on pendant polymer side chains, or on the polymer backbone[44]; and (iii) covalent binding of diazeniumdiolate groups to micro- or nanoparticles, and use of such particles as polymer fillers.[181] The half-life of NO release can be modulated by selecting different secondary amine structures,[182] and the NO flux can be tuned by changing the amount of diazeniumdiolate dopant, by the hydrophobicity of the polymer matrices, or by applying a polymeric coating to control the diffusion of water into the layer containing the NO-releasing polymer. The leaching of noncovalently bound small molecule diazeniumdiolates can be greatly reduced by using highly lipophilic diazeniumdiolates blended into the polymer matrix.[180]

The two most widely investigated NO donors for biomedical applications are RSNO and *N*-diazeniumdiolates (so-called NONOates). RSNOs can be prepared by reacting thiols with nitrous acid. *S*-Nitrosoglutathione (GSNO) and *S*-nitroso-*N*-acetyl-cysteine (SNAC) have been blended into various

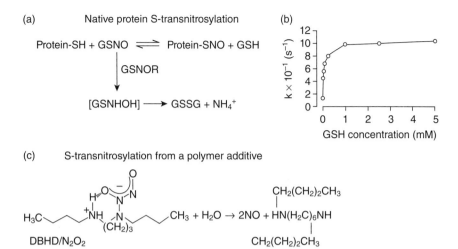

Figure 6.11 Prevention of inflammation on material surfaces by the production and release of NO. (a) "NO generation" that utilize endogenous RSNO species exist in physiological fluids as a continuously replenishing NO donor to generate enhanced NO levels at the blood/polymer interface, for example, nitrosoalbumin by transnitrosation. Transnitrosation reactions occur *in vivo* so that the nitroso-group can be transferred from one thiol to another.[173,174] (b) Denitrosation of N-acetyl-nitroso-Trp (NANT) by glutathione (GSH). The decomposition of NANT (100 mM) was followed spectrophotometrically at 335 nm upon incubation with increasing concentrations of GSH in 100 mM phosphate buffer (pH 7.4) containing 100 mM DTPA. NANT decay followed apparent first-order kinetics and NO flux for NANT decomposition was plotted as a function of (GSH). The values represent the mean of ($n = 4$). (c) Mechanism of NO release from DBHD/N_2O_2 a polymer additive (Z)-1-[*N*-methyl-*N*-[6-(*N*-butylammoniohexyl) amino]]-diazen-1-ium-1,2-diolate (DBHD/N_2O_2). The decomposition of the DBHD/N_2O_2 within the polymer film exposed to an aqueous environment, as found in tissue, releases two NO molecules.

polymers (e.g., poly(vinyl alcohol), poly(vinyl pyrrolidone), and PEG) for targeted delivery of NO or RSNOs.[183–185] It was also demonstrated that *S*-nitrosocysteine (CysNO) immobilized within a PEG hydrogel reduced platelet adhesion and smooth muscle cell proliferation *in vitro*.[186] Problems discussed in these studies were leaching of decomposition products such as free dimethylhexane diamine, which could react with labile nitrogen oxide species and form *N*-nitrosamines, which are carcinogenic. In addition, the leaching of NO donor into the aqueous phase would reduce the effectiveness of locally released NO to inhibit platelet adhesion/activation at the polymer/blood interface.[187]

An alternative concept of "NO generation" is to utilize endogenous RSNO species that exist in physiological fluids as a continuously replenishing NO donor to generate enhanced NO levels at the blood/polymer interface. RSNOs are regarded as a reservoir and carrier of NO in the body. The most abundant endogenous RSNOs are *S*-nitrosoalbumin (AlbSNO) and GSNO. Transnitrosation reactions occur *in vivo* so that the nitroso-group can be transferred from one thiol to another.[173,174] The cleavage of a S–NO bond in RSNOs to release NO can occur by three well-established mechanisms.[188] Copper ion-mediated catalytic decomposition requires reduction of Cu^{2+} to Cu^+. Cu^+ reacts with RSNO to liberate NO by transferring an electron, which forms a thiolate anion and regenerates Cu^{2+}. Under physiological conditions, ascorbate and thiolate anions are reducing agents to convert Cu^{2+} to Cu^+. The second RSNO decomposition pathway is through the reaction with high concentrations (>1 mM) of ascorbate to release NO and produces thiolate and dehydroascorbate.[189] The third decomposition mechanism of RSNOs consists of homolytic cleavage of the S–NO bond by light at 330–350 or 550–600 nm, yielding NO and the disulfide of the parent thiols.[190] The potential advantage of the NO-generation approach *in vivo* is the utilization of circulating RSNOs as an unlimited supply of NO at the polymer/blood interface. One study explored the possibility of generating NO by transnitrosation from endogenous RSNOs to L-cysteine immobilized on polymer surfaces.[191] They covalently attached L-cysteine to PU and PET and these L-cysteine-modified polymers reduced *in vitro* platelet adhesion by more than 50% when tested in plasma, but not with a platelet suspension in phosphate buffer.

Another study reported a lipophilic Cu(II)–cyclen-type complex to generate NO from RSNO and nitrite under physiological conditions.[192,193] PVC and PU films doped with this Cu(II) complex generated NO in the presence of reducing agents (e.g., ascorbate, cysteine, and glutathione) (Fig. 6.12). It was demonstrated that such polymers can generate NO with an apparent surface flux as high as 8×10^{-10} mol/cm^2/min from physiological levels of GSNO. The same polymer was also shown to generate NO from nitrite under physiological conditions in the presence of ascorbate.[187] As Cu^{2+} is cytotoxic and can leach, the question arises as to its biological effects when attempting to translate such approaches to the *in vivo* situation.

6.5.5.4   *Reduction of the Inflammatory Response by Increasing Hemocompatibility*   Blood-exposed medical devices such as casdiovascular or urethral stents, CPBs, heart valves, synthetic blood vessels, and others have been investigated extensively for hemocompatiblity, and many materials and surface treatments have been investigated in order to characterize adverse effects on blood, blood cells, and soluble proteins affecting downstream body responses such as inflammation. The most efficient coatings use heparin; however, polymer coatings as well as lipid-like surfaces coated with phosphorylcholine (PC) have also been described.[194,195]

Modification of a biomaterial surface by the addition of a heparin coating has improved the biocompatibility of extracorporeal devices.[196–199] Most often, heparin was physisorbed or covalently immobilized by end-point attachment, in which the reducing end of the linear heparin chain is depolymerized to yield a reactive aldehyde group that can then be conjugated to a primary amine on

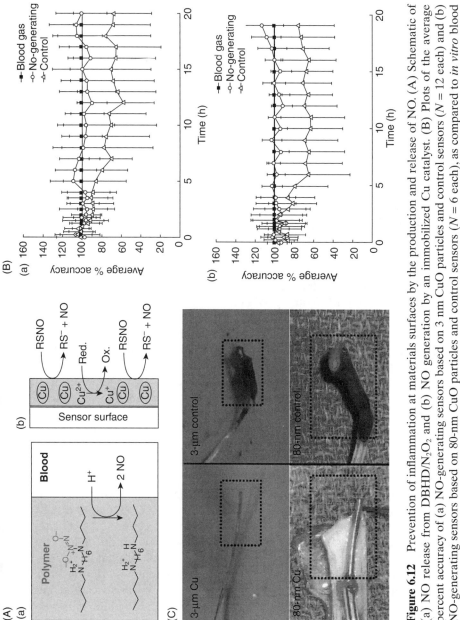

Figure 6.12 Prevention of inflammation at materials surfaces by the production and release of NO. (A) Schematic of (a) NO release from DBHD/N_2O_2 and (b) NO generation by an immobilized Cu catalyst. (B) Plots of the average percent accuracy of (a) NO-generating sensors based on 3 nm CuO particles and control sensors ($N = 12$ each) and (b) NO-generating sensors based on 80-nm CuO particles and control sensors ($N = 6$ each), as compared to in vitro blood gas analyzer. (C) Images of two representative pairs of NO-generating (left) and control sensors (right) after in vivo studies. The portions within the dotted boxes were exposed to blood. Adapted from Wu and Meyerhoff[187] with permission from Elsevier, © 2008.

a graft or stent surface. Heparin-coated stents were demonstrated to reduce platelet and endothelial activation when compared to bare metal controls by plasma sP-selectin and E-selectin assessment in a small human study.[200] The anticoagulant activity of surface-bound heparin is believed to depend largely on binding to antithrombin III (ATIII) and on subsequent inactivation of several key coagulation factors such as FIIa, FXa, and FIXa.[201] However, this mechanism is only one out of several responsible for the antithrombotic effects of immobilized heparin. Other potentially relevant biological effects may be selective adhesion and cleavage of serum proteins, cell activation mechanisms, and the subsequently release of coagulation factors, cytokines, and the expression of cellular adhesion proteins. The fact that heparin in solution does not catalyze antithrombin (AT)-mediated inhibition of surface-adsorbed FXIIa and FXIa and thus cannot effectively control the contact activation of the complement system[201] indicates a different anticoagulation mechanism between soluble heparin and immobilized heparin. Moreover, it has been shown that activation or denaturation of adsorbed plasma proteins play a key role in the adhesion and activation of blood cells.[202,203] It was shown that significant differences arise between adsorption patterns on heparin-coated and uncoated PVC surfaces. Fibronectin, fibrinogen, C3, and high-molecular-weight kininogen (HMWK) exhibited specific adsorption profiles depending on the heparin coating of the surface.[196,197] Comparing heparin-coated PVC tubing with noncoated PVC tubing for hemocompatibility over 5 hours, it was found that heparin coating of PVC tubing gave reduced platelet adhesion, leukocyte activation, and deposition of serum proteins.[199] Differences between heparin-coated and noncoated PVS appeared only after 2 hours' incubation with whole human blood, suggesting that long-term studies for hemocompatibility are required. Therefore, it is assumed that at least some of the improved hemocompatibility of heparin-coated surfaces may be ascribed to differences in adsorption of plasma proteins.

End-point-attached heparin coatings have been translated into clinical trials. Interestingly, clinical findings are highly controversial as a randomized, prospective clinical study of heparin-bonded Dacron grafts in the femoropopliteal position showed no significant improvement compared with uncoated ePTFE after 5 years.[204] In contrast, an ePTFE prosthesis coated with end-point immobilized heparin (Propaten graft, W. L. Gore & Associates, Flagstaff, AZ) was tested in a preclinical animal study in greyhounds, causing a significant reduction in acute and chronic thrombogenicity with retention of heparin bioactivity at 12 weeks.[205] Another study found reduction of platelet deposition and anastomotic neointimal hyperplasia in *ex vivo* femoral arteriovenous shunts and chronic aortoiliac bypass models.[206] However, it was also noted that neither covalently nor ionically bonded heparin-coated cardiopulmonary perfusion circuits reduced the rate of thrombin formation, protected platelets, or reduced postoperative bleeding or transfusion requirements. In general, heparin-coated circuits appear to reduce some biochemical aspects of the inflammatory response, but a clinical benefit has not been documented.[207]

PEO or PEG coatings have been used as surface coating (by physisorption or by covalent attachment via different linker molecules) since the 1970s as they efficiently reduce protein and cell adhesion.[208] This property was attributed to the presence of a hydrophilic ether oxygen in its structural repeat unit, $[CH_2–CH_2–O]_n$, which leads to a water-solvated structure that is capable of forming a "liquid-like" surface with highly mobile molecular chains that exhibit no systematic molecular order. In most cases, investigators have been able to demonstrate resistance to protein binding *in vitro*. *In vivo* results have been inconsistent, however, and clinical studies of a PEO-modified stent or graft have yet to be reported.

Albumin is the most abundant blood protein and binds to the glycocalyx of an intact endothelial cell layer, thus rendering it inert and thromboresistant.[209] When albumin is used as a coating on artificial surfaces, it induces significantly less platelet adhesion compared with other plasma proteins, including fibrinogen and γ-globulin.[210,211] Some have covalently grafted albumin to surfaces[212–214] or covalently attached monocolonal antibodies to attract and bind native albumin from blood.[215] The affinity of albumin to a dye, Cibacron Blue F3G-A, was used in another approach.[216] Others modified surfaces with long aliphatic chains (C8–C18) to increase selective affinity for endogenous albumin.[217,218] A glutaraldehyde-cross-linked albumin coating showed reduced platelet and leukocyte adhesion and aggregation, as well as reduced fibrin production *in vitro*.[219] A prosthesis thus coated was investigated in a thoracoabdominal bypass model in dogs and in clinical studies, but only small differences were observed between coated and uncoated grafts.[219,220]

Another approach used photochemically linked soluble and cross-linked poly(VPGVG)-peptides to silicone and demonstrated reduced fibrinogen and immunoglobulin adsorption *in vitro* as well as decreased release of proinflammatory cytokines released by monocytes.[221] A recombinant elastin polypeptide (EP20-24-24) consisting of exons 20, 21, 23, and 24 of the human elastin gene was passively adsorbed onto synthetic surfaces, which decreased platelet deposition and activation *in vitro* and delayed catheter occlusion *in vivo*.[222] Similarly, a novel recombinant elastin-mimetic protein polymer was synthesized and placed as a thin film on 4-mm-diameter ePTFE grafts. These grafts were analyzed in an acute primate *ex vivo* shunt model and were found to induce only minimal thrombogenicity.[195]

PC is a synthetic mimic of the cell membrane of the red blood cell and has been shown to limit protein and cell adhesion *in vitro*.[223–225] PC is thought to reduce protein and cell adhesion because of the zwitterionic nature of the PC head group, which is electrically neutral at physiological pH, though carrying both positively and negatively charged groups. Supported lipid films can be unstable as coatings form by self-assembly, but polymers with PC side groups overcome this problem. Methods have also been developed to create stable "membrane-mimetic" films using protein anchors,[226,227] heat stabilization,[228] and *in situ* polymerization of synthetically modified polymerizable phospholipids.[229–232] In a variety of animal models, PC has been shown to be biologically inert.[233,234] The integrity of the coating was confirmed following high-pressure deployment and at 12 weeks' postimplantation.[235] Experimentally, endothelialization was found to be similar in both PC-coated and uncoated stents.[233,234,236] However, platelet and endothelial activation was reduced compared to bare metal stents in a small human study.[237] A good summary of many clinical studies using PC coatings can be found in Reference 195.

6.6 CONCLUSIONS AND OUTLOOK

Literature reports describe a wide range of antibacterial material surfaces and coatings, but few strategies are designed on a biomolecular basis and with sufficient control to be called intelligent. The most abundant category concerns bactericidal materials or coatings containing silver ions, which are released over periods of days or weeks, and surfaces comprising quaternary amine compounds. Both approaches are effective against both gram-positive and gram-negative bacteria but also cause adverse effects on mammalian cells. The subject of damage to mammalian cells and tissue by silver is, however, the subject of much controversy. The reasons for the widely diverging literature reports on silver toxicity are not established but are likely to relate to different amounts and release rates of silver ions as well as differences in testing modalities. It is unfortunate that a standardized, widely accepted test protocol for establishing the severity of cytotoxicity to mammalian cells and tissue does not exist. There is not even a standard test protocol for testing antibacterial material surfaces; the standards used for testing antibiotics in solution do not apply well to testing of antibacterial materials. Different workers have used different protocols depending on their particular samples and study objectives.

Yet, despite literature controversies, silver-releasing products have entered the biomedical devices market, particularly in the form of wound dressings. The prevention of bacterial infection outweighs potential concerns about cytotoxicity, and clinical practice has demonstrated clear benefits from their use. This serves to reinforce the notion that materials, surfaces, and coatings need to be designed with the specific requirements of particular applications in mind; a universal antibacterial and "biocompatible" coating may not be achievable. Intelligent design of antibacterial biomaterials includes consideration of the specific biological environment and its interactions with the biomaterial surface.

Nonfouling surfaces have been shown to resist the attachment of bacteria and biofilm formation, and such coatings are of promise for some biomedical applications, such as contact lenses, but are less well suited to application with biomedical devices that need to achieve integration with cells and tissue.

The covalent grafting onto solid material surfaces of antibacterial molecules has received considerable attention, and some of those strategies may achieve the objective of combating biofilm formation while allowing attachment of human cells and tissue. None of these strategies appear to have attained trans-lation to clinical practice, but some appear to have considerable promise. The grafting of established antibiotics, for which the mechanism of action is known, onto biomaterial surfaces may be a route toward creating surfaces with pre-dictable biological consequences, provided that the antibiotic molecule can still exert activity when covalently immobilized. Steric hindrance of interfer-ence with the active part of the molecule may render it inactive, or a molecule, such as furanones, which mimics quorum sensing molecules secreted by bac-teria, may need to enter the bacterial cytoplasm, which it can no longer do when covalently grafted. Some of the most interesting strategies are based on natural biomolecular observations, for example, studies designing molecules that mimic natural host defense peptides.

While covalent grafting might be able to achieve long-term protection against biofilm formation, in other applications, it may be beneficial to release antibiotics over a limited period of time, but to do so in a stimulus-triggered fashion, for example, in response to a bacterial metabolic product signaling the onset of an infection. Such approaches are challenging in many ways, chemically, biologically, and in terms of engineering and manufacturing, and at present are at an early stage.

The inflammatory response is a highly complex set of reactions that occur at least as a transient phase upon injury and especially after implantation of medical implants. The severity and extent of the inflammatory response depend markedly on the surface chemistry and topography of the implanted medical device as well as on the surgical procedure. Unfortunately, systemic as well as local inflammatory processes are induced; therefore, treatment of excessive inflammation needs to comprise a combination of systemic treatment by injection of soluble medication such as corticosteroids, non-steroidal anti-inflammatory agents, or therapeutic proteins as well as by local inhibition of the inflammatory response. For this, intelligent surface coatings might be helpful.

Various strategies are feasible, as inflammation can be reduced by reducing contact activation of the complement system, for example, by the release of anti-inflammatory agents such as Compstatin, which inhibits the activation of C3, a key factor of the complement system cascade. Another approach is to prevent the foreign body reaction, thus reducing the induction of the inflam-matory response by preventing macrophage adhesion and fusion. Here, mac-rophage surface integrins can be a target, or inhibition of the migratory activity of macrophages can be addressed. Further indirect effects on the induction of the inflammatory reaction on material surfaces might be addressed by the release and/or production of NO that inhibits platelet adhesion and activation. Such surface modifications of medical implants might be very efficient and reduce platelet adhesion and activation; however, technically, it is challenging and cannot be applied onto surfaces where tight apposition between the adja-cent tissue and the biomaterial surface is desired. Therefore, such NO-producing or -releasing surfaces could be useful for sensors inserted into the blood stream, but they are not appropriate for hip, knee, and dental implants where direct and tight tissue contact is required.

An efficient way to reduce the inflammatory response upon the implantation of a medical implant would seem to be to render the surfaces as hemocompatible as possible. For this, a series of surface coatings have been explored, such as heparin, albumin, or lipid and polymer coatings, predominantly, PEO or PEG coatings. These various coatings seem to be efficient in the reduction of the inflammatory response; they also reduce activation of the complement system as well as reduce adhesion and activation of platelets and macrophages. Therefore, such well-established surface treatments might be, on the basis of present knowledge, the best prevention against excessive inflammation, extensive foreign body reaction, and contact activation of the complement system. Moreover, such general cell adhesion prevention strategies reduce bacterial adhesion and might, in the long run, be successful for both prevention of biofilm formation and reduction of chronic inflammation at the surface of an implanted device. Solutions that improve long-term biocompatibility are desirable while being straightforward to manufacture, easy to handle, and as inexpensive as possible to allow a large number of patients to benefit from such devices.

Given that infection increases inflammation and the need to control wound-healing responses, a highly desirable intelligent approach might be to equip the surface of a biomedical device with bioactives that can monitor and counteract both infection and excessive inflammation. Inflammation is part of the wound-healing response; thus, complete suppression would be detrimental, but a grafted layer of molecules that can deter bacterial colonization and at the same time downregulate excessive inflammation would seem a very worthwhile aim. Some molecules, for example, serrulatanes, possess antibacterial as well as anti-inflammatory activity *in vitro*, but it remains to be investigated clinically whether grafted layers on biomaterial surfaces can steer *in vivo* responses and whether a single molecule or a combination of multiple bioactives would be more effective. There is a clearly documented clinical need for such intelligent biomaterial surfaces, and there is plenty of scope for novel concepts and intelligently designed strategies to explore these aspects. Yet, the cytokine and cellular activities in inflammation are not just confined to biomaterial surfaces; they occur in a three-dimensional manner throughout nearby tissues. This raises a question regarding to what extent a biomaterial surface or a releasing coating might be able to regulate inflammation.

REFERENCES

1. Smith & Nephew. Acticoat: Antimicrobial barrier dressing. http://global.smith-nephew.com/master/ACTICOAT_27517.htm.
2. Kumar, V., Abbas, A.K., Fausto, N., & Mitchell, R.N. *Robbins Basic Pathology*, 8th edn. Philadelphia: Saunders Elsevier (2007). Ch. 2.

3. Costerton, J.W., Stewart, P.S., & Greenberg, E.P. Bacterial biofilms: a common cause of persistent infections. *Science* **284**, 1318–1322 (1999).

4. Darouiche, R.O. Current concepts—treatment of infections associated with surgical implants. *New England Journal of Medicine* **350**, 1422–1429 (2004).

5. Harris, L.G. & Richards, R.G. Staphylococci and implant surfaces: a review. *Injury* **37**, 3–14 (2006).

6. BD. Cell culture surfaces. http://www.bdbiosciences.com/cellculture/surfaces/surfacetypes/tc.jsp.

7. Nicolson, P.C. et al. Extended wear ophthalmic lens. U.S. Patent US 6,951,894 2005.

8. Costerton, J.W., Khoury, A.E., Ward, K.H., & Anwar, H. Practical measures to control device-related bacterial infections. *The International Journal of Artificial Organs* **16**, 765–770 (1993).

9. Cheng, G., Xue, H., Zhang, Z., Chen, S., & Jiang, S. A switchable biocompatible polymer surface with self-sterilizing and nonfouling capabilities. *Angewandte Chemie* **47**, 8831–8834 (2008).

10. Tiller, J.C., Liao, C.-J., Lewis, K., & Klibanov, A.M. Designing surfaces that kill bacteria on contact. *Proceedings of the National Academy of Sciences of the United States of America* **98**, 5981–5985 (2001).

11. Gottenbos, B., Grijpma, D.W., Van der Mei, H.C., Feijen, J., & Busscher, H.J. Initial adhesion and surface growth of *Pseudomonas aeruginosa* on negatively and positively charged poly(methacrylates). *Journal of Materials Science. Materials in Medicine* **10**, 853–855 (1999).

12. Martin, T.P., Kooi, S.E., Chang, S.H., Sedransk, K.L., & Gleason, K.K. Initiated chemical vapor deposition of antimicrobial polymer coatings. *Biomaterials* **28**, 909–915 (2007).

13. Ostuni, E., Chapman, R.G., Liang, M.N., Meluleni, G., Pier, G., Ingber, D.E., & Whitesides, G.M. Self-assembled monolayers that resist the adsorption of proteins and the adhesion of bacterial and mammalian cells. *Langmuir* **17**, 6336–6343 (2001).

14. Harris, L.G., Tosatti, S., Wieland, M., Textor, M., & Richards, R.G. *Staphylococcus aureus* adhesion to titanium oxide surfaces coated with non-functionalized and peptide-functionalized poly(L-lysine)-grafted-poly(ethylene glycol) copolymers. *Biomaterials* **25**, 4135–4148 (2004).

15. Kingshott, P., Wei, J., Bagge-Ravn, D., Gadegaard, N., & Gram, L. Covalent attachment of poly(ethylene glycol) to surfaces, critical for reducing bacterial adhesion. *Langmuir* **19**, 6912–6921 (2003).

16. Fundeanu, I., van der Mei, H.C., Schouten, A.J., & Busscher, H.J. Polyacrylamide brush coatings preventing microbial adhesion to silicone rubber. *Colloids and Surfaces. B, Biointerfaces* **64**, 297–301 (2008).

17. Rabea, E.I., Badawy, M.E.T., Stevens, C.V., Smagghe, G., & Steurbaut, W. Chitosan as antimicrobial agent: applications and mode of action. *Biomacromolecules* **4**, 1457–1465 (2003).

18. Boributh, S., Chanachai, A., & Jiraratananon, R. Modification of PVDF membrane by chitosan solution for reducing protein fouling. *Journal of Membrane Science* **342**, 97–104 (2009).

19. Salick, D.A., Kretsinger, J.K., Pochan, D.J., & Schneider, J.P. Inherent antibacterial activity of a peptide-based beta-hairpin hydrogel. *Journal of the American Chemical Society* **129**, 14793–14799 (2007).

20. Hetrick, E.M. & Schoenfisch, M.H. Reducing implant-related infections: active release strategies. *Chemical Society Reviews* **35**, 780–789 (2006).

21. Zilberman, M. & Elsner, J.J. Antibiotic-eluting medical devices for various applications. *Journal of Controlled Release* **130**, 202–215 (2008).

22. Wu, P. & Grainger, D.W. Drug/device combinations for local drug therapies and infection prophylaxis. *Biomaterials* **27**, 2450–2467 (2006).

23. Schnieders, J., Gbureck, U., Thull, R., & Kissel, T. Controlled release of gentamicin from calcium phosphate—poly(lactic acid-co-glycolic acid) composite bone cement. *Biomaterials* **27**, 4239–4249 (2006).

24. Alt, V., Bitschnau, A., Osterling, J., Sewing, A., Meyer, C., Kraus, R., Meissner, S.A., Wenisch, S., Domann, E., & Schnettler, R. The effects of combined gentamicin-hydroxyapatite coating for cementless joint prostheses on the reduction of infection rates in a rabbit infection prophylaxis model. *Biomaterials* **27**, 4627–4634 (2006).

25. Rauschmann, M.A., Wichelhaus, T.A., Stirnal, V., Dingeldein, E., Zichner, L., Schnettler, R., & Alt, V. Nanocrystalline hydroxyapatite and calcium sulphate as biodegradable composite carrier material for local delivery of antibiotics in bone infections. *Biomaterials* **26**, 2677–2684 (2005).

26. Jones, S.A., Bowler, P.G., Walker, M., & Parsons, D. Controlling wound bioburden with a novel silver-containing hydrofiber((R)) dressing. *Wound Repair and Regeneration* **12**, 288–294 (2004).

27. Shanmugasundaram, N., Sundaraseelan, J., Uma, S., Selvaraj, D., & Babu, M. Design and delivery of silver sulfadiazine from alginate microspheres-impregnated collagen scaffold. *Journal of Biomedical Materials Research. Part B, Applied Biomaterials* **77B**, 378–388 (2006).

28. Kumar, R. & Munstedt, H. Polyamide/silver antimicrobials: effect of crystallinity on the silver ion release. *Polymer International* **54**, 1180–1186 (2005).

29. Nablo, B.J., Rothrock, A.R., & Schoenfisch, M.H. Nitric oxide-releasing sol-gels as antibacterial coatings for orthopedic implants. *Biomaterials* **26**, 917–924 (2005).

30. Price, C.I., Horton, J.W., & Baxter, C.R. Topical liposomal delivery of antibiotics in soft tissue infection. *The Journal of Surgical Research* **49**, 174–178 (1990).

31. Stigter, M., Bezemer, J., de Groot, K., & Layrolle, P. Incorporation of different antibiotics into carbonated hydroxyapatite coatings on titanium implants, release and antibiotic efficacy. *Journal of Controlled Release* **99**, 127–137 (2004).

32. Joosten, U., Joist, A., Frebel, T., Brandt, B., Diederichs, S., & von Eiff, C. Evaluation of an in situ setting injectable calcium phosphate as a new carrier material for gentamicin osteomyelitis: studies in the treatment of chronic in vitro and in vivo. *Biomaterials* **25**, 4287–4295 (2004).

33. Liang, J., Chen, Y., Barnes, K., Wu, R., Worley, S.D., & Huang, T.S. N-halamine/quat siloxane copolymers for use in biocidal coatings. *Biomaterials* **27**, 2495–2501 (2006).

34. Makal, U., Wood, L., Ohman, D.E., & Wynne, K.J. Polyurethane biocidal polymeric surface modifiers. *Biomaterials* **27**, 1316–1326 (2006).

35. Mizerska, U., Fortuniak, W., Chojnowski Halasa, J.R., Konopacka, A., & Werel, W. Polysiloxane cationic biocides with imidazolium salt (ImS) groups, synthesis and antibacterial properties. *European Polymer Journal* **45**, 779–787 (2009).

36. Gaonkar, T.A., Caraos, L., & Modak, S.M. Efficacy of a silicone urinary catheter impregnated with chlorhexidine and triclosan against colonization with *Proteus mirabilis* and other uropathogens. *Infection Control and Hospital Epidemiology* **28**, 596–598 (2007).

37. Park, J.H. et al. Norfloxacin-releasing urethral catheter for long-term catheterization. *Journal of Biomaterials Science. Polymer Edition* **14**, 951–962 (2003).

38. Rossi, S., Azghani, A.O., & Omri, A. Antimicrobial efficacy of a new antibiotic-loaded poly(hydroxybutyric-co-hydroxyvaleric acid) controlled release system. *The Journal of Antimicrobial Chemotherapy* **54**, 1013–1018 (2004).

39. Katti, D.S., Robinson, K.W., Ko, F.K., & Laurencin, C.T. Bioresorbable nanofiber-based systems for wound healing and drug delivery: optimization of fabrication parameters. *Journal of Biomedical Materials Research. Part B, Applied Biomaterials* **70B**, 286–296 (2004).

40. Aviv, M., Berdicevsky, I., & Zilberman, M. Gentamicin-loaded bioresorbable films for prevention of bacterial infections associated with orthopedic implants. *Journal of Biomedical Materials Research. Part A* **83A**, 10–19 (2007).

41. Prabu, P., Dharmaraj, N., Aryal, S., Lee, B.M., Ramesh, V., & Kim, H.Y. Preparation and drug release activity of scaffolds containing collagen and poly(caprolactone). *Journal of Biomedical Materials Research. Part A* **79A**, 153–158 (2006).

42. Blanchemain, N., Haulon, S., Boschin, F., Marcon-Bachari, E., Traisnel, M., Morcellet, M., Hildebrand, H.F., & Martel, B. Vascular prostheses with controlled release of antibiotics—part 1: surface modification with cyclodextrins of PET prostheses. *Biomolecular Engineering* **24**, 149–153 (2007).

43. Charville, G.W., Hetrick, E.M., Geer, C.B., & Schoenfisch, M.H. Reduced bacterial adhesion to fibrinogen-coated substrates via nitric oxide release. *Biomaterials* **29**, 4039–4044 (2008).

44. Frost, M.C., Reynolds, M.M., & Meyerhoff, M.E. Polymers incorporating nitric oxide releasing/generating substances for improved biocompatibility of blood-contactincy medical devices. *Biomaterials* **26**, 1685–1693 (2005).

45. Rai, M., Yadav, A., & Gade, A. Silver nanoparticles as a new generation of antimicrobials. *Biotechnology Advances* **27**, 76–83 (2009).

46. Lansdown, A.B.G. *Issues in Toxicology No. 6, Silver in Healthcare: Its Antimicrobial Efficacy and Safety in Use*. Cambridge: Royal Society of Chemistry (2010).

47. Amberg, M., Grieder, K., Barbarodo, P., Heuberger, M., & Hegemann, D. Electromechanical behavior of nanoscale silver coatings on PET fibers. *Plasma Processes and Polymers* **5**, 874–880 (2008).

48. Ho, C.H., Tobis, J., Sprich, C., Thomann, R., & Tiller, J.C. Nanoseparated polymeric networks with multiple antimicrobial properties. *Advanced Materials* **16**, 957–961 (2004).

49. Lee, H., Lee, Y., Statz, A.R., Rho, J., Park, T.G., & Messersmith, P.B. Substrate-independent layer-by-layer assembly by using mussel-adhesive-inspired polymers. *Advanced Materials* **20**, 1619–1623 (2008).

50. Vasilev, K., Sah, V., Anselme, K., Ndi, C., Mateescu, M., Dollmann, B., Martinek, P., Ys, H., Ploux, L., & Griesser, H.J. Tunable antibacterial coatings that support mammalian cell growth. *Nano Letters* **10**, 202–207 (2010).

51. Poulter, N., Munoz-Berbel, X., Johnson, A.L., Dowling, A.J., Waterfield, N., & Jenkins, A.T.A. An organo-silver compound that shows antimicrobial activity against *Pseudomonas aeruginosa* as a monomer and plasma deposited film. *Chemical Communications* **47**, 7312–7314 (2009).

52. Vasilev, K., Cook, J., & Griesser, H.J. Antibacterial surfaces for biomedical devices. *Expert Review of Medical Devices* **6**, 553–567 (2009).

53. Gordon, O., Slenters, T.V., Brunetto, P.S., Villaruz, A.E., Sturdevant, D.E., Otto, M., Landmann, R., & Fromm, K.M. Silver coordination polymers for prevention of implant infection: thiol interaction, impact on respiratory chain enzymes, and hydroxyl radical induction. *Antimicrobial Agents and Chemotherapy* **54**, 4208–4218 (2010).

54. Schrand, A.M., Braydich-Stolle, L.K., Schlager, J.J., Dai, L., & Hussain, S.M. Can silver nanoparticles be useful as potential biological labels? *Nanotechnology* **19**, 1–13 (2008). Article No: 235104.

55. Stevens, K.N., Knetsch, M.L., Sen, A., Sambhy, V., & Koole, L.H. Disruption and activation of blood platelets in contact with an antimicrobial composite coating consisting of a pyridinium polymer and AgBr nanoparticles. *ACS Applied Materials & Interfaces* **1**, 2049–2054 (2009).

56. Vasilev, K., Griesser, S.S., Ys, H., Ndi, C., & Griesser, H.J. Mammalian cell responses to antibacterial coatings comprising silver nanoparticles in plasma polymers. Proceedings of the 20th Annual Meeting of the Australasian Society of Biomaterials and Tissue Engineering, Brisbane, Australia, February 10–12, 2010.

57. Riley, D.M., Classen, D.C., Stevens, L.E., & Burke, J.P. A large randomized clinical-trial of a silver-impregnated urinary catheter—lack of efficacy and Staphylococcal superinfection. *The American Journal of Medicine* **98**, 349–356 (1995).

58. Srinivasan, A., Karchmer, T., Richards, A., Song, X., & Perl, T.M. A prospective trial of a novel, silicone-based, silver-coated Foley catheter for the prevention of nosocomial urinary tract infections. *Infection Control and Hospital Epidemiology* **27**, 38–43 (2006).

59. RSC. Gallium-based antimicrobials. http://www.rsc.org/chemistryworld/news/2007/march/19030701.asp.

60. Kingshott, P., Thissen, H., & Griesser, H.J. Effects of cloud-point grafting, chain length, and density of PEG layers on competitive adsorption of ocular proteins. *Biomaterials* **23**, 2043–2056 (2002).

61. Kingshott, P., McArthur, S., Thissen, H., Castner, D.G., & Griesser, H.J. Ultrasensitive probing of the protein resistance of PEG surfaces by secondary ion mass spectrometry. *Biomaterials* **23**, 4775–4785 (2002).

62. Hamilton-Brown, P., Gengenbach, T., Griesser, H.J., & Meagher, L. End terminal, poly(ethylene oxide) graft layers: surface forces and protein adsorption. *Langmuir* **25**, 9149–9156 (2009).

63. Thissen, H., Gengenbach, T., du Toit, R., Sweeney, D., Kingshott, P., Griesser, H.J., & Meagher, L. Clinical observations of biofouling on PEO coated silicone hydrogel contact lenses. *Biomaterials* **31**, 5510–5519 (2010).

64. Saldarriaga Fernandez, C.I., van der Mei, H.C., Lochhead, M.J., Grainger, D.W., & Busscher, H.J. The inhibition of the adhesion of clinically isolated bacterial

strains on multi-component cross-linked poly(ethylene glycol)-based polymer coatings. *Biomaterials* **28**, 4105–4112 (2007).

65. Statz, A.R., Park, J.P., Chongsiriwatana, N.P., Barron, A.E., & Messersmith, P.B. Surface-immobilised antimicrobial peptoids. *Biofouling* **24**, 439–448 (2008).

66. Tiller, J.C., Liao, C.J., Lewis, K., & Klibanov, A.M. Designing surfaces that kill bacteria on contact. *Proceedings of the National Academy of Sciences of the United States of America* **98**, 5981–5985 (2001).

67. Harris, L.G. & Richards, R.G. Staphylococci and implant surfaces: a review. *Injury* **37**, 3–12 (2006).

68. Kugler, R., Bouloussa, O., & Rondelez, F. Evidence of a charge-density threshold for optimum efficiency of biocidal cationic surfaces. *Microbiology* **151**, 1341–1348 (2005).

69. Murata, H., Koepsel, R.R., Matyjaszewski, K., & Russell, A.J. Permanent, non-leaching antibacterial surfaces—2: how high density cationic surfaces kill bacterial cells. *Biomaterials* **28**, 4870–4879 (2007).

70. Wikipedia. Melittin. http://en.wikipedia.org/wiki/Melittin.

71. Thierry, B., Jasieniak, M., de Smet, L.C.P.M., Vasilev, K., & Griesser, H.J. Reactive epoxy-functionalized thin films by a pulsed plasma polymerization process. *Langmuir* **24**, 10187–10195 (2008).

72. Vreuls, C., Zocchi, G., Thierry, B., Garitte, G., Griesser, S.S., Archambeau, C., Van de Weerdt, C., Martial, J., & Griesser, H. Prevention of bacterial biofilms by covalent immobilization of peptides onto plasma polymer functionalized substrates. *Journal of Materials Chemistry* **20**, 8092–8098 (2010).

73. Glinel, K., Jonas, A.M., Jouenne, T., Leprince, J., Galas, L., & Huck, W.T.S. Antibacterial and antifouling polymer brushes incorporating antimicrobial peptide. *Bioconjugate Chemistry* **20**, 71–77 (2009).

74. Joerger, R.D., Sabesan, S., Visioli, D., Urian, D., & Joerger, M.C. Antimicrobial activity of chitosan attached to ethylene copolymer films. *Packaging Technology and Science* **22**, 125–138 (2009).

75. Tseng, H.J., Hsu, S.H., Wu, M.W., Hsueh, T.H., & Tu, P.C. Nylon textiles grafted with chitosan by open air plasma and their antimicrobial effect. *Fibers and Polymers* **10**, 53–59 (2009).

76. Abdou, E.S., Elkholy, S.S., Elsabee, M.Z., & Mohamed, E. Improved antimicrobial activity of polypropylene and cotton nonwoven fabrics by surface treatment and modification with chitosan. *Journal of Applied Polymer Science* **108**, 2290–2296 (2008).

77. Aumsuwan, N., Heinhorst, S., & Urban, M.W. The effectiveness of antibiotic activity of penicillin attached to expanded poly(tetrafluoroethylene) (ePTFE) surfaces: a quantitative assessment. *Biomacromolecules* **8**, 3525–3530 (2007).

78. Wach, J.-Y., Bonazzi, S., & Gademann, K. Antimicrobial surfaces through natural product hybrids. *Angewandte Chemie (International ed. in English)* **47**, 7123–7126 (2008).

79. Parvizi, J., Wickstrom, E., Zeiger, A.R., Adams, C.S., Shapiro, I.M., Purtill, J.J., Sharkey, P.F., Hozack, W.J., Rothman, R.H., & Hickok, N.J. Frank Stinchfield Award—titanium surface with biologic activity against infection. *Clinical Orthopaedics and Related Research* **429**, 33–38 (2004).

80. Shepherd, J., Sarker, P., Rimmer, S., Swanson, L., MacNeil, S., & Douglas, I. Hyperbranched poly(NIPAM) polymers modified with antibiotics for the reduction of bacterial burden in infected human tissue engineered skin. *Biomaterials* **32**, 258–267 (2011).

81. Ys, H. Antibacterial coatings for biomedical devices by covalent grafting of serrulatane diterpenes. PhD Thesis, University of South Australia. 2010.

82. Reece, R.J. & Maxwell, A. DNA-gyrase: structure and function. *Critical Reviews in Biochemistry and Molecular Biology* **26**, 335–375 (1991).

83. Berg, J.M., Tymoczko, J.L., & Stryer, L. *Biochemistry*, 6th edn. New York: W. H. Freeman (2007).

84. Caro, A., Humblot, V., Methivier, C., Minier, M., Salmain, M., & Pradier, C.-M. Grafting of lysozyme and/or poly(ethylene glycol) to prevent biofilm growth on stainless steel surfaces. *The Journal of Physical Chemistry B* **113**, 2101–2109 (2009).

85. Strömstedt, A.A., Ringstad, L., Schmidtchen, A., & Malmsten, M. Interaction between amphiphilic peptides and phospholipid membranes. *Current Opinion in Colloid and Interface Science* **15**, 467–478 (2010).

86. Porter, E.A., Weisblum, B., & Gellman, S.H. Mimicry of host–defense peptides by unnatural oligomers: antimicrobial beta-peptides. *Journal of the American Chemical Society* **124**, 7324–7330 (2002).

87. Mowery, B.P., Lee, S.E., Kissounko, D.A., Epand, R.F., Epand, R.M., Weisblum, B., Stahl, S.S., & Gellman, S.H. Mimicry of antimicrobial host-defense peptides by random copolymers. *Journal of the American Chemical Society* **129**, 15474–15476 (2007).

88. Mowery, B.P., Lindner, A.H., Weisblum, B., Stahl, S.S., & Gellman, S.H. Structure-activity relationships among random nylon-3 copolymers that mimic antibacterial host-defense peptides. *Journal of the American Chemical Society* **131**, 9735–9745 (2009).

89. Lee, M.-R., Stahl, S.S., Gellman, S.H., & Masters, K.S. Nylon-3 copolymers that generate cell-adhesive surfaces identified by library screening. *Journal of the American Chemical Society* **131**, 16779–16789 (2009).

90. Zhu, H., Kumar, A., Ozkan, J., Bandara, R., Ding, A., Perera, I., Steinberg, P., Kumar, N., Lao, W., Griesser, S.S., Britcher, L., Griesser, H.J., & Willcox, M.D.P. Fimbrolide-coated antimicrobial lenses: their in vitro and in vivo effects. *Optometry & Vision Science* **85**, 292–300 (2008).

91. Hume, E.B.H., Baveja, J., Muir, B., Schubert, T.L., Kumar, N., Kjelleberg, S., Griesser, H.J., Thissen, H., Read, R., Poole-Warren, L.A., Schindhelm, K., & Willcox, M.P.D. The control of *Staphylococcus epidermidis* biofilm formation and in vivo infection rates by covalently bound furanones. *Biomaterials* **25**, 5023–5030 (2004).

92. Rasmussen, T.B., Manefield, M., Andersen, J.B., Eberl, L., Anthoni, U., Christophersen, C., Steinberg, P., Kjelleberg, S., & Givskov, M. How *Delisea pulchra* furanones affect quorum sensing and swarming motility in Serratia liquefaciens MG1. *Microbiology* **146**, 3237–3244 (2000).

93. Al-Bataineh, S.A., Britcher, L.G., & Griesser, H.J. XPS characterization of the surface immobilization of antibacterial furanones. *Surface Science* **600**, 952–962 (2006).

94. Al-Bataineh, S.A., Britcher, L.G., & Griesser, H.J. Rapid radiation degradation in the XPS analysis of antibacterial coatings of brominated furanones. *Surface and Interface Analysis* **38**, 1512–1518 (2006).

95. Al-Bataineh, S., Jasieniak, M., Britcher, L., & Griesser, H.J. TOF-SIMS and principal component analysis characterization of the multilayer surface grafting of small molecules: antibacterial furanones. *Analytical Chemistry* **80**, 430–436 (2008).

96. Al-Bataineh, S.A. Spectroscopic characterisation of surface—immobilised antibacterial furanone coatings. PhD Thesis, University of South Australia, 2006.

97. Kuehl, R., Al-Bataineh, S., Gordon, O., Luginbuehl, R., Otto, M., Textor, M., & Landmann, R. Furanone at subinhibitory concentrations enhances staphylococcal biofilm formation by luxS repression. *Antimicrobial Agents and Chemotherapy* **53**, 4159–4166 (2009).

98. Ndi, C.P., Semple, S.J., Griesser, H.J., Pyke, S.M., & Barton, M.D. Antimicrobial compounds from the Australian desert plant *Eremophild neglecta*. *Journal of Natural Products* **70**, 1439–1443 (2007).

99. Ndi, C.P., Semple, S.J., Griesser, H.J., Pyke, S.M., & Barton, M.D. Antimicrobial compounds from *Eremophila serrulata*. *Phytochemistry* **68**, 2684–2690 (2007).

100. Cole, M.A., Voelcker, N.H., Thissen, H., & Griesser, H.J. Stimuli-responsive interfaces and systems for the control of protein-surface and cell-surface interactions. *Biomaterials* **30**, 1827–1850 (2009).

101. Gupta, B., Agarwal, R., & Alam, M.S. Textile-based smart wound dressings. *Indian J. of Fibre & Textile Research* **35**, 174–187 (2010).

102. Cosgrove, S.E. Evidence that prevention makes cents: costs of catheter-associated bloodstream infections in the intensive care unit. *Critical Care Medicine* **34**, 2243–2244 (2006).

103. Warren, D.K. et al. Attributable cost of catheter-associated bloodstream infections among intensive care patients in a nonteaching hospital. *Critical Care Medicine* **34**, 2084–2089 (2006).

104. Young, A.E. & Thornton, K.L. Toxic shock syndrome in burns: diagnosis and management. *Archives of Disease in Childhood—Education and Practice Edition* **92**, ep97–ep100 (2007).

105. Woodbridge, T.R., Weisfeld-Adams, J.D., Wilkins, E.C., Estela, C.M., & Young, A.E.R. Epidemiology and severity of paediatric burn injuries occurring during camping and caravanning holidays. *Burns* **36**, 1096–1100 (2010).

106. Poon, V.K.M. & Burd, A. In vitro cytotoxity of silver: implication for clinical wound care. *Burns* **30**, 140–147 (2004).

107. Russell, A.D. & Hugo, W.B. Antimicrobial activity and action of silver. In: Ellis, G.P. & Luscombe, D.K. (eds.), *Progress in Medicinal Chemistry*, pp. 351–369. Amsterdam: Elsevier Science (1994).

108. Asharani, P.V., Wu, Y.L., Gomg, Z.Y., & Valiyaveettil, S. Toxicity of silver nanoparticles in zebra fish models. *Nanotechnology* **19**, (2008). Article No: 255102.

109. Schreml, S., Szeimies, R.M., Karrer, S., Heinlin, J., Landthaler, M., & Babilas, P. The impact of the pH value on skin integrity and cutaneous wound healing. *Journal of the European Academy of Dermatology and Venereology* **24**, 373–378 (2010).

110. Garbern, J.C., Hoffman, A.S., & Stayton, P.S. Injectable pH- and temperature-responsive poly(N-isopropylacrylamide-co-propylacrylic acid) copolymers for delivery of angiogenic growth factors. *Biomacromolecules* **11**, 1833–1839 (2010).

111. Jenkins, A.T.A. & Young, A.E.R. Smart dressings for the prevention of infection in pediatric burns patients. *Expert Review of Anti-infective Therapy* **8**, 1063–1065 (2010).

112. Zhou, J., Loftus, A.L., Mulley, G.J., & Jenkins, A.T.A. A thin film detection/response system for pathogenic bacteria. *Journal of the American Chemical Society* **132**, 6566–6570 (2010).

113. Kolusheva, S., Wachtel, E., & Jelinek, R. Biomimetic lipid/polymer colorimetric membranes: molecular and cooperative properties. *Journal of Lipid Research* **44**, 65–71 (2003).

114. Wilson, G.S. & Gifford, R. Biosensors for real-time in vivo measurements. *Biosensors and Bioelectronics* **30**, 2388–2403 (2005).

115. Anderson, J.M., Rodriguez, A., & Chang, D.T. Foreign body reaction to biomaterials. *Seminars in Immunology* **20**, 86–100 (2008).

116. Anderson, J.M. Mechanisms of inflammation and infection with implanted devices. *Cardiovascular Pathology* **2**, S33–S41 (1993).

117. Nilsson, B. et al. The role of complement in biomaterial-induced inflammation. *Molecular Immunology* **44**, 82–94 (2007).

118. Ekdahl, K.N. & Nilsson, B. Phosphorylation of complement component C3 and C3 fragments by a human platelet protein kinase. Inhibition of factor I-mediated cleavage of C3b. *Journal of Immunology* **154**, 6502–6510 (1995).

119. Chenoweth, D.E. Complement activation produced by biomaterials. *Artificial Organs* **12**, 508–510 (1988).

120. Anderson, J. et al. Binding of C3 fragments on top of adsorbed plasma proteins during complement activation on a model biomaterial surface. *Biomaterials* **26**, 1477–1485 (2005).

121. Anderson, J. et al. C3 adsorbed to a polymer surface can form an initiating alternative pathway convertase. *Journal of Immunology* **168**, 5786–5791 (2002).

122. Nilsson, B. et al. Compstatin inhibits complement and cellular activation in whole bloodin two models of extracorporeal circulation. *Blood* **92**, 1661–1667 (1998).

123. Grailer, J.J., Kodera, M., & Steeber, D.A. L-selectin: role in regulating homeostasis and cutaneous inflammation. *Journal of Dermatological Science* **56**, 141–147 (2009).

124. Vroman, L. & Adams, A.L. Identification of rapid changes at plasma-solid interfaces. *Journal of Biomedical Materials Research* **3**, 43–67 (1969).

125. Jung, S.Y., Lim, S.M., Albertorio, F., Kim, G., Gurau, M.C., Yang, R.D., Holden, M.A., & Cremer, P.S. The Vroman effect: a molecular level description of fibrinogen displacement. *Journal of the American Chemical Society* **125**, 12782–12786 (2003).

126. Kao, W.J. et al. Role for interleukin-4 inforeign-body giant cell formation on a poly(etherurethane urea) in vivo. *Journal of Biomedical Materials Research* **29**, 1267–1275 (1995).

127. McNally, A.K. & Anderson, J.M. Interleukin-4 induces foreign body giant cells from human monocytes/macrophages. Differential lymphokine regulation of macrophage fusion leads to morphological variants of multinucleated giant cells. *American Journal of Pathology* **147**, 1487–1499 (1995).

128. Bown, M.J. et al. The systemic inflammatory response syndrome, organ failure, and mortality after abdominal aortic aneurysm repair. *Journal of Vascular Surgery* **37**, 600–606 (2003).

129. Raja, S.G. & Dreyfus, G.D. Modulation of systemic inflammatory response after cardiac surgery. *Asian Cardiovascular and Thoracic Annals* **13**, 382–395 (2005).

130. Laffey, J.G., Boylan, J.F., & Cheng, D.C. The systemic inflammatory response to cardiac surgery: implications for the anesthesiologist. *Anesthesiology* **97**, 215–252 (2002).

131. Levy, J.H. & Tanaka, K.A. Inflammatory response to cardiopulmonary bypass. *The Annals of Thoracic Surgery* **75**, S715–S720 (2003).

132. Rubens, F.D. & Mesana, T. The inflammatory response to cardiopulmonary bypass: a therapeutic overview. *Perfusion* **19**(Suppl 1), S5–12 (2004).

133. Bledsoe, R.K. et al. Crystal structure of the glucocorticoid receptor ligand binding domain reveals a novel mode of receptor dimerization and coactivator recognition. *Cell* **110**, 93–105 (2002).

134. Carrigan, A. et al. An active nuclear retention signal in the glucocorticoid receptor functions as a strong inducer of transcriptional activation. *The Journal of Biological Chemistry* **282**, 10963–10971 (2007).

135. De Bosscher, K. & Haegeman, G. Minireview: latest perspectives on antiinflammatory actions of glucocorticoids. *Molecular Endocrinology* **28**, 281–291 (2009).

136. Liberman, A.C. et al. Glucocorticoids in thex regulation of transcription factors that control cytokine synthesis. *Cytokine and Growth Factor Reviews* **18**, 45–56 (2007).

137. Hill, G.E. et al. Glucocorticoid reduction of bronchial epithelial inflammation during cardiopulmonary bypass. *American Journal of Respiratory and Critical Care Medicine* **152**, 1791–1795 (1995).

138. Kawamura, T. et al. Influence of methylprednisolone on cytokine balance during cardiac surgery (vol 27, P545). *Critical Care Medicine* **27**, 1404 (1999).

139. Wan, S. et al. Hepatic release of interleukin-10 during ardiopulmonary bypass in steroid-pretreated patients. *American Heart Journal* **133**, 335–339 (1997).

140. Singh, U. & Devaraj, S. Vitamin E: inflammation and atherosclerosis. *Vitamins and Hormones* **76**, 519–549 (2007).

141. De Backer, W.A. et al. N-acetylcysteine pretreatment of cardiac surgery patients influences plasma neutrophil elastase and neutrophil influx in bronchoalveolar lavage fluid. *Intensive Care Medicine* **22**, 900–908 (1996).

142. Calzada, C., Bruckdorfer, K., & Rice Evans, C. The influence of antioxidant nutrients on platelet function in healthy volunteers. *Atherosclerosis* **128**, 97–105 (1997).

143. Steiner, M. Effect of alpha tocopherol administration on platelet function in man. *Thrombosis and Haemostasis* **49**, 73–77 (1983).

144. Barter, P.J., Baker, P.W., & Rye, K.A. Effect of high-density lipoproteins on the expression of adhesion molecules in endothelial cells. *Current Opinion in Lipidology* **13**, 285–288 (2002).

145. Norata, G.D. & Catapano, A.L. Molecular mechanisms responsible for the antiinflammatory and protective effect of HDL on the endothelium. *Vascular Health and Risk Management* **1**, 119–129 (2005).

146. Nofer, J.R. et al. High density lipoproteinassociated lysosphingolipids reduce E-selectin expression in human endothelial cells. *Biochemical and Biophysical Research Communications* **310**, 98–103 (2003).

147. Barter, P.J., Nicholls, S., & Rye, K.A. Anti inflammatory properties of HDL. *Circulation Research* **95**, 764–772 (2004).

148. Mahdy, A.M. & Webster, N.F. Perioperative systemic haemostatic agents. *British Journal of Anaesthesia* **93**, 842–858 (2004).

149. Mannucci, P.M. Hemostatic drugs. *The New England Journal of Medicine* **339**, 245–253 (1998).

150. Diehl, M. & Fischer, M. T.c.P.r., Bayer temporarily suspends global Trasylol marketing. http://www.trasylol.com/Trasylol_11_05_07.pdf, (2007).

151. Davenpeck, K.L. et al. Inhibition of adhesion of human neutrophils and eosinophils to P-selectin by the sialyl Lewis(x) antagonist TBC-1269. Preferential activity against neutrophil adhesion in vitro. *The Journal of Allergy and Clinical Immunology* **105**, 769–775 (2000).

152. Kogan, T.P. et al. Novel synthetic inhibitors of selectin-mediated cell adhesion: synthesis of 1,6-bis[3-(3-carboxymethylphenyl)-4-(2-a-D-mannopyranosyloxy) phenyl]-hexane (TBC-1269). *Journal of Medicinal Chemistry* **41**, 1099–1111 (1997).

153. Hicks, A.E.R. et al. The anti inflammatory effects of a selectin ligandmimetic, TBC-1269, are not a result of competitive inhibition of leukocyte rolling in vivo. *Journal of Leukocyte Biology* **77**, 59–66 (2005).

154. Fitch, J.C. et al. Pharmacology and biological efficacy of a recombinant, humanized, single chain antibody C5 complement inhibitor in patients undergoing coronary artery bypass graft surgery with cardiopulmonary bypass. *Circulation* **100**, 2499–2506 (1999).

155. Ito, K., Chung, K.F., & Adcock, I.M. Update on glucocorticoid action and resistance. *The Journal of Allergy and Clinical Immunology* **117**, 522–543 (2006).

156. Bazzoni, F. & Beutler, B. The tumor necrosis factor ligand and receptor families. *The New England Journal of Medicine* **334**, 1717–1725 (1996).

157. Maini, R. et al. Infliximab (chimeric anti-tumour necrosis factor a monoclonal antibody) versus placebo in rheumatoid arthritis patients receiving concomitant methotrexate: a randomized phase III trial. *Lancet* **354**, 1932–1939 (1999).

158. Horsham, P. and Kenilworth, N.J. Remicade becomes first anti-TNF biologic therapy to treat one million patients worldwide. http://www.jnj.com/connect/ NewsArchive/all-news-archive/20071106_141812 (2007).

159. The Johns Hopkins Arthritis Center. Anti-TNF therapy for the treatment of rheumatoid arthritis. http://www.hopkins-arthritis.org/arthritis-info/rheumatoid-arthritis/tnf.html#development.

160. Janssen, B.J.C. et al. Structure of Compstatin in complex with complement component C3c reveals a new mechanism of complement inhibition. *The Journal of Biological Chemistry* **282**, 29241–29247 (2007).

161. Morikis, D. & Lambris, J.D. Structural aspects and design of low molecular-mass complement inhibitors. *Biochemical Society Transactions* **30**, 1026–1036 (2001).

162. Van Goethem, E. et al. Matrix architecture dictates three-dimensional migration modes of human macrophages: differential involvement of proteases and podosome-like structures. *Journal of Immunology* **184**, 1049–1061 (2010).

163. McNally, A.K., Macewan, S.R., & Anderson, J.M. Alpha subunit partners to beta1 and beta2 integrins during IL-4-induced foreign body giant cell formation. *Journal of Biomedical Materials Research. Part A* **82**, 568–574 (2007).

164. Keselowsky, B.G. et al. Role of plasma fibronectin in the foreign body response to biomaterials. *Biomaterials* **28**, 3626–3631 (2007).

165. Schmidt, D.R. & Kao, W.J. The interrelated role of fibronectin and interleukin-1 in biomaterial-modulated macrophage function. *Biomaterials* **28**, 371–382 (2007).

166. Anderson, J.M., Ziats, N.P., Azeez, A., Brunstedt, M.R., Stack, S., & Bonfield, T.L. Protein adsorption and macrophage activation on polydimethylsiloxane and silicone rubber. *Journal of Biomaterials Science. Polymer Edition* **7**, 159–169 (1995).

167. Bonfield, T.L. & Anderson, J.M. Functional versus quantitative comparison of IL-1 beta from monocytes/macrophages on biomedical polymers. *Journal of Biomedical Materials Research* **27**, 1195–1199 (1992).

168. Bonfield, T.L. et al. Cytokine and growth factor production by monocytes/macrophages on protein preadsorbed polymers. *Journal of Biomedical Materials Research* **26**, 837–850 (1992).

169. DeFife, K.M., Jenney, C.R., McNally, A.K., Colton, E., & Anderson, J.M. Interleukin-13 induces human monocyte/macrophage fusion and macrophage mannose receptor expression. *Journal of Immunology* **158**, 3385–3390 (1997).

170. Brodbeck, W.G. et al. Biomaterial surface chemistry dictates adherent monocyte/macrophage cytokine expression in vitro. *Cytokine* **18**, 311–319 (2002).

171. Ignarro, L.J. Nitric oxide as a unique signaling molecule in the vascular system: a historical overview. *Journal of Physiology and Pharmacology* **53**(4 Pt 1): 503–514 (2002).

172. Stamler, J.S. et al. Nitric oxide circulates in mammalian plasma primarily as an S-nitroso adduct of serum albumin. *Proceedings of the National Academy of Sciences of the United States of America* **89**, 7674–7677 (1992).

173. Hogg, N. Biological chemistry and clinical potential of S-nitrosothiols. *Free Radical Biology and Medicine* **28**, 1478–1486 (2000).

174. Jourd'heuil, D. et al. Dynamic state of S-nitrosothiols in human plasma and whole blood. *Free Radical Biology and Medicine* **28**, 409–417 (2000).

175. Alderton, W.K., Cooper, C.E., & Knowles, R.G. Nitric oxide synthases: structure, function and inhibition. *The Biochemical Journal* **357**, 593–615 (2001).

176. Wong, K. & Li, X.B. Nitric oxide infusion alleviates cellular activation during preparation, leukofiltration and storage of platelets. *Transfusion and Apheresis Science* **30**, 29–39 (2004).

177. Ramamurthi, A. & Lewis, R.S. Design of a novel apparatus to study nitric oxide (NO) inhibition of platelet adhesion. *Annals of Biomedical Engineering* **26**, 1036–1043 (1998).

178. Wallis, J.P. et al. Recovery from post-operative anaemia. *Transfusion Medicine* **15**, 413–418 (2005).

179. Vaughn, M.W., Kuo, L., & Liao, J.C. Estimation of nitric oxide production and reaction rates in tissue by use of a mathematical model. *American Journal of Physiology. Heart and Circulatory Physiology* **43**, H2163–H2176 (1998).

180. Batchelor, M.M. et al. More lipophilic dialkyldiamine-based diazeniumdiolates: synthesis, characterization, and application in preparing thromboresistant nitric oxide release polymeric coatings. *Journal of Medicinal Chemistry* **46**, 5153–5161 (2003).

181. Zhang, H.P. et al. Nitric oxide-releasing fumed silica particles: synthesis, characterization, and biomedical application. *Journal of the American Chemical Society* **125**, 5015–5024 (2003).

182. Hrabie, J.A. & Keefer, L.K. Chemistry of the nitric oxide-releasing diazeniumdiolate ("nitrosohydroxylamine") functional group and its oxygen-substituted derivatives. *Chemical Reviews* **102**, 1135–1154 (2002).

183. Shishido, S.M. & de Oliveira, M.H.G. Polyethylene glycol matrix reduces the rates of photochemical and thermal release of nitric oxide from S-nitroso-N-acetylcysteine. *Photochemistry and Photobiology* **71**, 273–280 (2000).

184. Seabra, A.B. et al. Solid films of blended poly(vinyl alcohol)/poly(vinyl pyrrolidone) for topical S-nitrosoglutathione and nitric oxide release. *Journal of Pharmaceutical Sciences* **94**, 994–1003 (2005).

185. Shishido, S.M. et al. Thermal and photochemical nitric oxide release from S-nitrosothiols incorporated in pluronic F127 gel: potential uses for local and controlled nitric oxide release. *Biomaterials* **24**, 3543–3553 (2003).

186. Bohl, K.S. & West, J.L. Nitric oxide-generating polymers reduce platelet adhesion and smooth muscle cell proliferation. *Biomaterials* **21**, 2273–2278 (2000).

187. Wu, Y. & Meyerhoff, M.E. Nitric oxide-releasing/generating polymers for the development of implantable chemical sensors with enhanced biocompatibility. *Talanta* **75**, 642–650 (2008).

188. Williams, D.L.H. The chemistry of S-nitrosothiols. *Accounts of Chemical Research* **32**, 869–876 (1999).

189. Holmes, A.J. & Williams, D.L.H. Reaction of ascorbic acid with S-nitrosothiols: clear evidence for two distinct reaction pathways. *Journal of the Chemical Society. Perkin Transactions 1* **33**, 1639–1644 (2000).

190. Singh, R.J. et al. Mechanism of nitric oxide release from S-nitrosothiols. *The Journal of Biological Chemistry* **271**, 18596–18603 (1996).

191. Duan, X.B. & Lewis, R.S. Improved haemocompatibility of cysteine-modified polymers via endogenous nitric oxide. *Biomaterials* **23**, 1197–1203 (2002).

192. Oh, B.K. & Meyerhoff, M.E. Spontaneous catalytic generation of nitric oxide from S-nitrosothiols at the surface of polymer films doped with lipophilic copper(II) complex. *Journal of the American Chemical Society* **125**, 9552–9553 (2003).

193. Oh, B.K. & Meyerhoff, M.E. Catalytic generation of nitric oxide from nitrite at the interface of polymeric films doped with lipophilic Cu(II)-complex: a potential route to the preparation of thromboresistant coatings. *Biomaterials* **25**, 283–293 (2004).

194. Lowe, R. et al. Coronary stents: in these days of climate change should all stents wear coats? *Heart* **91**, iii20–iii23 (2005).

195. Jordan, S.W. & Chaikof, E.L. Novel thromboresistant materials. *Journal of Vascular Surgery* **45**, 104A–115A (2007).

196. Weber, N., Wendel, H.P., & Ziemer, G. Quality assessment of heparin coatings by their binding capacities of coagulation and complement enzymes. *Journal of Biomaterials Applications* **15**, 8–22 (2000).

197. Weber, N., Wendel, H.P., & Ziemer, G. Hemocompatibility of heparin-coated surfaces and the role of selective plasma protein adsorption. *Biomaterials* **23**, 429–439 (2002).

198. Riedl, C.R. et al. Heparin coating reduces encrustation of ureteral stents: a preliminary report. *International Journal of Antimicrobial Agents* **19**, 507–510 (2002).

199. Stevens, K.N.J. et al. Bioengineering of improved biomaterials coatings for extracorporeal circulation requires extended observation of blood-biomaterial interaction under flow. *Journal of Biomedicine and Biotechnology* (2007). Article ID 29464.

200. Beaudry, Y. et al. Six-month results of small vessel stenting (2.0–2.8 mm) with the Biodiv Ysio SV stent. *The Journal of Invasive Cardiology* **13**, 628–631 (2001).

201. Sanchez, J., Elgue, G., Riesenfeld, J., & Olsson, P. Studies of adsorption, activation, and inhibition of factor XII on immobilized heparin. *Thrombosis Research* **89**, 41–50 (1998).

202. Sapatnekar, S., Kieswetter, K.M., Merritt, K., Anderson, J.M., Cahalan, L., Verhoeven, M., Hnedriks, M., Fouache, B., & Cahalan, P. Blood biomaterial interactions in a flow system in the presence of bacteria—effect of protein adsorption. *Journal of Biomedical Materials Research* **29**, 247–256 (1995).

203. Jenney, C.R. & Anderson, J.M. Adsorbed serum proteins responsible for surface dependent human macrophage behavior. *Journal of Biomedical Materials Research* **49**, 435–447 (2000).

204. Devin, C. & McCollum, C. Heparin-bonded Dacron or polytetrafluoroethylene for femoropopliteal bypass: five-year results of a prospective randomized multicenter clinical trial. *Journal of Vascular Surgery* **40**, 924–931 (2004).

205. Begovac, P.C. et al. Improvements in GORE-TEX vascular graft performance by Carmeda BioActive surface heparin immobilization. *European Journal of Vascular and Endovascular Surgery* **25**, 432–437 (2003).

206. Lin, P.H. et al. Small-caliber heparin-coated ePTFE grafts reduce platelet deposition and neointimal hyperplasia in a baboon model. *Journal of Vascular Surgery* **39**, 1322–1328 (2004).

207. Edmunds, L.H. & Colman, R.W. Thrombin during cardiopulmonary bypass. *The Annals of Thoracic Surgery* **82**, 15–22 (2006).

208. Lee, J.H., Lee, H.B., & Andrade, J.D. Blood compatibility of polyethylene oxide surfaces. *Progress in Polymer Science* **20**, 1043–1079 (1996).

209. Osterloh, K., Ewert, U., & Pries, A.R. Interaction of albumin with the endothelial cell surface. *American Journal of Physiology. Heart and Circulatory Physiology* **283**, H398–H405 (2002).

210. Lyman, D.J., Klein, K.G., Brash, J.L., Fritzinger, B.K., Andrade, J.D., & Bonomo, F.S. Platelet interaction with protein coated surfaces. *Thrombosis et Diathesis Haemorrhagica* **42**(Suppl), 109 (1970).

211. Park, K., Mosher, D.F., & Cooper, S.L. Acute surface-induced thrombosis in the canine ex vivo model—importance of protein-composition of the initial monolayer and platelet activation. *Journal of Biomedical Materials Research* **20**, 589–612 (1986).

212. Ishikawa, Y., Sasakawa, S., Takase, M., & Osada, Y. Effect of albumin immobilization by plasma polymerization on platelet reactivity. *Thrombosis Research* **35**, 193–202 (1984).

213. Kottke-Marchant, K., Anderson, J.M., Umemura, Y., & Marchant, R.E. Effect of albumin coating on the in vitro blood compatibility of Dacron arterial prostheses. *Biomaterials* **10**, 147–155 (1989).

214. Mulvihill, J.N., Faradji, A., Oberling, F., & Cazenave, J.P. Surface passivation by human albumin of plasmapheresis circuits reduces platelet accumulation and thrombus formation—experimental and clinical studies. *Journal of Biomedical Materials Research* **24**, 155–163 (1990).

215. McFarland, C.D., Jenkins, M., Griesser, H.J., Chatelier, R.C., Steele, J.G., & Underwood, P.A. Albumin-binding surfaces: synthesis and characterization. *Journal of Biomaterials Science. Polymer Edition* **9**, 1207–1225 (1998).

216. Martin, M.C.L., Naeemi, E., Ratner, B.D., & Barbosa, M.A. Albumin adsorption on Cibacron Blue F3G-A immobilized onto oligo(ethylene glycol)-terminated self-assembled monolayers. *Journal of Materials Science: Materials in Medicine* **14**, 945–954 (2003).

217. Nelson, K.D. et al. High affinity polyethylene oxide for improved biocompatibility. *ASAIO Journal* **42**, M884–M889 (1996).

218. Munro, M.S., Quattrone, A.J., Ellsworth, S.R., Kulkarni, P., & Eberhart, R.C. Alkyl substituted polymers with enhanced albumin affinity. *Transactions—American Society for Artificial Internal Organs* **27**, 499–503 (1981).

219. Marois, Y., Chakfe, N., Guidoin, R., Duhamel, R.C., Roy, R., Marois, M., King, M.W., & Douville, Y. An albumin-coated polyester arterial graft: in vivo assessment of biocompatibility and healing characteristics. *Biomaterials* **17**, 3–14 (1996).

220. Al-Khaffaf, H. & Charlesworth, D. Albumin-coated vascular prostheses: a five-year follow-up. *Journal of Vascular Surgery* **23**, 686–690 (1998).

221. DeFife, K.M. et al. Cytoskeletal and adhesive structural polarizations accompany IL-13-induced human macrophage fusion. *The Journal of Histochemistry and Cytochemistry* **47**, 65–74 (1999).

222. Woodhouse, K.A., Klement, P., Chen, V., Gorbet, M.B., Keeley, F.W., Stahl, R., Fromstein, J.D., & Bellingham, C.M. Investigation of recombinant human elastin polypeptides as non-thrombogenic coatings. *Biomaterials* **25**, 4543–4553 (2004).

223. Glasmastar, K. et al. Protein adsorption on supported phospholipid bilayers. *Journal of Colloid and Interface Science* **246**, 40–47 (2002).

224. Andersson, A.S. et al. Cell adhesion on supported lipid bilayers. *Journal of Biomedical Materials Research* **64A**, 622–629 (2003).

225. Vermette, P. et al. Albumin and fibrinogen adsorption onto phosphatidylcholine monolayers investigated by Fourier transform infrared spectroscopy. *Colloids and Surfaces. B, Biointerfaces* **29**, 285–295 (2003).

226. Kaladhar, K. & Sharma, C.P. Supported cell mimetic monolayers and their interaction with blood. *Langmuir* **20**, 11115–11122 (2004).

227. Kaladhar, K. & Sharma, C.P. Cell mimetic lateral stabilization of outer cell mimetic bilayer on polymer surfaces by peptide bonding and their blood compatibility. *Journal of Biomedical Materials Research. Part A* **79A**, 23–35 (2006).

228. Stine, R. et al. Heatstabilized phospholipid films: film characterization and the production of protein-resistant surfaces. *Langmuir* **21**, 11352–11356 (2005).

229. Orban, J.M. et al. Cytomimetic biomaterials. 4. In situ photopolymerization of phospholipids on an alkylated surface. *Macromolecules* **33**, 4205–4212 (2000).

230. Rogers, T.H. & Babensee, J.E. Altered adherent leukocyte profile on biomaterials in Toll-like receptor 4 deficient mice. *Biomaterials* **31**, 594–601 (2010).

231. Ross, E.E. et al. Planar supported lipid bilayer polymers formed by vesicle fusion. 1 Influence of diene monomer structure and polymerization method on film properties. *Langmuir* **19**, 1752–1765 (2003).

232. Kim, H.K., Kim, K., & Byun, Y.P. Preparation of a chemically anchored phospholipid monolayer on an acrylated polymer substrate. *Biomaterials* **26**, 3435–3444 (2005).

233. Whelan, D.M. et al. Biocompatibility of phosphorylcholine coated stents in normal porcine coronary arteries. *Heart* **83**, 338–345 (2000).

234. Kuiper, K.K.J. et al. Phosphorylcholine-coated metallic stents in rabbit iliac and porcine coronary arteries. *Scandinavian Cardiovascular Journal* **32**, 261–268 (1998).

235. Lewis, A.L., Tolhurst, L.A., & Stratford, P.W. Analysis of a phosphorylcholine-based polymer coating on a coronary stent pre- and post-implantation. *Biomaterials* **23**, 1697–1706 (2002).

236. Malik, N., Gunn, J., & Shepherd, L. Phosphorylcholine-coated stents in porcine coronary arteries: in vivo assessment of biocompatibility. *The Journal of Invasive Cardiology* **13**, 193–201 (2001).

237. Atalar, E., Haznedaroglu, I., & Aytemir, K. Effects of stent coating on platelets and endothelial cells after intracoronary stent implantation. *Clinical Cardiology* **24**, 159–164 (2001).

238. The Merck Manuals. http://www.merckmanuals.com/professional/immunology_allergic_disorders/biology_of_the_immune_system/complement_system.html.

CHAPTER 7

Intelligent Polymer Thin Films and Coatings for Drug Delivery

ALEXANDER N. ZELIKIN and BRIGITTE STÄDLER

7.1 INTRODUCTION

Past decades have witnessed the advent and accelerated development of biomedical engineering into a mature discipline that has already revolutionized health care and holds further promises for drug delivery, tissue engineering, and other biomedical applications with the ultimate goal of improving the quality of life. In turn, recent advances in tissue engineering and design of therapeutic implants called for the emergence of a novel research direction, namely, surface-mediated drug delivery. In a particular example of implants and stents, surface-mediated drug delivery enables greater control over tissue compatibility and tissue regeneration; for tissue engineering, controlled release of chemical stimuli and therapeutic cargo affords control over cell attachment, proliferation, and differentiation. Such applications require innovative strategies for a localized sustained drug release, and the challenge was recently addressed through the advent of intelligent polymer-based surface coatings for surface-mediated drug release. A particular success story relates to the sequential polymer deposition technique (layer by layer [LBL]), a strategy that enables the modification of virtually any unprepared surface with a polymer thin film of controlled thickness and functionality (see Methods Box 7.1). This technique exploits the interaction of macromolecules with their surface adsorbed complementary counterpart, for example, polymers with opposite charge, hydrogen-bonding donor–acceptor role, and reactive chemical moieties. Iterative repetition of this interaction leads to a buildup of a thin film, whereby the thickness of the film depends on the deposition conditions and the number of deposition steps. The process is typically all aqueous, which is highly favorable for drug loading and cargo stability and requires minimal,

Intelligent Surfaces in Biotechnology: Scientific and Engineering Concepts, Enabling Technologies, and Translation to Bio-Oriented Applications, First Edition.
Edited by H. Michelle Grandin and Marcus Textor.
© 2012 John Wiley & Sons, Inc. Published 2012 by John Wiley & Sons, Inc.

if any, surface preparation, the two characteristics making it highly attractive for biomedicine. Coupled with its instrumental simplicity, this has led to a sweeping development of LBL, and over the past two decades, the field has documented the use of commercial and custom-made polymers to meet virtually any demand for tuning and designing surface characteristics (Fig. 7.1). For biomedicine, the field offered the use of natural and biodegradable polymers and a suite of techniques for drug loading and controlled release, and, from proof-of-concept reports, this discipline has recently progressed to the first *in vivo* successes. The aim of this book chapter is therefore to present the potential held by the sequential polymer deposition technique as a tool in the design of intelligent polymer coatings for drug delivery.

METHODS BOX 7.1   ASSEMBLY OF MULTILAYERED POLYMER THIN FILMS ON PLANAR AND MACROSCOPIC SUBSTRATES

Substrate: Essentially no limit

Polymers: Essentially no limit, for typical candidate materials (see Fig. Box 7.1)

Protocol: In a typical procedure, a substrate is immersed into a 1 g/L solution of a polymer for 15 minutes to ensure adsorption and oversaturation of the surface with the polymer, followed by washing with copious amounts of water/buffer solution to remove the excess polymer. The substrate is then immersed in a solution of a complementary polymer (opposite charge, hydrogen-bonding donor–acceptor role, covalent linkage group, etc.) followed by washing. This completes the adsorption of one bilayer (one layer of each polymer) and can be repeated as necessary until the desired thickness of the film is attained.

Notes: The above exemplary protocol represents a typical procedure of coating of a substrate with a multilayered polymer film and, as such, is flexible in most constituting steps, namely, polymer concentration, presence of low-molecular-weight electrolytes, pH, duration of adsorption, and washing steps. Exposure of the substrate to polymers is commonly achieved via substrate immersion; however, other approaches are also employed, for example, spraying of solutions onto a substrate surface. The assembly of polymer multilayers commonly proceeds in either a "linear" fashion (with each adsorbed bilayer, the thickness increases with the same increment) or an "exponential" fashion (gradually increased thickness with each consecutive bilayer). At each step, a mixture of two or more polymers can be used to achieve their coadsorption and to form a "blended" layer of polymers.

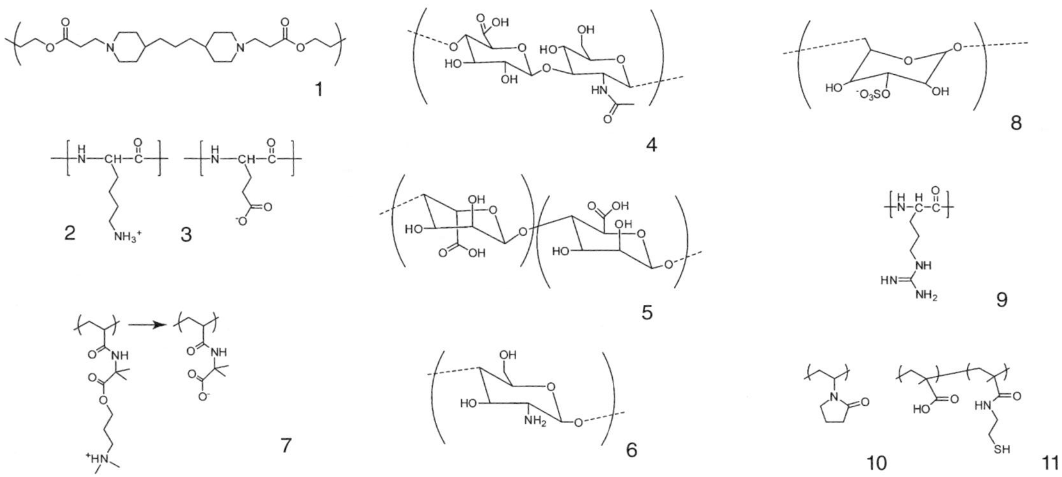

Figure 7.1 Candidate polymers for LBL: Multilayered polymer thin films for both surface-mediated drug delivery and assembly of polymer capsules employ various strategies to ensure a controlled degradation of the film and a controlled drug release. On planar substrates, successful candidate polymers include hydrolytically degradable poly(β-aminoesters) (1), enzymatically degradable (pseudo) natural peptides poly-L-lysine (2) and poly-L-glutamic acid (3), polysaccharides hyaluronic acid (4), alginic acid (5), and chitosan (6), as well as "charge-shifting" polymers (7). On colloidal substrates, the most successful examples of capsular drug carriers employ biodegradable polymers dextran sulfate (8) assembled with poly-L-arginine (9) and a hydrogen-bonded polymer pair, poly(vinyl pyrrolidone) (10) and thiolated poly(methacrylic acid) (11), the latter system giving rise to disulfide-stabilized single-component PMA hydrogel capsules.

245

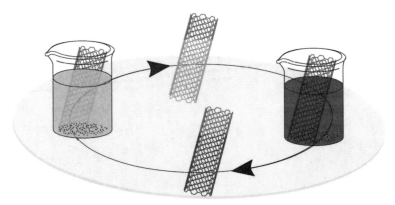

Figure Box 7.1 Schematic illustration of LBL performed via a repetitive adsorption of two interacting polymers and using a model macroscopic (planar) substrate. (See color insert.)

From a different perspective, the delivery of therapeutics using colloidal carriers is another avenue of research that benefits from the use of polymer coatings, specifically to modulate the carrier–tissue compatibility, to mask toxicity, and to achieve targeting. Some of the advanced opportunities in materials design offered by the LBL technique were adapted for implementation on colloidal particles, and the first successes of these undertakings in drug delivery are covered in the second part of this book chapter. Finally, the recent addition to the arsenal of colloidal drug carriers, namely, polymer capsules obtained via sequential polymer deposition on sacrificial colloidal templates, is briefly overviewed. Together with the concluding remarks on the plausible future developments of the field, this chapter provides a concise overview of the recent successes in the design of intelligent polymer films for drug delivery.

7.2 SURFACE-MEDIATED DRUG DELIVERY

Delivery of therapeutic cargo from the surface of a biomaterial is a facile and effective approach to modulate interaction of surfaces with adherent and suspension cells. As such, the use of polymer coatings to modulate cell adhesion is among the most well-established techniques with multiple polymer candidate materials and several polymer immobilization approaches readily available. A recent development in the field relates with the possibility of using these coatings to achieve both modulation of cell adhesion and controlled release of immobilized cargo for drug delivery, the latter being the main focus of this book chapter. Polymer adsorption and grafting are prominent techniques for the modulation of surface properties, yet to date, their utility in drug delivery has been limited. In contrast, sequential polymer deposition affords multilayered polymer architectures with controlled thicknesses, a possibility for spatial separation of drug reservoir layers and a surface to modulate inter-action with cells, a possibility of controlled degradation of the film, and controlled drug release. We believe that it is the combination of each of these factors in one technique that makes LBL such an attractive approach to surface modification and, in particular, the creation of intelligent polymer coatings for surface-mediated drug delivery.

7.2.1 Controlled Cell Adhesion and Proliferation

While an overall overview of biomaterial–cell interaction is beyond the scope of this chapter, in this section, we will briefly summarize the characteristics of LBL thin films toward modulation of cellular adhesion, specifically in the light of their potential use as drug depots. We emphasize that two independent modes of drug release are equally important and are clinically relevant with the use of polymer thin films, namely, (i) a gradual release of therapeutic molecules into the surrounding solution (a mimic of controlled drug release into the blood stream or surrounding tissue from a subcutaneously implanted carrier) and (ii) an uptake of the drug by adherent cells, possibly through substrate erosion or degradation facilitated by cells. In this regard, both cyto-phobic (cell adhesion resistant) and cytophilic (cell-adhesive) surfaces are important, and the overall goal is to gain control over biomaterial surface interaction with cells, coupled with a control over the kinetics of drug release. This part of the book chapter describes the properties of polymer thin films as substrates for cell adhesion and proliferation and then details the successes of this technique in the delivery of small molecule cargoes, peptide, and protein drugs, and finally, nucleic acid therapeutics.

The flexibility of the LBL technology and a wide array of available poly-mers with their inherent properties imply that multilayered polymer films can be tailored to exhibit cell-adhesive properties or to be cell resistant. This is indeed the case, and a multitude of cell types were successfully seeded on a variety of substrates coated with diverse polymer coatings; for a recent com-prehensive review, see Boudou et al.[1] As with other substrates, the "classical tools" of control over cell attachment, namely, surface coating using poly(ethylene glycol) (PEG) to prevent cell adhesion,[2–4] as well as the use of cell-adhesive proteins[5,6] and peptide sequences,[4,7] for example, arginyl-glycyl-aspartic acid (RGD), are all available in the context of LBL films. In either case, surface immobilization of PEG or RGD can be achieved without com-promising the bulk properties of the underlying (drug containing) polymer film. This approach to surface modification remains similar if applied to a polymer thin film or to a bare unprepared surface, and, as such, is extensively reviewed and updated. For this reason, we avoid a detailed discussion of this subject herein and instead focus on alternative strategies that are more unique to the multilayered polymer films.

During the past decade, the mechanical properties of substrates have been recognized as a factor with utmost importance in their interaction with adhering cells, and it has become a powerful addition to the arsenal of tools to gain control over cell–biomaterial interactions. The early observations were made using polyacrylamide gels with a gradient substrate rigidity achieved through a variation in an employed concentration of the cross-linker.[8] Remarkably, NIH 3T3 cells showed a distinct preference of more rigid areas of the gel surface and changed their migration direction to avoid the soft substrate.[8] This observation has led to a novel research direction attracting scientists from physics, biology, chemistry, and other areas of basic and applied science. Coincidently, around the same time, it was observed that the deposition of multi-layered polymer films can give rise to substrates that are effectively cytophobic, that is, those that support no cell adhesion.[9] This effect was achieved only upon the deposition of a certain number of poly-L-lysine (PLL)/alginate (ALG) polymer layers and was attributed to a gel-like, soft consistency of the thin film. These two reports, despite a very different background and research direction, effectively showed that substrate elasticity is pivotal for the adhesion of mammalian cells and their proliferation on the surfaces, and this finding has subsequently found extensive support within the field of multilayered polymer thin films.

A remarkable feature of the LBL technique, which is inherent with the sequential deposition employed to assemble the polymer film, is that this cytophobic–cytophilic property of the substrate can be effectively reversed via deposition of additional polymer layers. This was shown in 2003 by Rubner et al.[10] on substrates built using the polymers with pH-sensitive ionization behavior, poly(acrylic acid) (PAA) and poly(allylamine hydrochloride) (PAH). The deposition of PAA from its acidic solutions results in a thick polymer layer and, once transferred into pH 7, a polymer layer highly enriched with non-compensated charge, that is, reminiscent of an anionic hydrogel. In contrast, PAA deposition conducted from solutions with pH 6–7 yields polymer films with a well-compensated charge and a stiffer morphology. As a result, the former multilayers were effectively cytophobic and did not support cell adhesion; in contrast, the latter were quite similar in their ability to support cell adhesion to the tissue culture polystyrene (Fig. 7.2a). The design of these films employed the same two polymers, and thus biomaterial–cell interaction was modulated solely by the mechanical properties of the substrate, not the chemistry of polymer film. Furthermore, the deposition of films with "cytophilic" morphology on top of the "cytophobic" counterparts effectively reversed the performance of the biomaterial providing elegant proof of the facile and versatile nature of the LBL films as tools to modulate the properties of biomaterials. This example also suggests that the inner volume of the thin film can serve as a drug reservoir, while the subsequent layers independently serve the need to control the cellular adhesion. In a follow-up publication, Van Vliet et al.[11] further characterized the PAA/PAH system and established a correlation between mechanical compliance of the multilayered polymer film and its attractiveness to cells for attachment. The topmost layer of the multilayered film had a modest effect on cell adhesion. Remarkably, cell proliferation

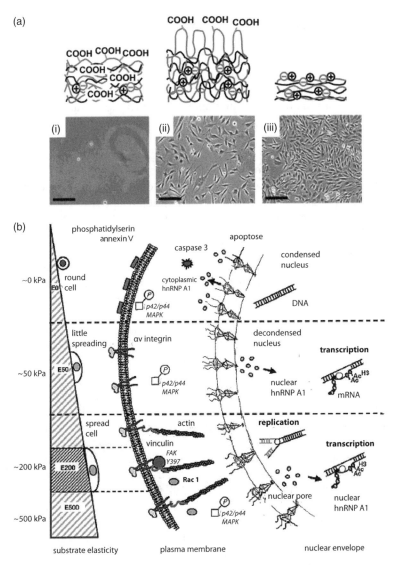

Figure 7.2 Effect of surface elasticity on cell adhesion: The mechanical properties of the substrate were recently recognized as a powerful tool to control cell adhesion and proliferation. (a) Intelligent polymer films allow for modulation of the mechanical compliance of the substrate using different polymers or, as in the presented case, via rational choice of polymer film assembly conditions. PAA/PAH multilayered films were constructed using adsorption solutions with varied pH to obtain "cytophobic" films with a gel-like morphology (i), coatings with increased stiffness and corresponding increased cell adhesiveness (ii), and polymer films well stitched through ionic bonds, which exhibited cell-adhesive properties similar to tissue culture polystyrene (iii). Adapted from Mendelsohn et al.,[10] American Chemical Society. © 2003. (b) Schematic illustration of cellular processes and cell adhesion behavior observed on substrates with varied mechanical compliance. Substrate elasticity has a complex and uncoupled influence on transcription and replication processes, a feature that may have significance for surface-mediated drug delivery, specifically to cell cycle-synchronized cells or cells with modulated cell activities. Adapted with permission from Kocgozlu et al.,[18] Company of Biologists Ltd. © 2010.

(division) was rather similar for all the substrates, and the final cell count was largely determined by the number of initially adhered cells.

Thus, mechanical properties of the substrate have become an important tool of control over the adhesion of mammalian cells to the surface of a biomaterial. In the examples above, substrate elasticity was modulated via the assembly conditions that led to an enrichment of the multilayered architecture with one of the constituents and a gel-like morphology of the resulting film. Another facile method of control over the mechanical properties of the films exploits cross-linking of the assembled films. In most cases, the polycationic component of the LBL film bares ionized (ionizable) amine groups (PLL and PAH), and the polyanionic counterpart has carboxylic functionalities (PAA, polyglutamic acid [PGA], and hyaluronic acid [HA]). These moieties can be cross-linked via amide linkages, for example, through a carbodiimide-mediated coupling, allowing a facile way of modulation of such properties of the thin film as degradation kinetics and, of importance for this discussion, mechanical properties. This approach is particularly important when applied to the thin films assembled using (pseudo)natural polymers, polypeptides, and polysaccharides, which often have a soft, gel-like morphology and therefore, as such, are poor substrates for cell adhesion. However, it is these films that hold immense potential as drug carrier films, and modulation of their cell-adhesive properties is therefore highly warranted.

Among the first examples, 1-ethyl-3-[3-dimethylaminopropyl]carbodiimide hydrochloride (EDC)-mediated cross-linking was employed to cross-link multilayered polymer films assembled using PLL and HA.[12] Pristine PLL/HA films, terminated with either PLL or HA, were poor substrates, and neither adhesion nor spreading of chondrosarcoma cells (HCS2/8) in culture over 2–6 days was observed. In contrast, when seeded on cross-linked thin films, the cells adhered and spread well and the cell density was comparable to that observed on uncoated glass slides. For this cross-linking route, EDC concentration and conjugation time present themselves as means to tweak the cross-linking density, and this was shown to affect the cell-adhesive properties of the film.[13] Furthermore, there was a correlation between Young's modulus of the thin film, and the observed cell spreading area, which further highlights the impact of the substrate elasticity on cell adhesion and proliferation. Similarly, skeletal smooth muscle cells (SMCs) exhibited preference to stiffer substrates (PLL/HA multilayers with a higher cross-linking density), which favored the formation of focal adhesion points, organization of cytoskeleton, and enhanced cell proliferation.[14] As with chondrosarcoma cells, softer substrates were poor substrates for adhesion of SMCs. In this work, the substrate elasticity was also found to affect the rate of cellular proliferation (measured by direct cell counting), as well as the kinetics of formation of myotubes, their detachment from the substrate, and also the morphology of the formed myotubes. Thus, substrate elasticity has a complex impact on the adhesion and subsequent proliferation of SMCs. Mesenchymal stem cells (MSCs)[15] and embryonic stem cells[16] (ESC), respectively, were also found to exhibit a preference toward cross-linked, stiffer PLL/HA films for adhesion and proliferation, and pristine films were found to support little, if any, cell adhesion. Chemical stimuli were then used for a successful differentiation of MSC into osteocytes and chondrocytes,[15] and for ESC, substrate mechanical properties influenced the differentiation of cells into an epiblast.[16] Cross-linking was also employed to modulate the properties of chitosan (CHI)/HA and CHI/ALG multilayered films toward their enhanced cell adhesiveness.[17]

Very recently, a more detailed analysis of the substrate elasticity on cell attachment and cell function was conducted using PtK2 epithelial cells and PLL/HA multilayers.[18] The substrate elasticity in this work was modulated via adsorption of additional layers of poly(styrene sulfonate) (PSS)/PAH, which further illustrates the flexibility of LBL as a technique to fabricate substrates with controlled mechanical elasticity and cell-adhesive properties. In agreement with the findings described earlier, pristine PLL/HA multilayered films were ill suited to support cell attachment, and an increase in the substrate rigidity was accompanied by a progressive increase in cell adhesion. This report further demonstrates that substrate elasticity has an influence on multiple intracellular processes and that this influence on transcription and on replication activities is uncoupled (Fig. 7.2b). On soft substrates, the cells had a morphology reminiscent of apoptotic cells. On substrates with an elastic modulus around 50 kPa, the cells were active in transcription, yet it took a further increase in substrate rigidity to ~200 kPa to observe initiation of cell replication. We believe that these findings can have a significant influence on the field of surface-mediated drug delivery, specifically for delivery to cells with synchronized cell cycles or modulated cell activities.

Other multilayered polymer films were also explored for their ability to support cell adhesion and proliferation. Thus, biodegradable PLL/PGA films with a promise for drug delivery applications were among the early candidate materials tested. While PLL-terminated polymer films supported the attachment of cells (melanoma[19] and chondrosarcoma[20]), their PGA-terminated counterpart were ill suited to support the attachment of chondrosacroma cells.[20] Different terminating layers (positively charged polyethyleneimine [PEI], PAH, PLL; negatively charged PGA and PSS) deposited on an underlying cushion of PSS/PAH film were tested for their ability to support adhesion of osteoblast-like SaOS-2 cells and human periodontal ligament (PDL) cells.[21] All candidate polymers were found to be well suited for this with the exception of PEI, the latter coatings being toxic to the cells. PSS- and PGA-terminated films exhibited good biocompatibility, as did PLL-terminated films toward SaOS-2 cells. When cultured on PGA- and PSS-terminated films, cells maintained the level of early osteoblast phenotypic markers over at least 48 hours, and none of the polyelectrolyte architectures tested in this work induced a production of tumor necrosis factor-α (TNF-α), indicating a lack of inflammatory responses mediated by the thin films. It was also observed that, at least for the systems studied, the cells did not detect the influence of the underlying polymer layers, not even the one immediately below the topmost layer, which suggests that the properties associated with the outer layer of the thin film play a decisive role.

Wittmer et al.[22] carried out a comprehensive study of polyelectrolyte multilayered coatings toward their hepatocellular applications and tested several polymer combinations for their ability to support attachment and proliferation of hepatocellular carcinoma cells (HepG2), adult rat hepatocytes (ARHs), and human fetal hepatoblasts (HFHbs). The films were assembled using synthetic polymers (PSS and PAH) as well as biodegradable polypeptides (PLL and PGA) and polysaccharides (CHI and ALG). One of the main findings of this report was that adhesiveness of a particular coating is cell type specific, and the same coating may not support attachment and proliferation of different cell types equally well. Further, of all the polymer film combinations tested, HepG2 cells reached confluency only when cultured on PSS-terminated PSS/PAH films and PLL-terminated cross-linked PLL/ALG films. It is surprising that thin films assembled using mimics of the extracellular matrix, that is, polysaccharides, did not support the attachment of HepG2 even when functionalized with galactose, a molecule that is used for specific recognition with hepatocytes. Overall, this work significantly contributes toward the identification of optimal candidate materials for liver tissue engineering applications. For the broad field of LBL coatings, it also demonstrates that cell surface interactions are to a great degree specific for a particular system and further highlights that these effects can be modulated via physicochemical approaches such as adsorption of proadhesive collagen coatings or cross-linking of the films.

One of the areas where controlled cell adhesion is of particular practical importance is cardivascular stenting and revascularization. In these applications, adhesion of endothelial cells is a desired effect, whereas adhesion of vascular cells, platelets, and growth of blood thrombi is undesired. To this end, Tabrizian et al. reported on polymer thin films consisting of CHI and HA, which were deposited on the internal surface of damaged aortic porcine arteries, and the polymer films effectively prevented platelet adhesion.[23] Incorporation of arginine, a precursor of nitric oxide, into the multilayered architecture further improved the performance of thin films, that is, decreased platelet adhesion. Coupled with drug loading and release techniques, as described further, this approach is highly promising for the creation of bioactive coatings. Polyelectrolyte thin films were also evaluated as tools to improve the mechanical properties of allografts during their cryopreservation. PSS/PAH films deposited in the luminal space of de-endothelialized arteries significantly enhanced their mechanical stability, rendering their performance similar to that of fresh arteries, and also resulted in an enhanced rate of re-endothelialization.[24] This approach for improved performance of small artery replacements was then tested *in vivo* and was proven to be highly promising with no detectable graft rejection and effective endothelialization of the thin film functionalized surface.[25] We expect that the performance of these

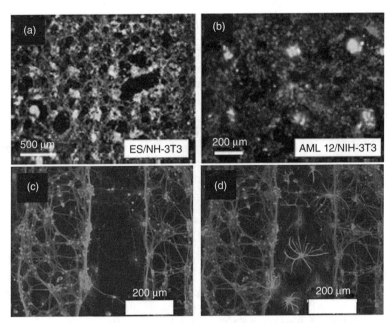

Figure 7.3   Patterning: Intelligent polymer thin films were used to achieve successful cell patterning and coculturing of multiple cell types, a significant step toward engineering of complex tissues with multiple cells. (a,b) Patterning and coculturing of embryonic cells (green, a) or hepatocytes (green, b) with fibroblasts (red, a,b) was achieved via seeding of primary cells on the surface with cell-resistant hualuronic acid islands. Subsequent coating of HA with fibronectin converted HA islets into cell-adhesive surfaces and allowed the seeding of secondary cells. Images reproduced from Fukuda et al.,[6] Elsevier. © 2006. (c,d) Patterning of neurons and astrocytes was achieved using synthetic polymers, PSS and poly(diallyldimethylammonium chloride) (PDADMAC), a multilayered polymer film with a surface patterned with PDDA via microcontact printing, and using a preference of neurons to adhere to a PSS-coated surface. Neurons were introduced first, and these cells occupied the PSS-coated surface; astrocytes were then introduced, and these adhered to the regions between neurons to give a final patterned surface for coculturing of these two cell types. Reprinted with permission from Kidambi et al.,[27] Wiley-VCH Verlag GmbH & Co. KGaA. © 2008. (See color insert.)

materials can be further improved when coupled with the drug release strategies discussed next.

Cell patterning and coculturing represents an approach toward the creation of multi-cell-type ensembles en route to complex tissue organization (Fig. 7.3). This has been realized on planar substrates employing multilayered polymer thin films using a cytophobic character of HA and the ease of reversal of this property by an added layer of PLL.[26] Thus, a fibronectin (FN)-coated glass surface was patterned using HA to produce non-cell-adhesive HA islets and to guide the attachment of the first cell type between the HA islets. Subsequent addition of PLL made the initially cytophobic HA islets cytophilic, and the introduced cells occupied the HA/PLL islets giving rise to a patterned multi-cell-type ensemble. This technique was then modified to achieve patterning of three components of the extracellular matrix, namely, FN, HA, and collagen.[6] In another report, patterning and coculturing of primary neurons and astrocytes was achieved on multilayered thin films using the synthetic polymers, PSS, and poly(diallyldimethylammonium chloride) (PDADMAC).[27] This work made use of a preference exhibited by neurons toward adhesion on PSS-coated surfaces, while astrocytes adhered well to surfaces coated with either polymer. First, polymer patterning was achieved via microcontact printing; neurons were then introduced and shown to adhere predominantly onto the PSS-coated surface. Subsequently, astrocytes were introduced and found to adhere between the neurons, thus giving rise to patterned cocultured cell architecture.

In three-dimensional (3-D) space, the multilayered architecture of films lends itself to obtain multistrata assemblies with individual or cocultured cells. To achieve this, a suitable separation polymer thin film has to be identified, taking into account the potential cytotoxic effects of polymers, especially that of polycations. Akashi et al.[5] have assembled four-layered architectures of fibroblast cells and have used FN and gelatin as constituents of the separation films. Both FN and gelatin are biocompatible and are negatively charged at physiological conditions, and their interaction to form a multilayered thin film relies on the collagen-binding domain on FN, that is, specific recognition. When deposited on the surface of an underlying cell sheet, at least 6-nm-thick FN/gelatin films are required to act as a suitable cell-adhesive surface for the attachment of the next cell layer. In another report, 3-D stratified films were assembled via a polymer/gel spraying technique employing a calcium ALG gel as a potential cell reservoir and layers of gel separated by PLL/HA polymer thin films.[28] We envision that the discussed efforts in cell patterning and 3-D organization will likely benefit from their coupling with drug delivery approaches, which will be discussed in the following section.

7.2.2 Small Cargo

Of the diverse candidate therapeutics for controlled release from the multi-layered polymer thin films, low-molecular-weight drugs are possibly the most challenging and thus remain the least explored. Polyelectrolyte multilayers are typically highly hydrated films with some examples even reminiscent of swollen hydrogels. As with most hydrogels, typical LBL films allow nearly unhindered diffusion of small molecules and are, therefore, ill suited for the confinement and controlled release of such therapeutics. However, a few notable exceptions can be mentioned here.

Impregnation of preformed multilayered thin films with a drug candidate, that is, adsorption of the drug from its solution into an assembled film, is one of the plausible approaches for drug entrapping in LBL films. Paclitaxel was introduced by this method into PLL/HA films, and the loading dose was under an effective control of the drug concentration in the solution used for impregnation.[29] Once absorbed, the drugs stayed in the film immersed in 0.15 M NaCl, pH 6.5, for at least 4 days without signs of passive desorption from the film. To allow cell adhesion, PLL/HA films were then capped with a layer of PSS or PSS/PAH multilayers, which also served the purpose of modifying the availability of paclitaxel to the cultured cells. The cytotoxic drug was effectively delivered to the cultured cells, reducing their viability and thus verifying the utility of this approach for a surface-mediated delivery of paclitaxel. Similarly, cross-linked CHI/HA and PLL/HA films were postloaded with diclofenac and paclitaxel for their delivery to the cultured cells.[30] Gentamicin, an aminoglycoside antibiotic, was loaded into a polymer thin film with HA and a biodegradable poly(β-aminoester) as the main structural constituents of the film.[31] This strategy afforded good control over the drug loading, and the release kinetics were defined by the choice of a degradable polycation. Released gentamicin effectively suppressed bacterial growth without altering the viability of model mammalian cells, thus making it a promising technique to obtain antibacterial coatings. An important step toward a controlled incorporation and release of small drugs from LBL films exploits a covalent conjugation of the drug candidate to a carrier polymer, which is then used in the construction of the thin film. To this end, paclitaxel was conjugated to HA and the polymer was incorporated into a multilayered film with CHI.[32] While pristine HA/CHI multilayers exhibited no cytotoxicity, the paclitaxel-functionalized counterpart displayed a ~95% decrease in viability of model cells. The above-mentioned examples illustrate that polymer films can be used to adsorb and subsequently release small cargo therapeutics. However, successes of these undertakings are few and are likely hard to be adapted for a broad range of low-molecular-weight drugs. Furthermore, it may be increasingly harder to engineer independent release profiles for multiple candidate drugs from the same coating. In this regard, we believe that incorporation of supramolecular drug carriers into the polymer thin films presents an opportunity to increase the scope and utility of these films for the delivery of small cargo.

Micelles and liposomes are among the best-performing and most well-established drug carriers. These carriers can accommodate the delivery of diverse cargo (hydrophilic, hydrophobic, etc.); the first micelle- and liposome-based products are already marketed, and more candidate formulations are currently in clinical trials. It can therefore be highly beneficial to incorporate these drug-loaded vehicles into the LBL multilayers for their sustained release or presentation to the cultured cells. To this end, micelles have been incorporated into polymer thin films through covalent,[33] electrostatic,[34] and hydrogen[35] bonding. Liposomes have also been introduced into polymer films via electrostatic interactions.[36-38] Recently, a noncovalent liposome anchoring strategy based on cholesterol-modified polymers was developed to facilitate embedding of liposomes into polymer films.[39,40] This approach is largely insensitive to the lipid composition of the liposomes or to the presence of other solutes in the medium, thus making it a convenient and facile technique. However, both the micelles and the liposomes as supramolecular carriers for surface-mediated drug delivery remain largely unexplored, with only a few successful examples having been reported.

Hydrogen-bonded polymer films constructed with the use of a polycarbox-ylic acid (PAA and polymethacrylic acid [PMA]) are attractive candidate materials in that they are inherently unstable in physiological conditions. These polymer films are typically assembled in acidic media and spontane-ously disintegrate when placed in a solution with a pH above the pKa of the polyacid. Covalent stabilization of these multilayers is often employed to render these films stable, and the kinetics of degradation of these films can be tuned via the choice of the cross-linking chemistry. For micelle-assisted surface-mediated delivery of triclosan, the hydrophobic internal volume of poly(ethylene oxide)-b-poly(ε-caprolactone) (PEO-PCL) micelles has been used as a drug reservoir, and the PEO corona facilitated the incorporation of the micelles into polymer films with a hydrogen-bonding donor, PAA.[41] As assembled, the films are unstable and their exposure to phosphate buffered saline (PBS) buffer (pH 7.4) results in a complete release of the drug within ~120 minutes. Thermal cross-linking of the films through anhydride linkages yields a much more stable yet biodegradable film, and the release profile for triclosan can be extended to almost 2 weeks and can further be tuned via the cross-linking conditions. In another report, micelle forming poly(propylene oxide)-function-alized poly(amidoamine) (PPO-PAMAM) dendrimers were used as positively charged components of a thin film with PAA as a negatively charged counter-part, and the inner micellar compartment was used to incorporate triclosan.[42] The cumulative drug loading was under an effective control of a number of deposited polymer–micelle layers, and the released drug was effectively inhib-iting bacterial growth. We expect that the use of supramolecular drug carriers as components of multilayered polymer films for surface-mediated drug deliv-ery will see a significant development in the upcoming future.

A facile alternative to both micelles and liposomes as hosts for small mol-ecule cargo is presented by cyclodextrins (CDs). Their potential in the context of multilayered polymer films was realized using PLL/PGA films and a nega-tively charged carboxymethylthio-β-cyclodextrin as a carrier for a non-steroidal anti-inflammatory drug, piroxicam.[43] Human THP-1 cells were first stimulated with lipopolysaccharide (LPS) to induce the production of proinflammatory cytokine, TNF-α. An inhibition of TNF-α production by THP-1 cells was used as a measure of bioactivity of the polymer films, and these were found to remain active for a period of at least 12 hours. Concurrently, another CD candidate was used with PLL/PGA multilayered films for the delivery of LPS, a reagent typically used to stimulate the production of cytokines.[44] This work highlights the importance of CD molecules in thin films: In the absence of CD, incorporated LPS was ineffective in stimulating the production of cytokines. In contrast, when exposed to films containing an inclusion complex of LPS with CD, the cells were producing TNF-α at a level comparable to that observed in cells exposed to LPS in solution. PLL/PGA films with embedded positively charged CDs were also effective carriers for lipid A antagonists and, similar to piroxicam-containing films, were effective in inhibiting the production of TNF-α by the THP-1 cells.[45] Bioconjugation of CD molecules to a carrier polymer chain has also been explored as a strategy for the controlled incorporation of these host molecules into drug-releasing polymer thin films, specifically for the incorporation of bisphosphonate drugs used in the prevention of bone metastasis.[46] A very recent example reported by the Hammond group further demonstrates the possibilities offered by these intelligent films, specifically for the controlled and timed release of non-steroidal anti-inflammatory drugs (flurbiprofen and diclofenac) and antibiotics (ciprofloxacin).[47] To achieve this, a negatively charged poly(carboxymethyl-β-cyclodextrin) was used as a host for small cargo and was incorporated into thin films with a hydrolytically degradable poly(β-aminoesters). Assembled films exhibited a negligible burst release of cargo and a near-linear release kinetics over at least 2 weeks. The use of CDs as hosts implied that, with the use of the same degradable polycation, drug release kinetics are largely independent of the nature of the drug and are similar for the tested compounds. This offers a simple way of delivering multiple therapeutic molecules from within the same polymer film with a well-controlled dosage of each component. This system takes further advantage of the multilayered architecture of the films and affords a surface erosion of the layers and a sequential release of associated drug molecules. The kinetics of this process is well defined by the choice of the poly(β-aminoester).

With the above-mentioned examples, we aimed to show that thin polymer films demonstrate potential for the delivery of small molecule drugs, specifically when these films act as hosts for supramolecular drug reservoirs. We believe this potential remains largely unrealized and expect that this research direction will receive considerable interest in the nearest future.

7.2.3   Delivery and Presentation of Protein and Peptide Cargo

Peptides and proteins are essential components of any living organism and exhibit diverse physiological properties with biomedical and clinical relevance. To name a few, controlled release and presentation of growth factors is pivotal in the design of tissue engineering matrices; delivery of anti-inflammatory peptides can aid in tissue regeneration; these candidate drugs are also used in guided cell differentiation; furthermore, cytokines are among the promising drugs in antiviral and anticancer treatment. While strategies of delivery of peptide and protein therapeutics are many, a significant benefit offered by the polymer thin films relates to a time-controlled, time-delayed delivery of drugs and a potential of delivery of multiple agents with individual release profiles. Some of these promises are yet to be delivered, while some have already been accomplished, and the first successes of the field are described further.

A small peptide hormone, α-melanocortin (α-MSH), stimulates melanogenesis in melanocytes and melanoma cells via binding to a specific receptor on the cell surface, which leads to an activation of adenylate cyclase and protein kinase A, resulting in the activation of tyrosinase and in the production of melanin. It is a convenient model system to test the presentation of peptide hormones, and both early and long-term effects can be monitored via the levels of cyclic adenosine monophosphate (cAMP) and melanin, respectively.[19] In an early report, Chluba et al.[19] conjugated α-MSH to a carrier polymer, PLL, and assembled multilayered polymer films with PGA as a negatively charged counterpart. The level of cAMP in the B16-F1 cells grown on multilayer films was comparable to that observed in cells in response to a soluble α-MSH analogue added in solution, demonstrating that peptide hormones can indeed be delivered to responding cells from multilayered polymer films. The levels of cAMP were different, depending on the position of PLL-α-MSH; that is, they could be controlled by the deposition of additional layers on top of the hormone-containing layer. Regardless of their position within the multilayered film, peptide hormone conjugates were effective in eliciting melanin production, thereby verifying the long-term effect of these films. The anti-inflammatory effect of α-MSH when delivered from PLL/PGA multilayered films was later tested using a PGA-α-MSH conjugate.[48] Human monocytes were stimulated with LPS to induce an inflammatory response, which is registered via the production of TNF-α. The anti-inflammatory action of α-MSH would be accompanied by a decrease in the cellular production of TNF-α and also by a secretion of interleukin-10 (IL-10), the latter being indicative of an anti-inflammatory response. Incorporation of PGA-α-MSH into a multilayered film afforded a durable response (longer reduction of TNF-α production as compared to a conjugate added in solution) and also a reduction in the delay in IL-10 production. This system was later tested for an *in vivo* performance in coatings for tracheal prosthesis.[49] PLL/PGA films containing a PGA-α-MSH conjugate were effective in eliciting production of IL-10 *in vivo*; that is, they retained their anti-inflammatory characteristic. Subsequently, as an important step toward mimicking a complex 3-D organization of tissues, PLL/PGA thin films with incorporated PGA-α-MSH conjugates were used to assemble a stratified architecture with cell-containing ALG gel layers surrounded by polymer thin films.[50] Incorporated melanocytes produced melanin in response to the peptide hormone, thus demonstrating the potential of polymer thin films as reservoirs for the delivery of peptides in diverse tissue engineering applications. PLL/PGA thin films have also been successfully used in an *in vivo* delivery of another peptide, an antifungal agent, chromofungin.[51]

Biodegradable polypeptide thin films based on PLL and PGA have also proven attractive for the delivery of intact proteins, specifically protein A[52] and growth factors.[53,54] In the latter case, two growth factors, bone morphogenic protein-2 (BMP-2) and TGF-β, were incorporated into the multilayered thin film for concurrent delivery to embryonic bodies and induced differentiation of the latter into cartilage and bone tissue.[54] While taken individually, neither of the proteins induced the desired effect; taken together, the two growth factors effectively stimulated cell differentiation, thus suggesting a possible synergistic effect. The mechanism of action is suggested to involve a contact between the cells and growth factors within multilayers rather than a release of proteins into bulk solution. In contrast, BMP-2 underwent a controlled release into bulk solution from the multilayered films constructed using DNA with poly-D-lysine or PAH, and the released protein also retained its biological activity.[55]

Other growth factors were also successfully incorporated into polymer thin films and were shown to retain their biological activity. Fibroblast growth factors (FGFs) are proteins with diverse biological responses (e.g., accelerated proliferation of fibroblasts) and a short half-life, which makes their controlled release strategies highly warranted. Acidic fibroblast growth factor (aFGF) was incorporated into thin films constructed using heparin and PEI, and this afforded an increased proliferation of cultured fibroblasts.[56] In contrast, this effect was not observed when aFGF was used with PEI only, that is, in the absence of heparin.[56] Basic fibroblast growth factor (bFGF) adsorbed on top of multilayered films also retained its activity, as suggested by an increased number of adsorbed responding cells and their proliferation.[57] Vascular endothelial growth factor (VEGF) was adsorbed onto PSS/PAH multilayers, and the resulting construct was proangiogenic; that is, it stimulated the proliferation of endothelial cells.[58] Remarkably, brain-derived neurotrophic factor (BDNF) and a chemorepulsive protein, semaphorin 3A (Sema 3A), retained their activity within nondegradable PSS/PAH thin films, and protein-functionalized multilayers exhibited a significant increase in the survival of neurons on BDNF-containing films and a decrease in survival on the Sema 3A-containing counterpart.[59]

Cross-linked PLL/HA thin films were explored as mimics for the extracellular matrix and were further functionalized with recombinant human bone morphogenic protein-2 (rhBMP-2).[60] This protein has a limited solubility at pH 7, which allowed its loading into preformed multilayers via absorption from a pH 3 protein solution. A subsequent change in pH resulted in loss of protein solubility and its effective entrapment in the polymer film. On pristine films, cultured myoblasts exhibited an expected proliferation and formation of myotubes. In contrast, rhBMP-2-functionalized films sustained the proliferation of myoblasts, which underwent differentiation into osteoblasts in a protein dose-dependent manner (Fig. 7.4). The bioactivity of the protein is suggested to arise from the contact between the cells and the functionalized polymer films, not from a slow protein release into bulk solution. The high protein loading levels coupled with good retention characteristics of the polymer films afforded a rhBMP-2 reservoir, which sustained at least three successive cell culture sequences. Subsequently, these authors showed that the use of heparin within these films did not provide added benefits in terms of protein incorporation and retention, and the protein activity was found to be insensitive to the film composition.[61]

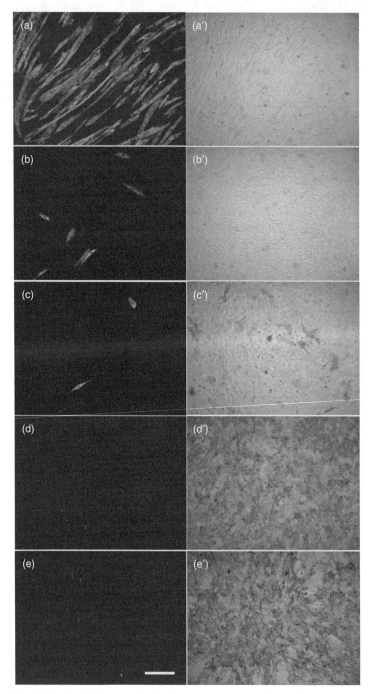

Figure 7.4 Surface-mediated delivery of growth factors: Intelligent polymer coatings are successful in presenting protein cargo, specifically growth factors, to the cultured cells. In this example, recombinant human bone morphogenic protein-2 (rhBMP-2) was incorporated into cross-linked PLL/HA multilayers and was used to induce a guided differentiation of cultured myoblasts into osteoblasts. This strategy of surface-mediated drug delivery was successful and proceeded in a dose-dependent manner (increasing concentration of rhBMP-2 from a to e), as evidenced by decreasing levels of a myogenic marker (troponin T, left column, immunochemical staining) and an accompanying increase in an osteogenic marker (alkaline phosphatase, right column, histochemical staining). Reprinted with permission from Crouzier et al.,[60] Wiley-VCH. © 2008. (See color insert.)

While most of the examples discussed earlier relate to the presentation of protein cargo by the functionalized substrate to the adhering cells, another possibility exists, namely, the release of the cargo into bulk solution. This approach also has clinical relevance and can be used to achieve a controlled release of the protein from a subcutaneously implanted depot into surrounding tissue (e.g., for vaccination applications) or from a stent into the blood stream (e.g., enzyme therapy). To this end, a promising opportunity is associated with the use of biodegradable synthetic polymers, specifically poly(β-aminoesters), to construct thin polymer films that undergo hydrolytic degradation and release their cargo. This was demonstrated using lysozyme as a model cargo and heparin or chondroitin sulfate as negatively charged counterparts to the protein and poly(β-aminoester).[62] A near-linear, sustained protein release was observed over at least 14 days, making this approach attractive for diverse biomedical applications and, specifically, drug delivery. While these experiments admittedly did not provide adequate simulation to an *in vivo* release environment and conditions, a steady release of an active protein achieved over such a significant time certainly makes this system highly attractive for further investigation and evaluation. Another promising approach to incorporate protein cargo into multilayered polymer films is its bioconjugation to a charged oligopeptide sequence, which facilitates protein deposition.[63] This was demonstrated on an example of RNase I conjugated to an oligoarginine sequence. The latter also promotes cellular uptake of the protein released from the surface; that is, it facilitates protein transduction.

7.2.4 Delivery of Gene Cargo

Controlled release and cellular uptake of DNA mediated by an intelligent surface is investigated within several research domains, specifically for the creation of DNA/cell arrays,[64,65] in tissue engineering,[66,67] and for the treatment of cardiovascular diseases.[68,69] In all of these cases, chemical or physical approaches are used to immobilize nucleic acids on the surface, which typically results in their high local concentration. Genetic material is then internalized by the cells cultured on top or in the near vicinity of the release sites, but it can also be released for circulation and delivery to distant sites. Various techniques have been developed for the immobilization of DNA for these applications, including the use of mineral nanocomposites,[70] adsorption of polyplexes[71,72] and lipoplexes,[72] immobilization using gelatin and a subsequent complexation with lipids,[65] and tethering within an adenoviral particle (Ad).[69] Upon its advent, sequential polymer deposition technique was recognized as a convenient, inexpensive, and facile tool to achieve surface immobilization of DNA, and the possibility to adsorb multiple layers of DNA makes it possible to create a very high concentration of nucleic acids on the surface of virtually any unprepared substrate. The examples of generic DNA used as a highly charged polyanion in the construction of polymer multilayered films are many and are not discussed herein. In a brief discussion below, we specifically focus on the successful examples of surface-mediated delivery of DNA or the systems that have a high potential to be successful in the near future.

Since 2004,[73] Lynn et al. have developed a robust technology for a surface-mediated controlled release of DNA with excellent control over the amount of nucleic acid immobilized on the surface and the kinetics of its release.[74–76] According to this method, hydrolytically degradable polycations, poly(β-aminoesters), are used as building blocks for a multilayered polymer film with DNA as a polyanion. Facile control over DNA loading is provided by the number of deposited polymer layers; gradual degradation of the polycations leads to a controlled release of nucleic acids, and the release profile can be tuned by the choice of the poly(β-aminoester). Released DNA was shown to be functional and was successfully used in transfection, specifically when the coated surface was placed in the vicinity of cultured cells.[77] From model substrates, these experiments were also transferred onto cardiovascular stents (Fig. 7.5a).[78] An important parameter of control over DNA release

---

Figure 7.5 Surface-mediated delivery of nucleic acids. Multilayered polymer coatings are successful in surface-mediated drug delivery and hold promise for diverse applications, specifically localized drug delivery achieved from the surface of cardiovascular stents for the prevention of restenosis. (a) Electron microscopy images show intravascular stents with DNA-containing multilayered polymer coatings for a surface-mediated gene delivery. Image (a,ii) shows a surface with a locally delaminated polymer film. Reprinted with permission from Jewell et al.,[78] American Chemical Society. © 2006. (b) Intelligent multilayered polymer coatings allow time-delayed delivery of multiple therapeutic molecules, a feature inherent with a sequential deposition approach and a possibility to incorporate cargo at different depths within the polymer film structure. In the example shown, two different plasmid nucleic acids (one encoding a nuclear transcription factor, Red, and another encoding a cytoplasmic protein, green) were sequentially released from the same polymer film and delivered to the cultured cells in a time-delayed manner. Reprinted with permission from Jessel et al.,[90] National Academy of Sciences, United States. © 2006. (c) The use of multilayered polymer films affords an increased deliverable payload via incorporation of cargo in multiple layers and a greater therapeutic response. Surface-mediated delivery of siRNA was shown to elicit a dose-dependent antiviral activity (1, 3, or 5 layers of HCV-specific siRNA, marked siHCV; effectiveness of delivery monitored via expression of viral proteins) and was more durable when compared to delivery of a corresponding amount of siRNA using PEI, liposomes (LT) or electroporation (EP) (c, top). Furthermore, this strategy of siRNA delivery elicited effective prevention of hepatitis C infection (monitored via the number of copies of viral RNA, image c, bottom) making it a highly promising tool for antiviral therapy. Reprinted with permission from Dimitrova et al.,[95] National Academy of Sciences, United States. © 2008. (See color insert.)

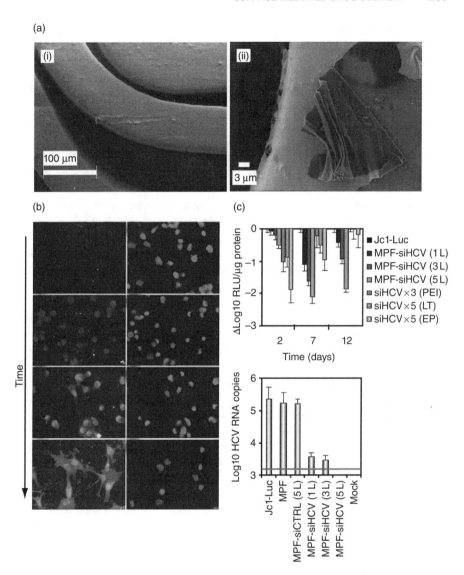

offered by this platform relates to the mechanism of degradation of the multilayered film, which depends on the structure of a particular poly(β-aminoester) used in the study. In a particularly important example, the rational choice of the poly(β-aminoester) afforded a surface erosion mechanism of degradation, which was imperative for a time-delayed release of multiple DNA molecules.[79] In this case, transfection of the cells with two nonidentical nucleic acids was achieved using the same intelligent polymer-coated surface. Another approach developed by Lynn et al. relates to the use of "charge-shifting" polymers,[80,81] that is, macromolecules that lose or reverse their charge upon a hydrolytic degradation of their side-chain functionalities (see Fig. 7.1). Compared to the poly(β-aminoesters) described earlier, the kinetics of degradation of these polymers is much slower and DNA is released over a considerably longer time period (up to 70 days).[80] These polymers were also successfully used to release two different plasmids in a time-delayed fashion.[81] Thus, these two developed platforms provide a means to control DNA incorporation and its release mediated from the surface of a biomaterial. An expected advancement for this research direction relates to the delivery of DNA to cells cultured directly on top of the DNA-containing films, possibly from surfaces with clinical relevance.

Other notable examples of nucleic acid incorporation and release from polymer thin films include multilayered assemblies of DNA and PLL, which release the nucleic acid upon digestion of the polypeptide with chymotrypsin.[82] The release and localized cellular internalization of RNA-containing complexes with PEI were also mediated from a surface of a hydrogen-bonded PAA–PEO film placed into a cell culture medium.[83] Finally, surface-mediated controlled release of antisense oligonucleotides was achieved using a phosphorylcholine containing polymer film.[84] To date and to the best of our knowledge, most of these and related approaches remain "proof of concept," and their implementation in a clinically relevant setting is yet to be performed. Another approach to a sustained DNA delivery relies on the release of DNA from a multilayered film with trans-activating transcriptional activator (TAT) oligopeptide cross-linked via disulfide linkages in response to reducing agents;[85] this work has recently seen a follow-up in vitro and in vivo characterization,[86] which will be discussed next.

The first successful transfection using a DNA-containing multilayered polymer film was reported in 2005 by Iwata et al.,[87] who used a DNA/PEI polymer film assembled on the surface of electrodes. In response to an electric pulse, multilayers released DNA and the cells cultured on the surface of the electrode were effectively transfected with high efficiency (percent of transfected cells). Flexibility of this platform was demonstrated using multiple cell lines (HEK293 and hyppocampal neurons) and using multiple plasmids for their coelectroporation into cells as well as site-specific parallel transfection of cells with multiple plasmids using a spotted array of DNA. This strategy was subsequently optimized for delivery of small interfering RNA (siRNA)[88] to achieve a dose-dependent gene silencing whereby siRNA loading is controlled by the number of deposited siRNA/PEI layers, and this strategy afforded ~80% reduction in the levels of the reporter gene. Another approach to surface-mediated gene delivery using polymer multilayered films was also introduced in 2005 and relies on the adsorption of DNA/PEI polyelectrolyte complexes onto or into polymer thin films.[89]

In 2006, the promise of thin polymer films as a platform for localized and time-delayed delivery of multiple DNA sequences was realized using PLL/PGA multilayered films and cationic cyclodextrin (cCD) as molecular chaperons to assist in transfection.[90] PGA-terminated thin films were used to adsorb cCD, which, in turn, sustained adsorption of DNA. Subsequent coating with another layer of cCD and additional PLL/PGA layers afforded the final architecture. Three cell types and two different plasmids, one expressing a nuclear transcription factor and one expressing a cytoplasmic protein, were used to demonstrate the flexibility of this delivery platform. The attained levels of transfection are quoted to be quantitative; that is, all of the cultured cells were expressing reporter genes when delivered from the polymer film-functionalized surfaces, which was in stark contrast with control methods (calcium phosphate precipitation and FuGENE 6 reagent). The proposed mechanism of action involves a local degradation of the polymer film by the cultured cells and not a passive release of DNA into bulk solution, as no DNA is detected in the supernatant solution above the multilayers. Two plasmids were incorporated at varied depths of the multilayered architecture, and both were successfully delivered to cells, as evidenced by the expression of the two proteins. Furthermore, this was achieved in a time-delayed fashion; that is, expression of a plasmid placed closer to the surface of the film precedes the expression of a plasmid placed deeper, further away from the surface of the film (Fig. 7.5b). We believe that this work reveals the potential of intelligent polymer films for surface-mediated delivery of gene cargo. Interestingly, this work also reports that in the absence of cCD, no transfection of cultured cells is observed, which highlights the importance of molecular chaperon activity for a successful transfection using this technique, but also puts into question the general applicability of this approach.

In a follow-up publication, a covalently coupled PLL-CD conjugate was used to interact with DNA in solution, and the resulting interpolyelectrolyte complex particle was incorporated into a multilayered PLL/HA film.[91] For all candidate vectors (PLL, CD, and PLL-CD), surface-mediated gene transfer was significantly higher when compared to a solution-based transfection, a significant finding for the overall attractiveness of this delivery paradigm. It is also suggested that cell entry proceeds via a nonendocytic pathway, and this factor is assigned as an underlying reason for the overall high level of transfection. We note that in contrast with the report discussed previously,[90] PLL-assisted delivery was successful in the absence of CD. Significant differences between the two studies include PLL/PGA versus PLL/HA multilayered films, and this may play an important role. However, a more likely explanation relates to the mode of DNA incorporation into the thin films, that is, naked[90] or precomplexed with PLL.[91] It is plausible that in the latter case, nucleic acids are released/taken up by cells within a polyelectrolyte complex particle with PLL, and the latter is likely to facilitate cellular internalization. This line of reasoning finds support in a publication by Cai et al.,[92] who studied surface-mediated DNA delivery using its multilayered films with galactosylated chitosan (G-CHI) and observed that the released DNA indeed appeared in the form of polyelectrolyte complex particles with G-CHI. A mechanism of transfection observed on PEI/CD multilayers with DNA also involved the release of DNA-containing polyelectrolyte complex particles with PEI/CD.[93] Another significant finding of Cai et al.[92] was that G-CHI/DNA thin films elicited similar transfection levels in HEK293 when compared to nongalactosylated CHI/DNA films. In contrast, a significant increase in transgene expression was observed for G-CHI/DNA films compared to their CHI/DNA counterpart when HepG2 cells were used, the latter expressing an asialoglycoprotein receptor that recognizes galactose. In other words, this report demonstrates an enhancement of transfection using the tools of drug targeting and, in doing so, significantly increases the intelligence of thin polymer films for surface-mediated gene transfer.

Another important recent finding in the field relates to the presentation of bioactive Ad.[94] While solution-based delivery of Ad requires that the cells have an appropriate receptor to facilitate viral cell entry, this was not the case for polymer thin film-assisted presentation of Ad, and with the latter approach, transduction proceeded even with cells that lack such receptors.[94] This team also pioneered the use of multilayered polymer films for a surface-mediated gene silencing, specifically RNA interference (RNAi) aimed to inhibit replication of the hepatitis C virus in infected cells (Fig. 7.5c).[95] To facilitate delivery, siRNA was incorporated into the structure of the films in a form of a polyelectrolyte complex particle with PEI. PEI–siRNA complexes were adsorbed onto a surface and were further coated with HA/CHI/HA polymer layers. For an increased incorporation of nucleic acids and an enhanced RNAi, this cycle was repeated up to five times. The results of RNAi using polymer films were compared side by side with alternative technologies, namely, electroporation, liposomal delivery, and PEI-assisted delivery. Solution-based methods yielded a faster response, but these peaked at day 5 and gradually decreased. In contrast, responses to a surface-mediated siRNA delivery were durable and sustained inhibition of viral replication for over 12 days. Remarkably, delivery of siRNA by this method also markedly decreased the level of infection of cells. In other words, cells that were grown on PEI–siRNA-functionalized polymer thin films were significantly resistant to the introduced viral particles and effectively withstood infection. We expect that this report will significantly boost the attractiveness of polymer thin films for surface-mediated drug delivery.

The described developments in the field have laid the foundation for diverse biomedical applications of intelligent multilayered polymer films. With equal importance, the first decade has delivered diverse protocols for the assembly of thin films and their drug loading, and also outlined the potential scope and utility of these films in biomedicine. Recently, the first *in vivo* successes have been described, and the field has also developed through the examples of codelivery of structurally and functionally diverse cargo as well as delved into unexplored territories, such as transcutaneous drug delivery. For example, Oupicky et al.[86] have demonstrated the potential of thin films constructed using DNA and bioreducible polycations, specifically hyperbranched poly(amidoamines), in surface-mediated gene delivery using a subcutaneously implanted substrate. The reporter plasmid encoded a secreted form of alkaline phosphatase (SEAP), which enables the measurement of the level of gene expression via plasma levels of SEAP. The drug level peaked at day 5 and, together with a half-life in blood of ~17 hours, this implies a sustained expression of the transgene. It is suggested that SEAP secretion occurs in the fibroblasts in the vicinity of the implant and also that further work will be required to attain a more durable response. Nevertheless, this work takes a significant step toward clinically relevant applications of surface-mediated gene transfer using thin polymer films.

An interesting strategy toward a guided differentiation of MSCs was reported by Hu et al.,[96] who used CHI/DNA multilayered films to deliver a plasmid encoding for the production of BMP-2, which, in turn, is a chemical stimulus for MSC toward their differentiation into osteoblasts. DNA is released from the multilayers upon incubation with PBS over a period of at least 7 days and the nucleic acid deliverable payload controlled by the number of deposited layers. In agreement with the previous reports from this group,[92] DNA is shown to be released from the films in a form of a polyelectrolyte complex with CHI, which is thought to facilitate the subsequent cell entry. Production of BMP-2 was ascertained through the levels of mRNA using RT-PCR, and this analysis revealed that surface-mediated transfection yielded a durable response with detectable levels of BMP-2 mRNA at day 7, which was not observed for control samples (transfection with lipofectamine 2000). At day 7, levels of alkaline phosphatase, a marker for early osteogenesis, were highest for the surface-mediated transfection sample, as were the levels of osteocantin, a marker indicating late-stage differentiation of osteoblasts, at day 14.

By design, multicomponent polymer films are well suited to carry multiple candidate therapeutics for their concurrent or sequential delivery from within the same film. Indeed, sequential incorporation of building blocks, universal and widely applicable forces facilitating the assembly (electrostatic interaction, hydrogen bonding, etc.), and the possibility to coadsorb more than one polymer type within the same layer make LBL films a flexible platform for surface-mediated codelivery of therapeutics for combination therapy. In a prominent example, Meyer et al.[97] described the codelivery of an oligopeptide hormone, α-MSH, for the stimulated production of melanin and a DNA plasmid for transfection, achieved using the same multilayered polymer film. In another report, Irvine et al.[98] take this concept further and describe biodegradable thin films that exploit poly(β-aminoesters) as a means of controlled degradation and carry two essential components for successful vaccination, a protein vaccine and an oligonucleotide adjuvant, for their time-controlled release. This report is also unique in that multilayered films are used for transcutaneous drug delivery, wherein the polymer film is assembled on the inner surface of a skin adhesive patch. Released therapeutic penetrates through the skin and is subsequently internalized by professional antigen-presenting cells (APCs), Langerhans cells.

Taken together, we believe the above-mentioned discussion outlines the tools and techniques offered by the field of multilayered polymers films for localized, sustained delivery of diverse therapeutic cargo. These intelligent polymer films are undergoing a transition from the proof-of-concept stage toward clinically relevant applications, and we expect that the upcoming years will witness an explosion of high-impact reports from this area of fundamental and applied science.

7.3 DRUG DELIVERY VEHICLES WITH FUNCTIONAL POLYMER COATINGS

The second part of this book chapter considers the drug delivery applications of intelligent polymer coatings assembled on micro- and nanoparticles as well as polymer capsules, that is, freestanding polymer multilayer films encapsulating a liquid-containing void (see Methods Box 7.2). For the purpose of this discussion, we define core–shell particles as a solid core coated with at least three layers of polymers; therefore, the large body of literature on (nano) particles coated with a single polymer layer to change the charge of the particle or to make them "stealth" via PEGylation is beyond the scope of this book chapter (for relevant reviews, refer to References 99–101).

In the following applications, functional polymer films can serve the purpose of governing the interaction with biological systems (e.g., blood residence time, selectivity, and efficiency of uptake by cells) as well as to provide control over payload release and activity. However, while on planar and macroscopic substrates LBL films appear to be quite unique and possibly constitute the most advanced strategy for surface-mediated drug delivery, successes of LBL films in the colloidal domain are largely shadowed by other techniques (e.g., polymers, liposomes, micelles, and microgel particles). Of the possibilities offered by multilayered films on planar substrates, namely, controlled interaction with cells, incorporation of small molecule cargo, presentation of peptide and protein drugs, and delivery of nucleic acids, only the latter has received considerable research attention employing LBL and core–shell particles. However, the field of multilayered intelligent polymer coatings on colloidal particles is blossoming, and this is largely due to an increased interest is hollow capsules obtained upon removal of the core particles. These carriers receive enhanced attention, and it is with them that the potential of polymer coatings, in a form of "freestanding" polymer coatings, is realized to a greater extent. These two strategies, drug delivery using core–shell particles and hollow capsules, are detailed next.

7.3.1 Core–Shell Particles

As with polymer films on planar substrates, their application on colloidal particles is expected to provide a controlled interaction with cells (targeting),

METHODS BOX 7.2   ASSEMBLY OF MULTILAYERED POLYMER THIN FILMS ON COLLOIDAL PARTICLES

Protocol: In a typical procedure, a 5% particle suspension is incubated in a 1 g/L polymer solution to ensure adsorption and oversaturation of the surface with the polymer, typically 15 minutes, followed by three centrifugal washing/redispersing steps to remove excess polymer. The particles are then suspended in a solution of a complementary polymer (opposite charge, hydrogen-bonding donor–acceptor role, covalent linkage group, etc.), followed by washing. This completes the adsorption of one bilayer (one layer of each polymer) and can be repeated as necessary until the desired thickness of the film of the core–shell particles is obtained. Polymer films can be further cross-linked to enhance their stability. In order to yield capsules, the template particles are removed with an appropriate etching reagent, and the capsules are washed and isolated via centrifugation.

Notes: The above-mentioned exemplary protocol represents a typical procedure of coating of a substrate with a multilayered polymer film and, as such, is flexible in most of the described steps, as mentioned in Methods Box 7.1.

Templates: SiO_2 (removed by HF), polystyrene (removed by tetrahydrofuran), melamine formaldehyde (removed by HCl), calcium carbonate (removed by EDTA or HCl); typical size range: from 500 nm to 6 µm in diameter, but both smaller (as little as 20 nm) and larger templates were employed.

Polymers: No fundamental restrictions (see Fig. Box 7.2), yet particle aggregation imposes a lower size limit of particles below which instrumental difficulties become arresting, and for most polymers, this limit is on the order of $1 \div 3$ µm.

Cargo Loading: Adsorption onto the template prior LBL (e.g., polymer–peptide conjugates, DNA, and loaded liposomes), cargo as part of the polymer multilayers (e.g., as building block, via covalent conjugation to a building block), loading during template formation (e.g., $CaCO_3$ coprecipitation with proteins), infiltration into a preformed capsule.

incorporation of diverse cargo, and an increased payload due to a possibility to assemble multiple layers of each constituent. Unfortunately, to date, the progress toward these goals is rather modest. A further significant limitation to these prospects is a loss of colloidal stability of particles upon polymer adsorption, a phenomenon that becomes more pronounced with decreased particle sizes and that tremendously limits the practical utility of this approach.

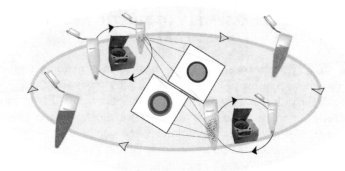

Figure Box 7.2 Schematic illustration of LBL performed via a repetitive adsorption of interacting polymers onto colloidal substrates with intermediate substrate washing achieved via multiple centrifugation-redispersion cycles. (See color insert.).

Targeting the core–shell particles to the desired cells constitutes a premier expectation associated with colloidal drug carriers. To this end, Cortez et al. coated 500-nm polystyrene particles with PAH/PSS multilayers and adsorbed a humanized A33 monoclonal antibody (HuA33) on the surface in order to investigate the targeting possibility of these core–shell particles with three different types of cells: A33 antigen-expressing LIM1215 cells, A33 antigen-expressing LIM1215 cells with blocked A33 antigen, and non-A33-antigen-expressing SW480 cells.[102] This strategy afforded an increased association of HuA33-modified particles with LIM1215 cells in comparison to SW480 cells. Also, a lower association with LIM1215 cells for particles without HuA33 or immunoglobulin G ligands in comparison to HuA33-coated ones was reported. In a follow-up study, this team confirmed that the same strategy also works for capsules and that selective binding efficiency depends on the size and dosage of particles (capsules).[103] Increasing the dosage led to a larger fraction of cells with associated particles, and larger particles were more prone to nonspecific interaction with cells then smaller ones. In another study, Zhou et al. coated 200- to 400-nm poly(DL-lactide-coglycolide) (PLGA) particles with CHI and ALG layers and compared the uptake of these particles by HepG2 cells depending on the presence of a targeting moiety, folic acid (FA).[104] FA is a suitable targeting ligand since it is known that cancer cells overexpress folate receptors. In this report, FA-modified nanoparticles were taken up with higher efficiency in comparison with the unmodified ones. However, the targeting of these particles to a specific cell type was not yet demonstrated.

A crucial aspect for drug delivery applications of the core–shell particles, specifically delivery of DNA, is the intracellular defoliation of the multilayers. In 2006, Reibetanz et al. were the first ones to demonstrate this effect.[105] The authors incorporated a plasmid DNA into the multilayer film assembled from protamine sulfate and dextran sulfate sodium salt (DXS) (the plasmid DNA replaced DXS in specific layers) and showed the cellular uptake of these 3-μm core–shell particles. Subsequent expression of the plasmid-encoded proteins in HEK293T cells was achieved, providing proof for defoliation and a release of the plasmid into the cytoplasm. Kakade et al. reported the multilayer assembly of DNA and PEI on the surface of 2 ÷ 6 μm PLGA particles and the subsequent transfection of macrophages.[106] However, the transfection efficiency of these core–shell particles was found to be lower than for PEI/DNA polyplexes. The likely limitation was the lack of obvious degradation of the coated particles, suggesting that the intracellular disassembly of the PEI/DNA films is highly inefficient. Saurer et al. presented an approach to fabricate erodible DNA-containing films on the surfaces of microparticles with the aim of delivering DNA to APCs.[107] While the erosive property of the multilayered film was successfully demonstrated in a test tube and the employed 6-μm core–shell particles were effectively internalized by cells, no transfection of the cells was observed.

From a different perspective, gold nanoparticles (AuNPs) have been employed in transfection as carriers for nucleic acids immobilized onto the particle surface in a number of reports.[108–111] It is therefore plausible that with a proper choice of particle size and a mechanism of nucleic acid release, it may become possible to increase the deliverable payload associated with nanoparticles using the sequential polymer deposition technique. To this end, Elbakry et al. suggested a coating for 20-nm gold colloids (AuNP) by assembling PEI/siRNA/PEI (Fig. 7.6).[112] The reported uptake of AuNP/PEI/siRNA was around four times higher in comparison with AuNP/PEI/siRNA/PEI. The nanoparticles were found to be nontoxic and largely localized in endocytic vesicles. The activity of the delivered siRNA was assessed upon internalization of the coated AuNP by CHO-K1 cells expressing enhanced green fluorescent protein (EGFP). Interestingly, while a dose-dependent knockdown was observed when AuNP/PEI/siRNA/PEI was used, no gene silencing was observed when the top PEI layer was missing.

7.3.2 Polymer Capsules

The third research direction based on the LBL technique considers the creation of freestanding polymer multilayered assemblies, polymer capsules. The polymer membrane is assembled via sequential deposition of interacting polymers and, as the final step, the sacrificial core particle is dissolved. The first polymer capsules were reported in 1998[113] and since then, there has been a significant amount of literature published on the assembly and the physical/chemical properties of these capsules,[114–117] techniques for drug encapsulation and mechanisms of cargo release,[118] their utility in drug delivery,[119] and applications in encapsulated catalysis and cell mimicry.[120] Expectations associated with these drug carriers are high due to an increased therapeutic payload and the adaptability of the polymer membrane, a possibility to assemble the capsules using biocompatible and/or biodegradable polymers, and to implement stimuli responsiveness. Further, the number of deposited polymer layers is a proposed tool of control over the capsule permeability and cargo release, while

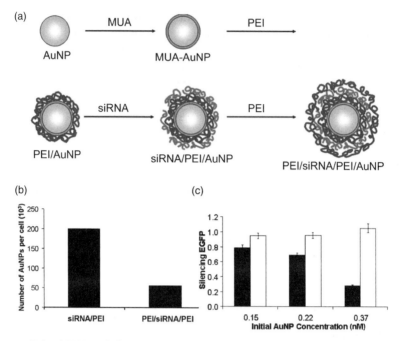

Figure 7.6 siRNA delivery using polymer-coated gold colloids: (a) 11-mercaptoundecanoic acid (MUA) was adsorbed onto ca. 15-nm gold colloids followed by the deposition of PEI, siRNA, and PEI. (b) Cellular uptake of the polymer-coated nanoparticles. The number of siRNA/PEI/AuNPs per cell was significantly higher as compared with PEI/siRNA/PEI/AuNPs. (c) Gene silencing of EGFP in CHO-K1 cells using different concentrations of PEI/siRNA/PEI/AuNPs coated with either siRNA against EGFP (black bars) or a nontargeted siRNA control (white bars). A dose-dependent specific knockdown was observed, and the cellular EGFP production was reduced to about 28% for the highest tested PEI/siRNA/PEI/AuNP concentration. Reprinted with permission from Elbakry et al.,[112], American Chemical Society. © 2009. (See color insert.)

the outermost layer of the film has the potential to be tuned to provide a suitable biointerface, that is, by employing PEGylation or targeting moieties.

Understanding the interaction between polymer capsules and cells is of utmost importance in order to deliver the payload in an efficient and controlled (targeted) manner. Efforts to achieve an understanding of this complex topic were started in 2005 and are still ongoing. It is evident today that micron-sized capsules are taken up by different cell lines regardless of the capsule size and without the need for specific ligands on their surface.[121–126] Nevertheless, the pivotal characteristics of these capsules as drug carriers, namely, uptake pathway, localization, deformation, or degradation kinetics, remain largely open. Flow cytometry, confocal laser scanning microscopy, and, to a lesser extent, transmission electron microscopy and atomic force microscopy are the predominant techniques employed to assess the uptake efficiency of the capsules by cells.

Ai et al. were among the first to study the uptake of polyelectrolyte capsules by cells.[127] They used 0.9-μm capsules assembled from PDDA and gelatin and different outermost layers (PEI, PLL, PDDA, PAH, PSS, albumin, PEG, or lipid bilayers) and monitored the capsule uptake by human MCF-7 breast cancer cells.[127] Regardless of the surface chemistry, it was observed that a large amount of capsules were taken up by the cells after 4 hours of incubation. Another conclusion from this work was that the interaction of capsules with serum proteins has to be taken into consideration. Surprisingly, the ability to implement low fouling and/or targeting molecules on the surface of polymer capsules still remains one of the core challenges in the field. While the idea of actively enhancing the uptake by a specific cell type over others is very appealing, the experimental proof remains undelivered. In fact, even successful PEGylation attempts, possibly the first crucial step to be considered when aiming at targeting, are few, for both core–shell particles[128] and capsules.[2,129,130]

The premier characteristic of drug carrier vehicles is their cytotoxicity, and this was evaluated for multiple candidate polymer capsules in several studies. However, due to a large variability in the capsule size and constituting polymers, as well as employed cell type and experimental protocols (cell confluency, incubation time, etc.), we feel it is premature to draw broad conclusions about capsule toxicity and safety. A general observation in the field is that at a low capsule-per-cell administered ratio, regardless of their size and composition, the capsules have an insignificant effect on cell viability; in contrast, an increased capsule-per-cell ratio typically leads to a decrease in the viability of cultured cells.[131–133] While low toxicity of capsules to cells at a low administered dose is encouraging, we believe these data should be interpreted with caution as these conditions likely imply a low uptake level and few cells contain internalized capsules. We strongly believe that to draw reliable conclusions, viability studies warrant an accompanying assay on efficiency in internalization to be conducted under the same experimental conditions. Nevertheless, PSS/PAH capsules (1.2- or 4.8-μm diameter, with or without PLL–PEG coating) were nontoxic to macrophages and dendritic cells (DCs) over 3 days' observation;[130] 3-μm-sized dextran sulfate/poly(arginine) capsules were moderately toxic toward DCs with ~80% remaining viable upon incubation with capsules at a 30:1 capsule-to-cell ratio;[132] 3-μm covalently stabilized PGA capsules elicited no decrease in cell viability when incubated at a 2:1 ratio with LIM1899 cells;[134] and covalently stabilized 800 nm poly(vinylpyrrolidone) (PVPON) capsules also exhibited a low level of cellular toxicity.[135] For large-sized capsules (e.g., 5-μm PSS/PAH capsules), their sedimentation onto cultured cells was proposed to be the reason for a deceased cell viability.[131] At similar administered ratios (~100 capsules per cell), 1- to 2-μm PSS/PAH capsules were significantly less toxic than their 8- to 10-μm counterparts.[133]

Single-component poly(methacrylic acid) capsules are obtained via sequential adsorption of thiolated PMA and PVPON in acidic pH, a process facilitated by hydrogen bonding of the two polymers.[136,137] While pristine capsules are inherently unstable at physiological pH due to the ionization of PMA, oxidation of the thiols into bridging disulfide linkages affords disulfide-stabilized capsules, which, upon the ionization of PMA, release PVPON and become single-component polymethacrylic acid hydrogel capsules (PMA HCs). We have developed a protocol that allows a reliable assembly of PMA HC using monodisperse silica template particles with sizes as low as 300 nm and tested these capsules for their toxicity in multiple cell lines[124,138,139] toward their applications in drug delivery. In a recent systematic study,[140] we screened a panel of mammalian cells (muscle NR6, ovary CHO, neuronal M17, kidney HEK, macrophage P388D1) and varied the capsules to cell feed ratio up to 1000 capsules per cell. For 500-nm capsules and for all cell types tested, these experimental conditions afforded at least a 70% fraction of cells with internalized capsules and only an insignificant decrease in cell viability. In other words, we showed that internalized PMA HCs are nontoxic to mammalian cells, which makes them superior candidate carriers for biomedical applications.

The uptake pathway of capsules by cells is of central interest when aiming to use these capsules as drug delivery vehicles. Identifying the uptake pathway will not only help in designing more advanced vehicles, but it is also involved in determining the localization of the delivery vehicle and the fate of the payload within the cell. However, we are only beginning to glean the first insights into this complex topic. Kreft et al.[141] reported a localization of capsules in acidic intracellular compartments, that is, endo/lysosomes. While lysosomal trafficking is typically assessed by staining techniques, an interesting alternative has been suggested, which considered using capsules loaded with SNARF, a dye that has a pH-dependent emission shift. This approach made it possible to distinguish between capsules attached to the cell membrane versus capsules internalized by cells using both microscopy[141] and flow cytometry.[125] De Geest et al. used ~3-μm dextran sulfate/poly-L-arginine capsules and employed selective uptake inhibitors to study the uptake pathway of capsules by cells,[121] and caveola-mediated endocytosis (CvME) was suggested as the uptake pathway for the tested VERO-1 cells. In a follow-up work, the mechanism of uptake of these capsules by DCs was shown to be a combination of CvME and macropinocytosis (MP) with subsequent retention of the capsules in the endolysosomal vesicles where their shell is ruptured to release the encapsulated cargo.[122] Our recent study with PMA HCs revealed that regardless of the capsule size (300 and 500 nm and 1 μm) and cell type (with an exception of RAMOS B cells), the internalization of capsules is significantly inhibited by chlorpromazine, an inhibitor of clathrin-mediated endocytosis.[140] This observation is unexpected as this mechanism was not implicated in cell entry for other capsule types, as discussed earlier. A plausible explanation for this phenomenon considers the inherent softness of PMA HCs, rendering them significantly different from other tested capsules, for example, dextran sulfate/poly-L-arginine. Indeed, this characteristic has recently been recognized as pivotal in the interaction of biomaterials with cells,[18,142] and to probe this directly, we compared PMA HC and PMA-coated silica particles. In the latter case, levels of cellular uptake were not significantly affected by the presence of chlorpromazine, providing initial proof for the hypothesis put forward. We do, however, acknowledge that inhibitor studies as described earlier do not rule out the possibility of other cell entry mechanisms and that the discovered effect of chlorpromazine may not imply the classic clathrin-mediated endocytosis as a mechanism of cell entry for PMA HC. A more detailed study into PMA HC cell entry is currently underway.

Overall and despite some promising reports, the papers describing successful drug delivery achieved with multilayered polymer capsules are few. One of the reasons for this is the poor colloidal stability of the capsules, which leads a majority of studies to consider large-sized carriers. The second significant limitation is that, despite numerous reports in the field, only a few examples demonstrate controlled dosage and controlled release of the drugs from the capsules. Among the few examples detailed next, the majority of reports relate to delivery of cytotoxic drugs or vaccination studies.

For anticancer therapy, accumulation of a cytotoxic drug within a carrier is employed to overcome a dilution of the therapeutic, to reduce side effects, to improve the solubility and half-life time of the drug, and to achieve an uptake of a greater deliverable payload by cells. If successful, this strategy dramatically increases the concentration of the drug inside the cell and thus increases the therapeutic effect. This has been demonstrated in a number of reports using LBL-derived polymer capsules, both *in vitro*[143–145] and even *in vivo* using intratumoral injection.[146] We believe that these reports are significant for the development of the field of LBL capsules but in their current form are unlikely to be clinically warranted: The large size of the capsules employed (typically 3–5 μm) significantly limits the choice of routes of administration, and the drug-loading technique, association with preformed capsules via a nonspecific absorption, implies poor control over drug loading, retention, and release. As a step toward a better control over drug loading, retention, and release, Ochs et al. conjugated doxorubicin (Dox) to PGA and assembled multilayered polymer thin films via click chemistry using this conjugate as a polymer membrane constituent (Fig. 7.7a).[134] This strategy afforded a fine control over the amount of loaded drug, and this formulation yielded a reduction in the viability of LIM1899 cells induced by the 3-μm capsules containing a specific concentration of Dox. In a different approach, Wang et al.[147] assembled drug-loaded sub-micron-sized capsules by a slightly different method than LBL but worth mentioning in this context due to its potential for intravenous administration. A PGA–Dox conjugate was infiltrated into custom-made solid core/mesoporous shell particles (ca. 400 nm in diameter) and was cross-linked using a disulfide-containing spacer, cystamine, to produce hollow capsules upon silica removal. This drug formulation afforded a much lower viability of LIM1215 human colorectal tumor cells when compared to the free

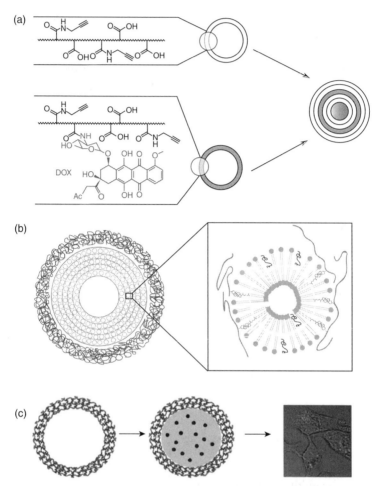

Figure 7.7 Approaches to formulate anticancer drugs using polymer capsules: (a) conjugation of the drug to a polymer, which is then used as in the capsule assembly. Reprinted with permission from Ochs et al.,[134] American Chemical Society. © 2010. (b) Incorporation of the drug into liposomes, which are then confined within polymer capsules;[40] and (c) solubilization of the lipophilic anticancer therapeutic in an oil phase and encapsulation of the emulsion droplets within the carrier capsules. Reprinted with permission from Sivakumar et al.,[138] Wiley-VCH. © 2009. (See color insert.)

drug–polymer conjugate or capsules without drug. While no enhancement in cytotoxicity was demonstrated for the Dox-containing capsules over free Dox, these capsules can prove relevant due to their small size and ease in preparation, as well as possibilities of coloading and further conjugation opportunities using the remaining free carboxyl groups.

Finally, the greatest control over drug loading and retention, a controlled drug release in response to a chemical stimulus with intracellular relevance, and the most pronounced therapeutic benefit offered by multilayered polymer capsules, was reported by Sivakumar et al.[138] In this report, disulfide-stabilized PMA HC were used for their structural stability and their mechanism of degradation in the presence of glutathione (GSH), a natural thiol-containing tripeptide with an increased intracellular concentration. These capsules were dehydrated and backfilled with an oil phase containing solubilized lipophilic anticancer drugs, Dox and 5-fluorouracil (5-FU) (Fig. 7.7c). This strategy affords a facile control over capsule loading through the choice of drug concentration in the oil phase, and the resulting capsules exhibited negligible passive release of Dox upon incubation in PBS. In contrast, in the presence of an intracellular concentration of GSH, the capsules released over 80% of Dox within 4–6 hours with a near-linear release kinetics. While pristine capsules and oil-filled capsules exhibited no cytotoxic effect, 500-nm Dox-oil-filled capsules exhibited a high antiproliferative activity which far exceeded that of free Dox administered in an equivalent amount in solution. In a follow-up publication, this effect was quantified and it was shown that PMA HC with a Dox-oil phase interior offer at least a 5000-fold decrease in the IC_{50} value compared to the free Dox.[124] A good control over drug loading, retention of the therapeutic with no passive leakage, and release in response to a stimulus with intracellular relevance makes this example the most well-characterized system offered by the field of multilayered polymer capsules for anticancer therapy.

One of the characteristic features of multilayered polymer capsules is their high permeability to low-molecular-weight molecules, which is attractive for diverse applications yet also significantly decreases the value of LBL-derived capsules for encapsulation and delivery of small drugs. One of the proposed ways to overcome this considers a capsule-templated assembly of a lipid bilayer, that is, assembly of an impermeable shell around a polymer capsule.[148–151] From a different standpoint, we hypothesized that a combination of liposomes and polymer capsules can lead to novel opportunities in biomedical design and to the creation of novel drug carriers in particular. To this end, we introduced capsosomes,[36,39] intact liposomal subcompartments confined within a polymer carrier capsule. In this context, degradable polymer capsules are employed as carriers, while the liposomes serve as entrapped drug deposits (Fig. 7.7b). While the core strength of capsosomes is expected to be in cell mimicry,[152,153] we have also demonstrated the potential of capsosomes for intracellular drug delivery by entrapping thiocoraline (TC), a small, hydrophobic antitumoral peptide, into the membrane of the liposomes. The successful delivery of TC-loaded capsosomes to LIM1899 cells was shown by a reduction in cell viability, while pristine capsosomes did not show cytotoxicity.[40]

While an overall majority of drug delivery applications would suffer from the large size of the multilayered polymer capsules, this factor may turn out to be beneficial for their utility in vaccination through an enhanced uptake by APCs. De Rose et al. screened a panel of 1-μm-sized capsules for their uptake by APCs in whole human blood and showed that, regardless of their chemistry, multilayered polymer capsules were effectively internalized by white blood cells, including DCs.[123] For vaccination, we developed a strategy for encapsulation of oligopeptide antigens, specifically a model HIV vaccine peptide, KP9. To achieve efficient encapsulation and to engineer a means of drug release, the oligopeptide was conjugated to a carrier polymer through a biodegradable

(a)

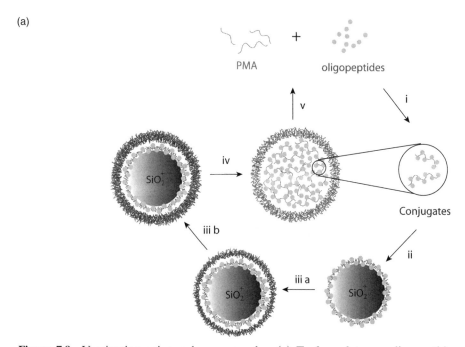

Figure 7.8 Vaccination using polymer capsules: (a) To formulate an oligopeptide vaccine with polymer capsules, the peptide is conjugated to an anchoring polymer through a biodegradable disulfide linkage (i); this is followed by the adsorption of the conjugates onto a template particle (ii), sequential deposition of PVPON and PMA$_{SH}$ (iii), cross-linking of the polymer film, and removal of the template (iv). In a reducing environment such as that experienced upon cellular internalization, degradation of disulfide linkages results in a release of the oligopeptide cargo (v). (b) Confocal laser scanning microscopy images of the capsules internalized by (i) dendritic cells and (ii) monocytes (green: capsules, red: cell membrane, blue: nuclei. (c) The immunostimulatory capability of peptide-loaded capsules was demonstrated via incubation of the capsules in whole blood and monitoring the production of IFN-γ and TNF-α by KP9-specific T cells: (i) control (unstimulated), (ii) free peptide (positive control), (iii) 500-nm empty PMA HC, and (iv) 500-nm KP9-loaded capsules. Production of cytokines by KP9-specific T cells indicates that the capsules were effectively internalized by the antigen-presenting cells and underwent intracellular processing to release the oligopeptide antigen. The latter is then trafficked to the surface and presented to the T cells within major histocompatibility complex (MHC) molecules class I to elicit an immune response. © 2009. Images (a) and (c) reprinted with permission from Chong et al.,[154] Elsevier. Image (b) reprinted with permission from De Rose et al.,[123] Wiley-VCH. © 2008. (See color insert.)

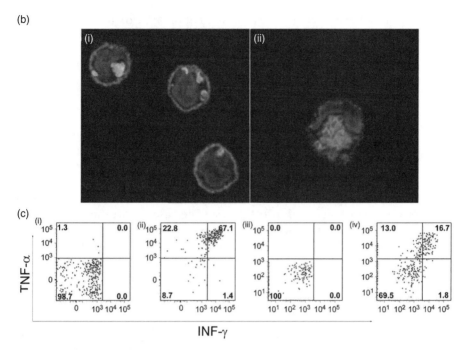

Figure 7.8 (*Continued*)

linkage, and the resulting peptide–polymer conjugate was encapsulated into PMA HC (Fig. 7.8a).[154] The capsules were successfully internalized by the APCs, which was followed by an intracellular release and processing of the antigen, its presentation within MHC-I to responding primate lympho-cytes, and a resulting immune response (Fig. 7.8b,c). This study was also impor-tant in that we were able to demonstrate fine control over peptide loading and retention as well as a triggered cargo release in response to an intracellular chemical stimulus. In a follow-up publication, we reported on using PMA HC for the delivery of full protein ovalbumin (OVA) and immunogenic OVA-derived peptide sequences to APCs and showed a successful stimulation of OVA-specific CD4 and CD8 T cells *in vitro*.[139] Moreover, following intravenous vaccination of mice with OVA protein- and OVA peptide-loaded PMA HCs, OVA-specific CD4 and CD8 T cells were also effectively stimulated to proliferate *in vivo*, and in both cases the encapsulated OVA was found to be more efficient in comparison to free OVA. De Koker and coworker also reported on the OVA delivery to DCs and efficient stimulation of CD4 and CD8 T-cell proliferation *in vitro* using capsules assembled from dextran sulfate and poly-L-arginine.[122] In a follow-up study, these authors also demonstrated *in vivo* that these microcapsules, when delivered to the lung, exhibit adjuvant activity.[155] Thus, vaccination appears to be a successful area of application for polymer capsules obtained using multilayered polymer films.

7.4 CONCLUDING REMARKS

Over the past decade, the field of multilayered polymer films has undergone a rapid development, from fundamental insights into their assembly to becoming a powerful biomedical platform with potential clinical relevance. In the case of surface-mediated drug delivery, this technology has delivered unprecedented opportunities and, in our opinion, is unsurpassed in terms of its versatility, flexibility, and effectiveness. The discussed examples demonstrate that, currently, the field is well fit to solve practical biomedical challenges. Mechanical properties of the polymer coatings are suitable to guide cell proliferation and differentiation. Intelligent multilayered substrates are able to control the drug release, for example, for transfection purposes or for the delivery of growth factors. We expect that the initial successes, together with the simplicity and adaptability of this approach, would provide a driving force for further development of this field with the aim to be applied in routine medical care. In other words, the perspectives for this field look bright, and it will benefit even further from a closer alignment with biomedical scientists and clinicians. On the other hand, successful and diverse applications of LBL coatings on micro- and nanoparticles and that of polymer capsules still require significant further research and development. We believe, however, that as such, the current state of the art makes this research direction highly promising. When carefully designed and with due consideration of particular applications in mind, LBL capsules could become a platform well competing with liposomes or micelles due to their nearly unlimited flexibility/adaptability in design. To sum up, this chapter presented polymer multilayered films, the ways these films equip surfaces with intelligent coatings, and their relevance in biomedicine, specifically in drug delivery.

REFERENCES

1. Boudou, T., Crouzier, T., Ren, K.F., Blin, G., & Picart, C. Multiple functionalities of polyelectrolyte multilayer films: new biomedical applications. *Advanced Materials* **22**, 441–467 (2010).

2. Heuberger, R., Sukhorukov, G., Voros, J., Textor, M., & Mohwald, H. Biofunctional polyelectrolyte multilayers and microcapsules: control of non-specific and bio-specific protein adsorption. *Advanced Functional Materials* **15**, 357–366 (2005).

3. Boulmedais, F. et al. Polyelectrolyte multilayer films with pegylated polypeptides as a new type of anti-microbial protection for biomaterials. *Biomaterials* **25**, 2003–2011 (2004).

4. Kinnane, C.R., Wark, K., Such, G.K., Johnston, A.P.R., & Caruso, F. Peptide-functionalized, low-biofouling click multilayers for promoting cell adhesion and growth. *Small* **5**, 444–448 (2009).

5. Matsusaki, M., Kadowaki, K., Nakahara, Y., & Akashi, M. Fabrication of cellular multilayers with nanometer-sized extracellular matrix films. *Angewandte Chemie (International ed. in English)* **46**, 4689–4692 (2007).

6. Fukuda, J. et al. Micropatterned cell co-cultures using layer-by-layer deposition of extracellular matrix components. *Biomaterials* **27**, 1479–1486 (2006).

7. Berg, M.C., Yang, S.Y., Hammond, P.T., & Rubner, M.F. Controlling mammalian cell interactions on patterned polyelectrolyte multilayer surfaces. *Langmuir* **20**, 1362–1368 (2004).

8. Lo, C.M., Wang, H.B., Dembo, M., & Wang, Y.L. Cell movement is guided by the rigidity of the substrate. *Biophysical Journal* **79**, 144–152 (2000).

9. Elbert, D.L., Herbert, C.B., & Hubbell, J.A. Thin polymer layers formed by poly-electrolyte multilayer techniques on biological surfaces. *Langmuir* **15**, 5355–5362 (1999).

10. Mendelsohn, J.D., Yang, S.Y., Hiller, J., Hochbaum, A.I., & Rubner, M.F. Rational design of cytophilic and cytophobic polyelectrolyte multilayer thin films. *Biomacromolecules* **4**, 96–106 (2003).

11. Thompson, M.T., Berg, M.C., Tobias, I.S., Rubner, M.F., & Van Vliet, K.J. Tuning compliance of nanoscale polyelectrolyte multilayers to modulate cell adhesion. *Biomaterials* **26**, 6836–6845 (2005).

12. Richert, L., Engler, A.J., Discher, D.E., & Picart, C. Elasticity of native and cross-linked polyelectrolyte multilayer films. *Biomacromolecules* **5**, 1908–1916 (2004).

13. Schneider, A. et al. Polyelectrolyte multilayers with a tunable Young's modulus: influence of film stiffness on cell adhesion. *Langmuir* **22**, 1193–1200 (2006).

14. Ren, K.F., Crouzier, T., Roy, C., & Picart, C. Polyelectrolyte multilayer films of controlled stiffness modulate myoblast cell differentiation. *Advanced Functional Materials* **18**, 1378–1389 (2008).

15. Semenov, O.V., Malek, A., Bittermann, A.G., Voros, J., & Zisch, A.H. Engineered polyelectrolyte multilayer substrates for adhesion, proliferation, and differentiation of human mesenchymal stem cells. *Tissue Engineering Part A* **15**, 2977–2990 (2009).

16. Blin, G. et al. Nano-scale control of cellular environment to drive embryonic stem cells selfrenewal and fate. *Biomaterials* **31**, 1742–1750 (2010).

17. Hillberg, A.L., Holmes, C.A., & Tabrizian, M. Effect of genipin cross-linking on the cellular adhesion properties of layer-by-layer assembled polyelectrolyte films. *Biomaterials* **30**, 4463–4470 (2009).

18. Kocgozlu, L. et al. Selective and uncoupled role of substrate elasticity in the regulation of replication and transcription in epithelial cells. *Journal of Cell Science* **123**, 29–39 (2010).

19. Chluba, J. et al. Peptide hormone covalently bound to polyelectrolytes and embedded into multilayer architectures conserving full biological activity. *Biomacromolecules* **2**, 800–805 (2001).

20. Richert, L. et al. Cell interactions with polyelectrolyte multilayer films. *Biomacromolecules* **3**, 1170–1178 (2002).

21. Tryoen-Toth, P. et al. Viability, adhesion, and bone phenotype of osteoblast-like cells on polyelectrolyte multilayer films. *Journal of Biomedical Materials Research* **60**, 657–667 (2002).

22. Wittmer, C.R. et al. Multilayer nanofilms as substrates for hepatocellular applications. *Biomaterials* **29**, 4082–4090 (2008).

23. Thierry, B., Winnik, F.M., Merhi, Y., & Tabrizian, M. Nanocoatings onto arteries via layer-by-layer deposition: toward the in vivo repair of damaged blood vessels. *Journal of the American Chemical Society* **125**, 7494–7495 (2003).

24. Kerdjoudj, H. et al. Re-endothelialization of human umbilical arteries treated with polyelectrolyte multilayers: a tool for damaged vessel replacement. *Advanced Functional Materials* **17**, 2667–2673 (2007).

25. Kerdjoudj, H. et al. Small vessel replacement by human umbilical arteries with polyelectrolyte film-treated arteries in vivo behavior. *Journal of the American College of Cardiology* **52**, 1589–1597 (2008).

26. Khademhosseini, A. et al. Layer-by-layer deposition of hyaluronic acid and poly-L-lysine for patterned cell co-cultures. *Biomaterials* **25**, 3583–3592 (2004).

27. Kidambi, S., Lee, I., & Chan, C. Primary neuron/astrocyte co-culture on polyelectrolyte multilayer films: a template for studying astrocyte-mediated oxidative stress in neurons. *Advanced Functional Materials* **18**, 294–301 (2008).

28. Mjahed, H. et al. Micro-stratified architectures based on successive stacking of alginate gel layers and poly(L-lysine)-hyaluronic acid multilayer films aimed at tissue engineering. *Soft Matter* **4**, 1422–1429 (2008).

29. Vodouhe, C. et al. Control of drug accessibility on functional polyelectrolyte multilayer films. *Biomaterials* **27**, 4149–4156 (2006).

30. Schneider, A. et al. Multifunctional polyelectrolyte multilayer films: combining mechanical resistance, biodegradability, and bioactivity. *Biomacromolecules* **8**, 139–145 (2007).

31. Chuang, H.F., Smith, R.C., & Hammond, P.T. Polyelectrolyte multilayers for tunable release of antibiotics. *Biomacromolecules* **9**, 1660–1668 (2008).

32. Thierry, B. et al. Delivery platform for hydrophobic drugs: prodrug approach combined with self-assembled multilayers. *Journal of the American Chemical Society* **127**, 1626–1627 (2005).

33. Emoto, K., Iijima, M., Nagasaki, Y., & Kataoka, K. Functionality of polymeric micelle hydrogels with organized three-dimensional architecture on surfaces. *Journal of the American Chemical Society* **122**, 2653–2654 (2000).

34. Ma, N., Zhang, H.Y., Song, B., Wang, Z.Q., & Zhang, X. Polymer micelles as building blocks for layer-by-layer assembly: an approach for incorporation and controlled release of water-insoluble dyes. *Chemistry of Materials* **17**, 5065–5069 (2005).

35. Zhu, Z.C. & Sukhishvili, S.A. Temperature-induced swelling and small molecule release with hydrogen-bonded multilayers of block copolymer micelles. *ACS Nano* **3**, 3595–3605 (2009).

36. Stadler, B., Chandrawati, R., Goldie, K., & Caruso, F. Capsosomes: subcompartmentalizing polyelectrolyte capsules using liposomes. *Langmuir* **25**, 6725–6732 (2009).

37. Volodkin, D.V., Schaaf, P., Mohwald, H., Voegel, J.C., & Ball, V. Effective embedding of liposomes into polyelectrolyte multilayered films: the relative importance of lipid-polyelectrolyte and interpolyelectrolyte interactions. *Soft Matter* **5**, 1394–1405 (2009).

38. Michel, M. et al. Layer-by-layer self-assembled polyelectrolyte multilayers with embedded liposomes: immobilized submicronic reactors for mineralization. *Langmuir* **22**, 2358–2364 (2006).

39. Chandrawati, R. et al. Cholesterol-mediated anchoring of enzyme-loaded liposomes within disulfide-stabilized polymer carrier capsules. *Biomaterials* **30**, 5988–5998 (2009).

40. Hosta-Rigau, L. et al. Capsosomes with multilayered subcompartments: assembly and loading with hydrophobic cargo. *Advanced Functional Materials* **20**, 59–66 (2010).

41. Kim, B.S., Park, S.W., & Hammond, P.T. Hydrogen-bonding layer-by-layer assembled biodegradable polymeric micelles as drug delivery vehicles from surfaces. *ACS Nano* **2**, 386–392 (2008).

42. Nguyen, P.M., Zacharia, N.S., Verploegen, E., & Hammond, P.T. Extended release antibacterial layer-by-layer films incorporating linear-dendritic block copolymer micelles. *Chemistry of Materials* **19**, 5524–5530 (2007).

43. Benkirane-Jessel, N. et al. Buildup of polypeptide multilayer coatings with anti-inflammatory properties based on the embedding of piroxicam-cyclodextrin complexes. *Advanced Functional Materials* **14**, 174–182 (2004).

44. Jessel, N.B. et al. Pyridylamino-beta-cyclodextrin as a molecular chaperone for lipopolysaccharide embedded in a multilayered polyelectrolyte architecture. *Advanced Functional Materials* **14**, 963–969 (2004).

45. Gangloff, S.C. et al. Biologically active lipid A antagonist embedded in a multilayered polyelectrolyte architecture. *Biomaterials* **27**, 1771–1777 (2006).

46. Daubine, F. et al. Nanostructured polyelectrolyte multilayer drug delivery systems for bone metastasis prevention. *Biomaterials* **30**, 6367–6373 (2009).

47. Smith, R.C., Riollano, M., Leung, A., & Hammond, P.T. Layer-by-layer platform technology for small-molecule delivery. *Angewandte Chemie (International ed. in English)* **48**, 8974–8977 (2009).

48. Benkirane-Jessel, N. et al. Control of monocyte morphology on and response to model surfaces for implants equipped with anti-inflammatory agents. *Advanced Materials* **16**, 1507–1511 (2004).

49. Schultz, P. et al. Polyelectrolyte multilayers functionalized by a synthetic analogue of an anti-inflammatory peptide, alpha-MSH, for coating a tracheal prosthesis. *Biomaterials* **26**, 2621–2630 (2005).

50. Grossin, L. et al. Step-by-step buildup of biologically active cell-containing stratified films aimed at tissue engineering. *Advanced Materials* **21**, 650–655 (2009).

51. Etienne, O. et al. Antifungal coating by biofunctionalized polyelectrolyte multilayered films. *Biomaterials* **26**, 6704–6712 (2005).

52. Jessel, N. et al. Bioactive coatings based on a polyelectrolyte multilayer architecture functionalized by embedded proteins. *Advanced Materials* **15**, 692–695 (2003).

53. Nadiri, A. et al. Cell apoptosis control using BMP4 and noggin embedded in a potyetectrotyte multilayer film. *Small* **3**, 1577–1583 (2007).

54. Dierich, A. et al. Bone formation mediated by synergy-acting growth factors embedded in a polyelectrolyte multilayer film. *Advanced Materials* **19**, 693–697 (2007).

55. van den Beucken, J.J.J.P. et al. Functionalization of multilayered DNA-coatings with bone morphogenetic protein 2. *Journal of Controlled Release* **113**, 63–72 (2006).

56. Mao, Z.W., Ma, L., Zhou, J., Gao, C.Y., & Shen, J.C. Bioactive thin film of acidic fibroblast growth factor fabricated by layer-by-layer assembly. *Bioconjugate Chemistry* **16**, 1316–1322 (2005).

57. Tezcaner, A. et al. Polyelectrolyte multilayer films as substrates for photoreceptor cells. *Biomacromolecules* **7**, 86–94 (2006).

58. Muller, S. et al. VEGF-functionalized polyelectrolyte multilayers as proangiogenic prosthetic coatings. *Advanced Functional Materials* **18**, 1767–1775 (2008).

59. Vodouhe, C. et al. Effect of functionalization of multilayered polyelectrolyte films on motoneuron growth. *Biomaterials* **26**, 545–554 (2005).

60. Crouzier, T., Ren, K., Nicolas, C., Roy, C., & Picart, C. Layer-by-layer films as a biomimetic reservoir for rhBMP-2 delivery: controlled differentiation of myoblasts to osteoblasts. *Small* **5**, 598–608 (2009).

61. Crouzier, T., Szarpak, A., Boudou, T., Auzely-Velty, R., & Picart, C. Polysaccharide-blend multilayers containing hyaluronan and heparin as a delivery system for rhBMP-2. *Small* **6**, 651–662 (2010).

62. Macdonald, M., Rodriguez, N.M., Smith, R., & Hammond, P.T. Release of a model protein from biodegradable self assembled films for surface delivery applications. *Journal of Controlled Release* **131**, 228–234 (2008).

63. Jewell, C.M., Fuchs, S.M., Flessner, R.M., Raines, R.T., & Lynn, D.M. Multilayered films fabricated from an oligoarginine-conjugated protein promote efficient surface-mediated protein transduction. *Biomacromolecules* **8**, 857–863 (2007).

64. Yamauchi, F., Kato, K., & Iwata, H. Micropatterned, self-assembled monolayers for fabrication of transfected cell microarrays. *Biochimica et Biophysica Acta* **1672**, 138–147 (2004).

65. Ziauddin, J. & Sabatini, D.M. Microarrays of cells expressing defined cDNAs. *Nature* **411**, 107–110 (2001).

66. Shea, L.D., Smiley, E., Bonadio, J., & Mooney, D.J. DNA delivery from polymer matrices for tissue engineering. *Nature Biotechnology* **17**, 551–554 (1999).

67. Saltzman, W.M. & Olbricht, W.L. Building drug delivery into tissue engineering. *Nature Reviews. Drug Discovery* **1**, 177–186 (2002).

68. Klugherz, B.D. et al. Gene delivery from a DNA controlled-release stent in porcine coronary arteries. *Nature Biotechnology* **18**, 1181–1184 (2000).

69. Fishbein, I. et al. Bisphosphonate-mediated gene vector delivery from the metal surfaces ot stents. *Proceedings of the National Academy of Sciences of the United States of America* **103**, 159–164 (2006).

70. Shen, H., Tan, J., & Saltzman, W.M. Surface-mediated gene transfer from nanocomposites of controlled texture. *Nature Materials* **3**, 569–574 (2004).

71. Bielinska, A.U. et al. Application of membrane-based dendrimer/DNA complexes for solid phase transfection in vitro and in vivo. *Biomaterials* **21**, 877–887 (2000).

72. Rea, J.C., Gibly, R.F., Davis, N.E., Barron, A.E., & Shea, L.D. Engineering surfaces for substrate-mediated gene delivery using recombinant proteins. *Biomacromolecules* **10**, 2779–2786 (2009).

73. Zhang, J.T., Chua, L.S., & Lynn, D.M. Multilayered thin films that sustain the release of functional DNA under physiological conditions. *Langmuir* **20**, 8015–8021 (2004).

74. Jewell, C.M. & Lynn, D.M. Multilayered polyelectrolyte assemblies as platforms for the delivery of DNA and other nucleic acid-based therapeutics. *Advanced Drug Delivery Reviews* **60**, 979–999 (2008).

75. Lynn, D.M. Layers of opportunity: nanostructured polymer assemblies for the delivery of macromolecular therapeutics. *Soft Matter* **2**, 269–273 (2006).

76. Jewell, C.M. & Lynn, D.M. Surface-mediated delivery of DNA: cationic polymers take charge. *Current Opinion in Colloid and Interface Science* **13**, 395–402 (2008).

77. Jewell, C.M., Zhang, J.T., Fredin, N.J., & Lynn, D.M. Multilayered polyelectrolyte films promote the direct and localized delivery of DNA to cells. *Journal of Controlled Release* **106**, 214–223 (2005).

78. Jewell, C.M. et al. Release of plasmid DNA from intravascular stents coated with ultrathin multilayered polyelectrolyte films. *Biomacromolecules* **7**, 2483–2491 (2006).

79. Zhang, J.T., Montanez, S.I., Jewell, C.M., & Lynn, D.M. Multilayered films fabricated from plasmid DNA and a side-chain functionalized poly(beta-amino ester): surface-type erosion and sequential release of multiple plasmid constructs-from surfaces. *Langmuir* **23**, 11139–11146 (2007).

80. Zhang, J.T. & Lynn, D.M. Ultrathin multilayered films assembled from "charge-shifting" cationic polymers: extended, long-term release of plasmid DNA from surfaces. *Advanced Materials* **19**, 4218–4223 (2007).

81. Liu, X.H., Zhang, J.T., & Lynn, D.M. Ultrathin multilayered films that promote the release of two DNA constructs with separate and distinct release profiles. *Advanced Materials* **20**, 4148–4153 (2008).

82. Ren, K.F., Ji, J., & Shen, J.C. Construction and enzymatic degradation of multilayered poly-L-lysine/DNA films. *Biomaterials* **27**, 1152–1159 (2006).

83. Mehrotra, S., Lee, I., & Chan, C. Multilayer mediated forward and patterned siRNA transfection using linear-PEI at extended N/P ratios. *Acta Biomaterialia* **5**, 1474–1488 (2009).

84. Zhang, Z.Q. et al. Controlled delivery of anti-sense oligodeoxynucleotide from multilayered biocompatible phosphorylcholine polymer films. *Journal of Controlled Release* **130**, 69–76 (2008).

85. Blacklock, J. et al. Disassembly of layer-by-layer films of plasmid DNA and reducible TAT polypeptide. *Biomaterials* **28**, 117–124 (2007).

86. Blacklock, J., You, Y.Z., Zhou, Q.H., Mao, G.Z., & Oupicky, D. Gene delivery in vitro and in vivo from bioreducible multilayered polyelectrolyte films of plasmid DNA. *Biomaterials* **30**, 939–950 (2009).

87. Yamauchi, F., Kato, K., & Iwata, H. Layer-by-layer assembly of poly(ethyleneimine) and plasmid DNA onto transparent indium-tin oxide electrodes for temporally and spatially specific gene transfer. *Langmuir* **21**, 8360–8367 (2005).

88. Fujimoto, H., Kato, K., & Iwata, H. Layer-by-layer assembly of small interfering RNA and poly(ethyleneimine) for substrate-mediated electroporation with high efficiency. *Analytical and Bioanalytical Chemistry* **397**, 571–578 (2010).

89. Meyer, F., Ball, V., Schaaf, P., Voegel, J.C., & Ogier, J. Polyplex-embedding in poly-electrolyte multilayers for gene delivery. *Biochimica et Biophysica Acta* **1758**, 419–422 (2006).

90. Jessel, N. et al. Multiple and time-scheduled in situ DNA delivery mediated by beta-cyclodextrin embedded in a polyelectrolyte multilayer. *Proceedings of the National Academy of Sciences of the United States of America* **103**, 8618–8621 (2006).

91. Zhang, X. et al. Transfection ability and intracellular DNA pathway of nanostruc-tured gene-delivery systems. *Nano Letters* **8**, 2432–2436 (2008).

92. Cai, K.Y. et al. Cell-specific gene transfection from a gene-functionalized poly(D,L-lactic acid) substrate fabricated by the layer-by-layer assembly technique. *Ange-wandte Chemie (International ed. in English)* **47**, 7479–7481 (2008).

93. Hu, Y., Cai, K.Y., Luo, Z., & Hu, R. Construction Of polyethyleneimine-beta-cyclodextrin/pDNA multilayer structure for improved in situ gene transfection. *Advanced Functional Materials* **12**, B18–B25 (2010).

94. Dimitrova, M. et al. Adenoviral gene delivery from multilayered polyelectrolyte architectures. *Advanced Functional Materials* **17**, 233–245 (2007).

95. Dimitrova, M. et al. Sustained delivery of siRNAs targeting viral infection by cell-degradable multilayered polyelectrolyte films. *Proceedings of the National Academy of Sciences of the United States of America* **105**, 16320–16325 (2008).

96. Hu, Y. et al. Surface mediated in situ differentiation of mesenchymal stem cells on gene-functionalized titanium films fabricated by layer-by-layer technique. *Bio-materials* **30**, 3626–3635 (2009).

97. Meyer, F. et al. Relevance of bi-functionalized polyelectrolyte multilayers for cell transfection. *Biomaterials* **29**, 618–624 (2008).

98. Su, X.F., Kim, B.S., Kim, S.R., Hammond, P.T., & Irvine, D.J. Layer-by-layer-assembled multilayer films for transcutaneous drug and vaccine delivery. *ACS Nano* **3**, 3719–3729 (2009).

99. Hillaireau, H. & Couvreur, P. Nanocarriers' entry into the cell: relevance to drug delivery. *Cellular and Molecular Life Sciences* **66**, 2873–2896 (2009).

100. Owens, D.E. & Peppas, N.A. Opsonization, biodistribution, and pharmacokinetics of polymeric nanoparticles. *International Journal of Pharmaceutics* **307**, 93–102 (2006).

101. Pasut, G. & Veronese, F.M. PEG conjugates in clinical development or use as anticancer agents: an overview. *Advanced Drug Delivery Reviews* **61**, 1177–1188 (2009).

102. Cortez, C. et al. Targeting and uptake of multilayered particles to colorectal cancer cells. *Advanced Materials* **18**, 1998–2003 (2006).

103. Cortez, C. et al. Influence of size, surface, cell line, and kinetic properties on the specific binding of A33 antigen-targeted multilayered particles and capsules to colorectal cancer cells. *ACS Nano* **1**, 93–102 (2007).

104. Zhou, J. et al. Layer by layer chitosan/alginate coatings on poly(lactide-co-glycolide) nanoparticles for antifouling protection and folic acid binding to

achieve selective cell targeting. *Journal of Colloid and Interface Science* **345**, 241–247 (2010).

105. Reibetanz, U., Claus, C., Typlt, E., Hofmann, J., & Donath, E. Defoliation and plasmid delivery with layer-by-layer coated colloids. *Macromolecular Bioscience* **6**, 153–160 (2006).

106. Kakade, S., Manickam, D.S., Handa, H., Mao, G.Z., & Oupicky, D. Transfection activity of layer-by-layer plasmid DNA/poly(ethylenimine) films deposited on PLGA microparticles. *International Journal of Pharmaceutics* **365**, 44–52 (2009).

107. Saurer, E.M., Jewell, C.M., Kuchenreuther, J.M., & Lynn, D.M. Assembly of erodible, DNA-containing thin films on the surfaces of polymer microparticles: toward a layer-by-layer approach to the delivery of DNA to antigen-presenting cells. *Acta Biomaterialia* **5**, 913–924 (2009).

108. Rosi, N.L. et al. Oligonucleotide-modified gold nanoparticles for intracellular gene regulation. *Science* **312**, 1027–1030 (2006).

109. Lee, S.H., Bae, K.H., Kim, S.H., Lee, K.R., & Park, T.G. Amine-functionalized gold nanoparticles as non-cytotoxic and efficient intracellular siRNA delivery carriers. *International Journal of Pharmaceutics* **364**, 94–101 (2008).

110. Giljohann, D.A., Seferos, D.S., Prigodich, A.E., Patel, P.C., & Mirkin, C.A. Gene regulation with polyvalent siRNA-nanoparticle conjugates. *Journal of the American Chemical Society* **131**, 2072–2073 (2009).

111. Kirkland-York, S. et al. Tailored design of Au nanoparticle-siRNA carriers utilizing reversible addition—fragmentation chain transfer polymers. *Biomacromolecules* **11**, 1052–1059 (2010).

112. Elbakry, A. et al. Layer-by-layer assembled gold nanoparticles for siRNA delivery. *Nano Letters* **9**, 2059–2064 (2009).

113. Donath, E., Sukhorukov, G.B., Caruso, F., Davis, S.A., & Mohwald, H. Novel hollow polymer shells by colloid-templated assembly of polyelectrolytes. *Angewandte Chemie International Edition* **37**, 2202–2205 (1998).

114. Johnston, A.P.R., Cortez, C., Angelatos, A.S., & Caruso, F. Layer-by-layer engineered capsules and their applications. *Current Opinion in Colloid & Interface Science* **11**, 203–209 (2006).

115. del Mercato, L.L. et al. LbL multilayer capsules: recent progress and future outlook for their use in life sciences. *Nanoscale* **2**, 458–467 (2010).

116. Kharlampieva, E., Kozlovskaya, V., & Sukhishvili, S.A. Layer-by-layer hydrogen-bonded polymer films: from fundamentals to applications. *Advanced Materials* **21**, 3053–3065 (2009).

117. Quinn, J.F., Johnston, A.P.R., Such, G.K., Zelikin, A.N., & Caruso, F. Next generation, sequentially assembled ultrathin films: beyond electrostatics. *Chemical Society Reviews* **36**, 707–718 (2007).

118. De Geest, B.G., Sanders, N.N., Sukhorukov, G.B., Demeester, J., & De Smedt, S.C. Release mechanisms for polyelectrolyte capsules. *Chemical Society Reviews* **36**, 636–649 (2007).

119. De Geest, B.G., Sukhorukov, G.B., & Mohwald, H. The pros and cons of polyelectrolyte capsules in drug delivery. *Expert Opinion on Drug Delivery* **6**, 613–624 (2009).

120. Stadler, B. et al. Polymer hydrogel capsules: en route toward synthetic cellular systems. *Nanoscale* **1**, 68–73 (2009).

121. De Geest, B.G. et al. Intracellularly degradable polyelectrolyte microcapsules. *Advanced Materials* **18**, 1005–1009 (2006).

122. De Koker, S. et al. Polyelectrolyte microcapsules as antigen delivery vehicles to dendritic cells: uptake, processing, and cross-presentation of encapsulated antigens. *Angewandte Chemie International Edition* **48**, 8485–8489 (2009).

123. De Rose, R. et al. Binding, internalization, and antigen presentation of vaccine-loaded nanoengineered capsules in blood. *Advanced Materials* **20**, 4698–4703 (2008).

124. Yan, Y. et al. Uptake and intracellular fate of disulfide-bonded polymer hydrogel capsules for doxorubicin delivery to colorectal cancer cells. *ACS Nano* **4**, 2928–2936 (2010).

125. Semmling, M. et al. A novel flow-cytometry-based assay for cellular uptake studies of polyelectrolyte microcapsules. *Small* **4**, 1763–1768 (2008).

126. Price, A.D., Zelikin, A.N., Wark, K.L., & Caruso, F.A. Biomolecular "ship-in-a-bottle": continuous RNA synthesis within hollow polymer hydrogel assemblies. *Advanced Materials* **22**, 720–723 (2010).

127. Ai, H., Pink, J.J., Shuai, X.T., Boothman, D.A., & Gao, J.M. Interactions between self-assembled polyelectrolyte shells and tumor cells. *Journal of Biomedical Materials Research Part A* **73A**, 303–312 (2005).

128. Ochs, C.J., Such, G.K., Stadler, B., & Caruso, F. Low-fouling, biofunctionalized, and biodegradable click capsules. *Biomacromolecules* **9**, 3389–3396 (2008).

129. Qi, W. et al. The lectin binding and targetable cellular uptake of lipid-coated polysaccharide microcapsules. *Journal of Materials Chemistry* **20**, 2121–2127 (2010).

130. Wattendorf, U., Kreft, O., Textor, M., Sukhorukov, G.B., & Merkle, H.P. Stable stealth function for hollow polyelectrolyte microcapsules through a poly(ethylene glycol) grafted polyelectrolyte adlayer. *Biomacromolecules* **9**, 100–108 (2008).

131. Kirchner, C. et al. Cytotoxicity of nanoparticle-loaded polymer capsules. *Talanta* **67**, 486–491 (2005).

132. De Koker, S. et al. In vivo cellular uptake, degradation, and biocompatibility of polyelectrolyte microcapsules. *Advanced Functional Materials* **17**, 3754–3763 (2007).

133. An, Z.H., Kavanoor, K., Choy, M.L., & Kaufman, L.J. Polyelectrolyte microcapsule interactions with cells in two- and three-dimensional culture. *Colloid and Surfaces. B, Biointerfaces* **70**, 114–123 (2009).

134. Ochs, C.J., Such, G.K., Yan, Y., van Koeverden, M.P., & Caruso, F. Biodegradable click capsules with engineered drug-loaded multilayers. *ACS Nano* **4**, 1653–1663 (2010).

135. Kinnane, C.R. et al. Low-fouling Poly(N-vinyl pyrrolidone) capsules with engineered degradable properties. *Biomacromolecules* **10**, 2839–2846 (2009).

136. Zelikin, A.N., Li, Q., & Caruso, F. Disulfide-stabilized poly(methacrylic acid) capsules: formation, cross-linking, and degradation behavior. *Chemistry of Materials* **20**, 2655–2661 (2008).

137. Becker, A.L., Zelikin, A.N., Johnston, A.P.R., & Caruso, F. Tuning the formation and degradation of layer-by-layer assembled polymer hydrogel microcapsules. *Langmuir* **25**, 14079–14085 (2009).

138. Sivakumar, S. et al. Degradable, surfactant-free, monodisperse polymer-encapsulated emulsions as anticancer drug carriers. *Advanced Materials* **21**, 1820–1824 (2009).

139. Sexton, A. et al. A protective vaccine delivery system for in vivo t cell stimulation using nanoengineered polymer hydrogel capsules. *ACS Nano* **3**, 3391–3400 (2009).

140. Zelikin, A.N., Breheney, K., Robert, R., Tjipto, E., & Wark, K. Cytotoxicity and Internalization of Polymer Hydrogel Capsules by Mammalian Cells. *Biomacromolecules* **11**, 2123–2129 (2010).

141. Kreft, O., Javier, A.M., Sukhorukov, G.B., & Parak, W.J. Polymer microcapsules as mobile local pH-sensors. *Journal of Materials Chemistry* **17**, 4471–4476 (2007).

142. Wong, J.Y., Leach, J.B., & Brown, X.Q. Balance of chemistry, topography, and mechanics at the cell-biomaterial interface: issues and challenges for assessing the role of substrate mechanics on cell response. *Surface Science* **570**, 119–133 (2004).

143. Liu, X.Y., Gao, C.Y., Shen, J.C., & Mohwald, H. Multilayer microcapsules as anti-cancer drug delivery vehicle: deposition, sustained release, and in vitro bioactivity. *Macromolecular Bioscience* **5**, 1209–1219 (2005).

144. Tao, X., Chen, H., Sun, X.J., Chen, H.F., & Roa, W.H. Formulation and cytotoxicity of doxorubicin loaded in self-assembled bio-polyelectrolyte microshells. *International Journal of Pharmaceutics* **336**, 376–381 (2007).

145. Wang, K.W. et al. Encapsulated photosensitive drugs by biodegradable microcapsules to incapacitate cancer cells. *Journal of Materials Chemistry* **17**, 4018–4021 (2007).

146. Han, B.S. et al. Layered microcapsules for daunorubicin loading and release as well as in vitro and in vivo studies. *Polymers for Advanced Technologies* **19**, 36–46 (2008).

147. Wang, Y.J., Bansal, V., Zelikin, A.N., & Caruso, F. Templated synthesis of single-component polymer capsules and their application in drug delivery. *Nano Letters* **8**, 1741–1745 (2008).

148. Katagiri, K. & Caruso, F. Functionalization of colloids with robust inorganic-based lipid coatings. *Macromolecules* **37**, 9947–9953 (2004).

149. Katagiri, K. & Caruso, F. Monodisperse polyelectrolyte-supported asymmetric lipid-bilayer vesicles. *Advanced Materials* **17**, 738–743 (2005).

150. Li, J.B., Möhwald, H., An, Z.H., & Lu, G. Molecular assembly of biomimetic microcapsules. *Soft Matter* **1**, 259–264 (2005).

151. Moya, S. et al. Lipid coating on polyelectrolyte surface modified colloidal particles and polyelectrolyte capsules. *Macromolecules* **33**, 4538–4544 (2000).

152. Chandrawati, R. et al. Engineering advanced capsosomes: maximizing the number of subcompartments, cargo retention, and temperature-triggered reaction. *ACS Nano* **4**, 1351–1361 (2010).

153. Stadler, B. et al. A Microreactor with thousands of subcompartments: enzyme-loaded liposomes within polymer capsules. *Angewandte Chemie (International ed. in English)* **48**, 4359–4362 (2009).

154. Chong, S.F. et al. A paradigm for peptide vaccine delivery using viral epitopes encapsulated in degradable polymer hydrogel capsules. *Biomaterials* **30**, 5178–5186 (2009).

155. De Koker, S. et al. Biodegradable polyelectrolyte microcapsules: antigen delivery tools with Th17 skewing activity after pulmonary delivery. *Journal of Immunology* **184**, 203–211 (2010).

Micro- and Nanopatterning of Active Biomolecules and Cells

DANIEL AYDIN, VERA C. HIRSCHFELD-WARNEKEN, ILIA LOUBAN, and JOACHIM P. SPATZ

8.1 INTRODUCTION

Patterning of biomolecules has been mainly driven by the development of biosensors and the need to place even more features on the same surface area. As a side effect, the advance in micro- and nanofabrication technology has paved the way for studying complex problems in cell biology by the application of biomimetic surfaces. Answering questions that relate to the spatial distribution of proteins and lipids within the cell membrane and their interaction with and subsequent modulation of the cytoskeleton has been the objective of many studies.[1]

In this chapter, we will first introduce chemical approaches for immobilizing biomolecules. This section is followed by a general overview of the most commonly applied patterning techniques for proteins and an introduction to block copolymer micelle nanolithography (BCML) and its variations. In the last part of this chapter, we will show examples of the use of nanostructured surfaces in cell biology.

8.2 CHEMICAL APPROACHES FOR PROTEIN IMMOBILIZATION

Immobilization chemistry represents a major challenge when patterning biomolecules on a surface. Proteins, in particular, are very sensitive to the applied immobilization method. Activity and proper function of proteins immobilized on a surface strongly depend on their orientation and ability to bind their cognate receptor in the right conformation. Generally, proteins can be immobilized in a site-directed fashion or at random orientation; the interaction of

Intelligent Surfaces in Biotechnology: Scientific and Engineering Concepts, Enabling Technologies, and Translation to Bio-Oriented Applications, First Edition.
Edited by H. Michelle Grandin and Marcus Textor.

TABLE 8.1 Covalent Protein Immobilization—Reactive Groups

Functional Group	Amino Acid	Surface	Product
R-NH$_2$	Lys, Arg, Glu	N-hydroxysuccinimide (NHS), ester, tetrafluorophenyl (TFP) ester, epoxide aldehyde, isothiocyanate	Amide, β-aminoalcohol, imine, thiourea
R-SH	Cys	Maleimide, pyridyl disulfide, vinylsulfone	Thioether, disulfide, β-sulfonyl thioether
R-CO$_2$H	Asp, Glu	Amine	Amide
R-OH	Ser, Thr, Tyr	Epoxide	Ether

protein and surface can be covalent or noncovalent.[2] Here, we briefly introduce common coupling schemes used for immobilizing biomolecules with a
clear focus on protein coupling.

In the simplest case, proteins are immobilized either by physisorption via
hydrophobic or polar interactions or by covalent coupling of functional groups
present in the amino acid sequence of the protein. The most commonly targeted amino acid side chains bear hydroxyl, sulfhydryl, amine, or carboxyl
groups. The latter two functionalities are also found in the N- and C-termini,
respectively. For a selection of the most frequently used functional surfaces
and the respective amino acid targets, see Table 8.1.

Another very prominent approach is to covalently attach biotin to one of
the functional amino acids mentioned earlier. Biotin is a high-affinity binding
partner for avidin or streptavidin (SAv) ($K = 10^{-15}$ M), proteins that can be
coated to a surface by simple physisorption. The advantage of this method is
a reduced interaction of the coupled protein with the surface and, as a result,
enhanced activity. However, all approaches lead to a random orientation of
the protein on the surface, which may drastically lower the activity of the
molecule.[3] Unspecific protein adsorption suffers additionally from the potential detachment of proteins from the surface when buffers and, consequently,
surface charges are changed.

Site-directed immobilization of proteins can either be covalent or can take
advantage of high-affinity molecular interactions between a tag and a specific
molecule on the surface. However, in both cases, the protein has to be specifically tagged at the desired site in order to obtain proper orientational binding.
Thus, even when using chemical reactions during the conjugation procedure,
the respective tag is usually introduced by recombinant protein engineering.
Here, the DNA encoding for the protein of interest (POI) is modified such
that in the expressed protein, another peptide sequence, the tag, is fused to
the POI.[4-7] The most common recombinantly introduced tags are listed in
Table 8.2.

Some of these tags can either be modified by a small molecule or directly
coupled to the respective binding partner. For example, proteins bearing an
intein tag have specifically been biotinylated at the tag and coupled to

TABLE 8.2   Protein Tags

Tag	Capture Reagent	Affinity Constant	Reference
Glutathione S-transferase (GST)	Glutathione	10^{-9} M	4
Maltose-binding protein (MBP)	Maltose	10^{-7}–10^{-6} M	5
Hexahistidine tag (his$_6$)	NTA, aa-tacn, tris-NTA	10^{-9}–10^{-5} M	12 and 99
FLAG peptide	Anti-FLAG M2	$1.5 \cdot 10^{-8}$ M	100
Fc-tag, IgG	Protein A, protein G	Dependent on isotype/species	101
Intein	N-terminal cysteine	Covalent	8 and 102
CVIA peptide	Farnesyl	Covalent	9, 103, and 104

streptavidin-coated surfaces in a site-directed fashion.[8] In another approach, azide-derivatized isoprenoid diphosphates were enzymatically linked to a C-terminal CVIA tag followed by a Cu(I) catalyzed (3 + 2) cycloaddition to an alkyne-containing immobilized linker molecule on the surface.[9] This so-called click reaction converts only chemical functionalities not found in nature and thereby renders the reaction highly specific. Azide-labeled proteins have also been coupled to phosphinothioester-functionalized surfaces in a traceless Staudinger reaction.[10] However, these recently developed site-specific reactions have only partially found their way into commercial products or academic research. Glutathione S-transferase (GST) and FLAG are standard tags for protein pull-down experiments, while maltose-binding protein (MBP), Fc-tag and his$_6$ are well established for the purification of recombinantly expressed proteins. These tag systems have been available for almost two decades now, and a huge toolbox has been developed ranging from appropriate expression systems and sensor chips to affinity resins and chemicals. The most prominent one, the his$_6$-tag, relies on the coordination of the imidazole moiety in the side chain of histidine to a chelated transition metal ion. A commonly used chelator is nitrilotriacetic acid (NTA), a tetradentate ligand that binds to Ni or Cu ions. In this octahedral complex, the two remaining sites are occupied by water, which are then replaced by histidine. The dative nature of the bond is responsible for the reversibility of the interaction, which is an advantage for transient immobilization as desired for purification purposes. However, the affinity between Ni-NTA and his$_6$ does not reach high values like biotin-SAv, for example, and potentially leads to undesired protein dissociation. At the same time, unspecific protein adsorption may occur. Other chelator systems have been developed in order to tackle these drawbacks, including multivalent NTAs[11,12] and aa-tacn,[13,14] a macrocycle with enhanced affinity to histidine in octahedral complexes with Ni(II).[15]

The immobilization chemistry has to be chosen depending on the molecule and the technique used in the patterning process. Important criteria include the need for orientation of the molecule, the stability of immobilization chemistry, and whether direct or indirect patterning is used.

8.3 BIOMOLECULE PATTERNING BY "TOP-DOWN" TECHNIQUES

In the following, we introduce methods used for the patterning of active biomolecules, in particular, proteins, on solid substrates. The selection presented in this chapter is far from being complete and is supposed to give a short overview of the most commonly used and the most promising new technologies.

8.3.1 Microcontact Printing (μCP)

μCP has originally been developed by Kumar and Whitesides to structure self-assembled monolayers (SAMs) of thiols on gold surfaces.[16] Nowadays, μCP is widely applied to structure many different molecules including DNA, virus particles, vesicles, or proteins.[17] First, a polymeric stamp—usually poly(dimethylsiloxane) (PDMS)—is fabricated by replica molding from a master. This master can be produced by standard photolithography. In a second step, the stamp is "inked" with the molecule by simple incubation of the respective solution and the pattern is printed onto the surface. Protein features as small as 40 nm have been reported in the literature.[18] Therefore, the process is sometimes also referred to as nanocontact printing (nCP). Also, more complex patterns can be printed by a combination of inking and subtraction.[19] Being a parallel process, μCP is the method of choice for the patterning of micrometer-sized features when large surface areas are required. The basic process is easy to perform, cheap, and fast. Only for the fabrication of casting molds are cleanroom facilities needed; all other steps can be performed by using standard laboratory equipment. Even though it is technically more demanding in terms of alignment of the different patterns, the stamping of multiple proteins is possible.

8.3.2 Nanoimprint Lithography (NIL)

NIL also takes advantage of a patterned stamp. However, in this case, it is not a material that is transferred to the substrate, but the whole topography is negatively replicated.[20,21] The stamp is brought into contact with a polymer layer that is consequently heated above its glass transition temperature. After cooling, the stamp is removed and the negative remains imprinted into the polymer layer; the process is similar to the fabrication of stamps in μCP. Falconnet et al. applied NIL to arrange SAv in lines and dot structures.[22,23] To this end, poly(methyl metacrylate) (PMMA) was patterned by a silicon stamp and was subjected to an anisotropic oxygen plasma treatment until reaching the underlying niobium oxide surface. Bare areas were filled with poly(L-lysine)-

graft-poly(ethylene glycol) (PLL-*g*-PEG)-biotin followed by lifting off of the PMMA layer and backfilling with nonfunctional protein-repellent PLL-*g*-PEG. After incubation with SAv, the imprinted structures were replicated. Similar approaches have also been reported by others.[24,25] The process is parallel and shares the advantages of µCP. The resolution of polymer imprint lithography has been brought down to feature sizes of 10 nm[26,27]; however, only the molecular composition of the polymer layer is theoretically limiting the resolution.[28] Protein nanopatterns in this regime have not been demonstrated thus far.

8.3.3 Electron Beam Lithography (EBL)

EBL is a well-established technology in the semiconductor industry. A modification of standard EBL has been applied by Denis et al. to generate lines of aligned collagen bundles. In this case, the electron-sensitive PMMA resist was used to pattern silicon wafers, followed by the gas-phase deposition of a CH_3-terminated SAM, PMMA removal, passivation of SiO_2 by protein-repellent poly(ethylene glycol) (PEG), and protein deposition at the irradiated sites.[29] However, direct patterning of SAMs has also been employed to generate structures at the submicrometer length scale.[30,31] For example, Turchanin et al. irradiated 4'-nitro-1-1'-biphenyl-4-thiol (NBPT) SAMs with electrons to selectively reduce nitro moieties to amines, which then served as anchor group for the attachment of proteins.[30] Protein features with dimensions smaller than 100 nm can easily be produced by EBL. Even protein multiplexing has been reported recently,[32] but the number of different proteins is limited to the number of different chemical functionalities and protein immobilization strategies, which can be addressed simultaneously—most likely, not more than three or four. The major drawback of this method is the relatively slow process speed and consequently the small surface areas, which can be patterned in a reasonable amount of time. Additionally, the equipment is relatively expensive when compared to other patterning techniques.

8.3.4 Dip-Pen Nanolithography (DPN)

DPN, like µCP, was first used to pattern SAMs of thiols on gold surfaces by the Mirkin Group.[33] The basic principle is very similar to that of a pen writing over a piece of paper. In DPN, the pen is an atomic force microscopy (AFM) cantilever, the paper is the surface, and the so-called ink is the material that is delivered from the tip of the cantilever through the liquid meniscus to the surface. The driving force is the chemical gradient that develops between the tip and the surface. DPN is probably the most flexible process to structure all kinds of molecules or supramolecular structures[34] including polymers,[35] colloidal particles,[36] DNA,[37] and proteins.[38–40] Indirect processes write a pattern of SAMs like 16-hexadecanoic acid onto gold surfaces and take advantage of well-established surface chemistry to couple the desired molecule.[41] Here, structure sizes down to 15 nm have been reported. Recent reports aimed at a massive parallelization of the process by using arrays composed of up to 55,000 cantilevers.[42,43] Lately, Huo et al. reported on the fabrication and successful application of an array of 11,000,000 pyramid-shaped polymeric PDMS pens.[44] These arrays allow for the patterning of square centimeter-sized surface areas within hours. Moreover, strategies for multiplexed patterning are being developed at the moment.[45] However, direct protein patterning is technically more demanding than writing thiol SAMs. Up to now, the minimal feature size of 45 nm has been reached by Lee et al. when directly patterning lysozyme or rabbit IgG.[38]

Modifications of the DPN process are achieved by nanoshaving and by the very similar technique of nanografting.[46] Here, an AFM cantilever is moved over a thiol SAM on a gold surface, selectively removing molecules at the desired sites; this process is called nanoshaving. In a variation, the blank parts of the surface are directly backfilled with a different thiol; this process is called nanografting. For example, Staii et al. applied nanografting to produce 100×100 nm^2 squares of double cystein-terminated MBP embedded in a undecanethiol-tri(ethylene glycol) SAM.[47]

Depending on the application, each of the different techniques has its advantages and drawbacks. When large surface areas are needed, parallel processes like µCP or NIL are usually favorable. However, regarding the flexibility to pattern multiple proteins, attainable feature size and pattern geometry, serial processes such as EBL, DPN, or nanografting are more competitive. Nevertheless, the surface areas that are patterned are usually relatively small in size.

This drawback can be circumvented by a technique that takes advantage of a self-assembly-based process to produce hexagonally ordered arrays of gold nanoparticles with a size of usually 4–8 nm. By combination with top-down processes, patterns of nanostructures can be obtained with feature sizes down to 100 nm, so-called micro-nanostructures. The gold nanoparticles serve as anchor points to immobilize recombinant proteins in a site-directed manner. Protein patches with a size down to 4 nm—the size of a single protein—can be fabricated. However, the pattern is always hexagonal, while the space between the proteins can be varied from 20 to 250 nm. Thus, arbitrary patterns cannot be achieved on the nanometer scale by this method, but the micro-nanostructuring process gives full flexibility on the patterning at the micrometer and hundreds of nanometer scale. In the following, we will describe BCML, its variations, and a set of applications.

8.4 BIOMOLECULE NANOARRAYS BY BLOCK COPOLYMER NANOLITHOGRAPHY

In this section, we will introduce simple block copolymer nanolithography as well as more advanced variations of this technique. Moreover, we show

how these templates can be addressed in order to specifically immobilize proteins.

8.4.1 Block Copolymer Nanolithography

Self-assembly-based methods, so-called bottom-up techniques, are considered an alternative concept for nanofabrication in the sub-100-nm regime.[48] Well-established techniques capable of producing such small features like EBL or X-ray lithography demand expensive instrumentation, whereas the technical requirements of self-assembly-based methods are usually comparably low. Block copolymers, in particular, feature many interesting characteristics; for example, the length scale of their microdomains is in the range of tens of nanometers, as well as the different chemical and physical properties of the different polymer blocks. Moreover, shape and size are relatively easy to tune by changing the molecular weight and composition of the building blocks. In the simplest case, a block copolymer consists of two chemically distinct polymer coils A and B, which are covalently connected to each other. As a consequence of the differences in chemistry, the two blocks tend to segregate into two microdomains held together by the covalent connection only. Two competing effects determine to which extent this separation can take place. Entropically, the polymer favors building a random coil structure while at the same time the area between the two phases is minimized to lower the interfacial energy.[49] Periodic, nanoscale microdomain structures are obtained by the interplay of these driving forces. Spherical micelles from diblock copolymers consisting of nonpolar polystyrene (PS) and polar poly(vinyl pyridine) (PVP) can be used for the templated synthesis of hexagonally ordered arrays of gold nanoparticles on solid inorganic surfaces. Here, interparticle spacing and size of gold nanoclusters are tunable depending on experimental conditions. PS-*b*-PVP diblock copolymer is dissolved in toluene. Above a certain concentration threshold, the so-called critical micelle concentration (CMC), the diblock copolymer chains start to assemble into spherical micelles. Increasing the concentration above the CMC does not change the number of free polymer chains in solution, but rather, all excessive polymers accumulate in micelles (see Fig. 8.1a).[50–52] As toluene is a more selective solvent for PS, the PS blocks form the outer shell of the micelle preventing an energetically unfavorable contact of the PVP block with the solvent.[53] The polar PVP core can now be used to incorporate metal precursor salt into the micelle. This process shifts the thermodynamic equilibrium between free polymer chains and assembled micelles toward the latter and decreases the CMC at the same time.[54] $HAuCl_4$ diffuses into the micelles and protonates the PVP. The negatively charged Au(III) complex $AuCl_4^-$ represents the counterion stabilizing the micellar core.

A micellar monolayer is formed either by a spin-coating or a dip-coating process. Therefore, a previously cleaned substrate like a glass coverslip or a cut silicon wafer chip is dipped into a gold-loaded micellar solution and is

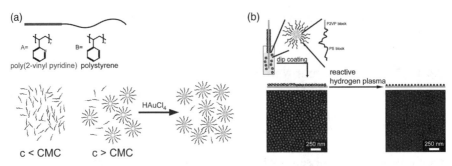

Figure 8.1 Block copolymer micelle nanolithography. (a) The diblock copolymer consists of one polystyrene and one poly(vinylpyridine) block. Below the critical micelle concentration (CMC), the polymer does not aggregate; the solution consists only of free chains. Above the CMC, micelles form, and only a constant number of molecules are in a free state. Upon the addition of HAuCl₄, micelles are stabilized and the thermodynamic equilibrium is shifted toward the micelles. (b) The substrate is retracted with a certain velocity from the micellar solution; micelles assemble on the surfaces in a hexagonal order. The scanning electron micrographs on the bottom show a coated substrate before (left side) and after exposure to hydrogen plasma (right side). Adapted from Aydin et al.[105] by permission of Carl Hanser Verlag, © 2011. (See color insert.)

retracted with a defined velocity. In solution, the micelles do not adsorb onto the surface; only during retraction do the micelles assemble on the substratum at the air–solvent–substrate interface. The driving force is the evaporation of the solvent at this interface. The quality of the resulting hexagonal order and packing of the micelles on the surfaces is governed by numerous parameters including the molecular weight of the polymer shell,[55] the retraction velocity,[56,57] the concentration of polymer in solution,[48] and the properties of the solvent like polarity, surface tension, vapor pressure, viscosity, and temperature.[58] These parameters strongly influence the formation of the micelle-containing solvent film and thereby the resulting attractive capillary and repulsive electrostatic and steric forces. In the next step, substrates bearing the freshly formed micellar monolayer are exposed to a reactive gas plasma. During the plasma etching, the metal precursor salt, in this case HAuCl₄, is reduced to spherical elemental gold nanoparticles, and the polymer shell is removed. The structuring process is schematically depicted in Figure 8.1b.

The particle size is restricted to a rather small size by the initial loading parameter. In order to control the particle diameter at a larger scale, an additional growing or postloading step is needed. Hydroxylamine seeding is capable for the selective enlargement of colloidal Au particles in solution and on rigid substrates. In order to preserve the spatial orientation of the nanopattern, nanoparticles were embedded into a matrix of alkylsiloxane or the diblock copolymer matrix itself was directly used as a stabilizing template.[59] Particle size can be precisely tuned by the reaction time and is only limited by the instability of large particles (>50 nm).

As mentioned earlier, interparticle distances depend on many parameters. Using a set of micellar solution with different block copolymers at different concentrations, the spacing can be seamlessly varied between 20 and 300 nm.

8.4.2 Biofunctionalization of Nanostructures

In order to selectively anchor proteins to gold nanoparticle arrays, interparticle areas have to be passivated against nonspecific protein adsorption. Two different approaches have been successfully employed. First, PEG thin films known to efficiently reduce protein surface interaction are grafted to plasma-activated glass surfaces.[60] In the second approach, gold nanoparticle arrays are transferred to polymeric PEG-diacrylate hydrogels, which are inherently protein repellent.[61,62] This technique allows for additionally controlling the stiffness of the nanostructured material as will be described in more detail later.

In the next step, gold nanoparticles are specifically addressed with the desired biomolecule. Short peptides can be directly coupled to gold nanoparticles via a terminal cystein or a thiolated linker,[63] while full-length proteins are coupled in a site-directed fashion using an NTA/his-tag system as depicted in Figure 8.2a.[64,65] Atomic force micrographs and the respective height line scans, as shown in Figure 8.2b, revealed that gold nanoparticles can be occupied by single his-green fluorescent protein (his-GFP) molecules. Maximum heights in the line scans increase from 4.5 nm without GFP to 9 nm when GFP is bound; the difference is exactly representing the height of the GFP molecule. This approach can be extended to pattern antibodies through their Fc portion to immobilized his-tagged protein A. To our knowledge, block copolymer

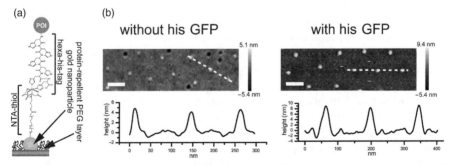

Figure 8.2 Protein immobilization. (a) Schematic of single-protein immobilization. Gold nanoparticles are embedded in a protein-repellent PEG matrix and are functionalized with a thiol-terminated NTA as an acceptor molecule for his-tagged proteins. (b) Atomic force micrographs of a gold nanoparticle surface before and after immobilization of his-GFP. The height rises from 4.5 to 9.0 nm; the difference corresponds to the size of the his-GFP molecule. The scale bar is 100 nm. Adapted from Aydin et al.[64] (See color insert.)

nanolithography combined with the above-described biofunctionalization scheme is currently the only method to provide nanometer controlled ligand interaction of a surface with a single receptor.

8.4.3 Hierarchically Nanostructured Biomolecule Arrays

Various techniques have been published describing the fabrication of micro-nanostructured surfaces. These approaches include the localized irradiation of a micellar monolayer by electrons,[66,67] UV light,[68] or focused ions[69] followed by selective removal of unmodified regions as exemplified in Figure 8.3a for micellar EBL. Moreover, micelles have successfully been transferred to designated regions by means of µCP.[70] However, all these approaches are either too slow to produce a sufficiently large surface area in a reasonable amount of time or result in inhomogeneously structured nanoparticles. Gold nanoparticle arrays as anchor points for active single biomolecules represent a very powerful tool to tackle open fundamental questions in cell biology. The micrometer-scale control over these structures is a crucial part of the tool box. However, the lack of high-quality micro-nanostructured surfaces over areas >1 cm^2 hampered the applicability of BCML templated protein arrays for cell biological research. Recently, two different methods have been shown to overcome this limitation.

The first is using a microcontact deprinting approach.[71] Here, a micellar monolayer is deposited on the substrate surface covered with a PS stamp that carries the desired structure and is shortly heated above the glass transition temperature of PS. After cool down, the stamp is peeled away, stripping the micelles at areas where the substrate had contact with the PS stamp. The following plasma treatment yields patches of hexagonally ordered gold nanoparticle arrays in a pattern that reproduces the structure on the stamp. Transfer of structures in the submicron regime has been demonstrated and, being a parallel process sample processing, is relatively fast.

The second approach combines the fast process speed of conventional photo- or electron beam resist lithography with the nanometer precision of block copolymer micellar nanolithography (BCMN) (Fig. 8.3b).[64] Therefore, novolak-based photo- or electron beam resist is coated on top of an extended gold nanoparticle surface. After irradiation of the resist material and the development of the structure, gold nanoparticles that are not protected by resists are dissolved by applying an ultrasound treatment in an aqueous solution of cysteamine. In the last step, the protecting resist layer is removed by simple rinsing in organic solvent, and the resulting micro-nanostructured surface is plasma cleaned. EBL was able to fabricate patches with features down to a size of 100 nm on conductive silicon chips, which is approximately 200 times faster than micellar EBL. However, photolithography could reach a resolution down to 1 µm, independent of the conductive properties of the surface.

Based on the specifications of the surface that has to be structured and the throughput time, the appropriate technique has to be selected. Serial processes

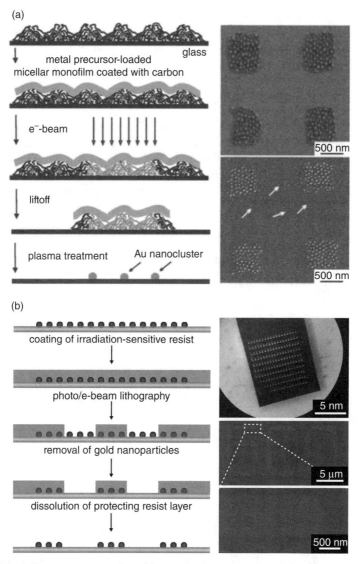

Figure 8.3 Micro-nanopatterning. (a) A micellar monolayer is irradiated at certain regions with focused electrons from a scanning electron microscope that cross-link the micelles at these spots. Nonirradiated parts are removed by sonication in organic solvents, and the substrate is exposed to the usual plasma process to obtain gold nanoparticles and to remove the polymer. Reproduced from Glass et al.[55] by permission of IOP Publishing Ltd., doi:10.1088/0957-4484/14/10/314. (b) An extended nanostructure is coated with an irradiation-sensitive resist, illuminated at desired sites by electrons from a scanning electron microscope (SEM->electron beam lithography) or UV light (->photolithography), and the structure is then developed. Gold nanoparticles that are not protected by the resist are removed, and the resist is subsequently dissolved leaving the micro-nanostructure. Adapted from Aydin et al.[105] by permission of Carl Hanser Verlag, © 2011.

such as electron beam or focused ion beam lithography are capable of fabricating super structures in the 100-nm regime but are comparably slow. In contrast, parallel processes allow for very fast sample processing; however, feature resolution is decreased.

8.4.4 Fabrication of Nanoscale Distance Gradients

As mentioned earlier, the thickness of the micellar film during the retraction process critically influences the interparticle distance on the processed substrate. To form distance gradients within one substrate, the film height has to be tuned during the retraction process.

The thickness of the film is determined by viscosity and capillarity, which play opposing roles. As the static meniscus is perturbated by the film dragged along, a dynamic meniscus forms. If the substrate is pulled slowly enough, the film it drags is adequately thin. Due to the liquid's viscosity, the meniscus moves at the same velocity as the substrate. However, the liquid/vapor interface is distorted by the film; thus, surface tension opposes this movement to maintain a static meniscus. Gravitation also opposes the upward dragging but is negligible compared to surface tension for low capillary numbers.[72] The ratio of viscous force to surface tension force acting across the liquid/vapor interface is described by the capillary number Ca. It represents the mobility potential of a liquid and is defined as $Ca = \mu U / \sigma$, where μ is the viscosity of the liquid, U is a characteristic velocity, and σ is the surface tension. Landau, Levich, and Derjaguin were the first who related the maximum height h_∞ for film thickness of Newtonian fluids to a functional form of the capillary number Ca of the following form:[73,74]

$$h_\infty = 0.94 \sqrt{\frac{\sigma}{\rho g}} \cdot Ca^{\frac{2}{3}} = 0.94 \frac{(\mu U)^{\frac{2}{3}}}{(\rho g)^{\frac{1}{2}} \sigma^{\frac{1}{6}}},$$

where Ca denotes the capillary number and g the gravitation acceleration (9.81 m/s^2); U is the retraction speed of the substrate from the micellar solution; and μ, σ, and ρ denote liquid viscosity, surface tension, and density, respectively. This relation is valid for low capillary number ($Ca = \mu U / \sigma \ll 1$) since the viscous contribution to the normal pressure is neglected.[75] As a consequence, the film height is orders of magnitude lower than the capillary length at the meniscus. When Ca approaches unity, both the thickness and the extent of the dynamic meniscus tend to the capillary length.[72] In that case, gravity becomes the dominant force and limits the thickness of the film layer. Another important aspect influencing the film height is the angle of the substrate toward the solution during the emersion process.[73] In the presence of an inclination angle, the film layer will be different for the front and rear of the substrate.

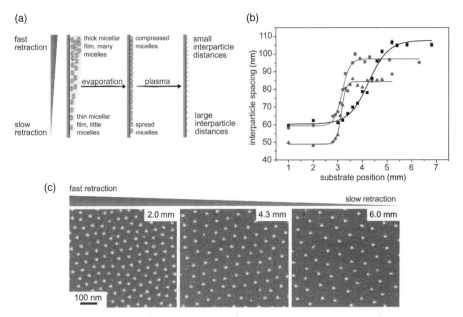

Figure 8.4   Nanoparticle spacing gradients by micellar nanolithography. (a) Particle distance gradient formation: A gradient in film height evolves due to the gradient in retraction velocity of the sample; after evaporation, a gradient in micelle density forms, which transforms into a gradient in gold nanoparticle distances after plasma treatment. (b) Plots of particle spacing gradients with varying gradient strengths (e.g., black and blue plots) and varying interparticle distances (e.g., blue and red plots). (c) Scanning electron micrographs of regions along a gradient on a single substrate. Adapted with permission from Aydin et al.[105] by Carl Hanser Verlag, © 2011. (See color insert.)

A gradient in film thickness that corresponds to a density gradient of the periodic pattern can be achieved by retracting the substrate with an accelerating or decelerating velocity (Fig. 8.4a). Practically, minimal and maximal values of interparticle spacing are limited by the dewetting properties of the solution and the micelles' ability to compress. Within this range, the interparticle distance can be adjusted by the retraction velocity with a variation of Δ 20–50 nm per substrate starting from 30- up to 250-nm interparticle distance, depending on the molecular weight of the applied polymer (Fig. 8.4b). The slope of the gradient is controlled by the gradient length and the time window in which the retraction velocity is accelerated or decelerated, respectively.

8.4.5   Soft Polymeric Biomolecule Arrays

Polymeric materials are not suitable for BCML; however, nanoparticles prepared on supports like glass or silicon can be transferred to polymeric, flexible substrates via transfer lithography (Fig. 8.5a), where gold nanoparticle structures are functionalized with an unsaturated thiolated linker molecule.[61,62] In

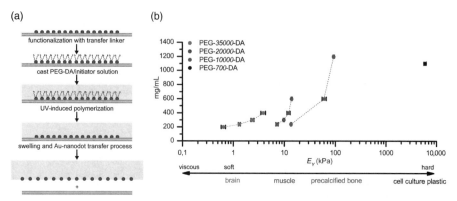

Figure 8.5 Transfer nanolithography. (a) Scheme of the transfer process. Nanoparticles are covalently functionalized with an unsaturated linker molecule. The PEG-DA prepolymer solution and the radical starter are cast over the sample and are irradiated with UV light. The radical polymerization cross-links the meshwork and copolymerizes the nanoparticles covalently into the top layer of the hydrogel. During swelling, the particles are detached from the template, and gel and support separate. (b) Young moduli (E_Y) of PEG-DA hydrogels derived from polymers of different sizes and polymer contents in the casting solution. As a reference, the Young moduli of different tissues are shown. Adapted from Aydin et al.[61] (See color insert.)

the following, the polyethylene glycol-diacrylate (PEG-DA) prepolymer solution is cast on top, cured with UV to copolymerize gold nanoparticles into the PEG-DA meshwork and left to swell for 2 days. During the swelling process, lateral forces detach the particles from the solid template and the structure is replicated on the polymer surface, which separates from the solid template. The resulting nanostructured gel can be rendered bioactive by the same functionalization schemes presented earlier.

Soft, nontoxic, and protein-repellent PEG-DA hydrogels are of special interest for biological applications. The mechanical properties of the substrate have been shown to strongly influence cellular behavior when cells are in contact with the material.[76,77] The Young moduli of different PEG-DA hydrogels are presented in Figure 8.5b. As illustrated, the stiffness of the gels can be arbitrarily adjusted across four orders of magnitude (0.6 kPa $\leq E_Y$ (M_W, C_{H2O}) $\geq$ 6 MPa), covering the range of all tissues that are found in the human body. Moreover, quasi-three-dimensional tubelike structures within PEG-DA hydrogels could be fabricated by the transfer of gold nanoparticles from structured glass fibers.[62] These tubes feature a size that is comparable to that of capillary blood vessels.

The flexibility in terms of varying surface structure, patterning at the nanometer length scale, and compliance makes these polymeric hydrogels a valuable tool to study cells interacting with their environment.

8.5 APPLICATION OF NANOSTRUCTURED SURFACES TO STUDY CELL ADHESION

8.5.1 Mimicking the Extracellular Environment

All tissue cells depend on contacts to the extracellular matrix (ECM) or surrounding cells.[78] Cell adhesion at these cell junctions is mediated by cell surface receptors, which have two basic functions. First, they provide physical support, and second, they function as signaling hubs to sense and to respond to external cues. Adhesion-dependent cells that fail to form external contacts die from anoikis, a form of apoptosis resulting from loss of anchorage.[78]

The primary cell adhesion mediating transmembrane receptors are members of the integrin family. Integrins are heterodimers that bind to ECM proteins such as fibronectin, vitronectin, or laminin and that mediate strong cell adhesion mainly via the ubiquitously found arginine-glycine-aspartate (RGD) tripeptide epitope. Intracellularly, the adhesion of a tissue cell depends on the formation of micrometer-sized protein clusters termed focal adhesions (FAs) linking the integrins to the cytoskeletal actin network. This configuration enables FAs to provide information on the cell's location, local environment, adhesive state, and surrounding matrix, which is important in processes like embryogenesis, cell differentiation, immune response, wound healing, hemostasis, and cancer.[79–81]

Only in recent years has it become apparent that this communication goes far beyond chemical ligand recognition and also encompasses physical cues such as internal sensing or externally applied forces.[82,83] Therefore, integrins are also known as natural biomechanical sensors, being able to convert mechanical forces into biochemical signaling. Based on today's knowledge, we can summarize that cells can process information regarding different properties of the ECM including the topography,[84,85] rigidity,[79] and the specific chemical signal, even anisotropies in ligand spacing.[56,86]

The complexity of the natural ECM demands novel tools that allow simplifying the system and varying factors independently from one another. Combining technologies from the fields of materials science, surface chemistry, and molecular cell biology allows for designing bioactive interfaces with defined molecular composition of ligands, ordered spatial arrangement, and tunable surface elasticity. Such biomimetic surfaces are valuable tools to gain insight into the complicated processing of the environmental sensing of a cell.

8.5.2 Nanoscale Control of Cellular Adhesion

A key question in cell biology is how the spatial arrangement of signaling cues at different length scales affects cell response. It has been shown at the macro- and micrometer length scale that chemical composition and topography drastically influence cell behavior.[1] However, only little is known about how cells react on the nanometer scale. High-resolution microscopy images of ECM molecules revealed highly organized submicrometer structures.[87,88] Further-more, many cellular signaling events are initiated through the recruitment and clustering of nanometer-sized transmembrane receptors. For example, the size of a single integrin receptor is estimated to range from 8 to 12 nm.[89,90] A pre-requisite for FA formation and thus stable cell adhesion is the close proximity of integrins for receptor multimerization.[91] The density of these receptor clus-ters, which is preset by the ligand density, determines the size and composition of the FA protein plaque and the adhesive state of the cell. This ECM ligand–integrin–FA–actin complex is substantial and functions bidirectionally; that is, it transmits chemical signals from inside out and from outside in.[91] Therefore, spatial control of the spacing of single-ligand molecules is critical for control-ling receptor clustering and understanding receptor-mediated signaling.

The few systematic investigations of cellular interaction with patterned structures at the nanometer scale indeed established an extraordinarily high sensitivity of cells to differentiate in nanometer-defined environments. A basic approach to nanopatterning is to coat a substrate with a nonadhesive layer to which proteins cannot adsorb and to incorporate adhesive epitopes into this background that selectively interact with one type of receptor. By applying functionalized star-shaped polymers bearing an RGD-containing pentapep-tide over a nonadhesive background, Maheshwari et al. were able to show that presentation of the peptide in clusters of at least five peptides per star led to the development of well-formed actin stress fibers and mature FAs. This was not the case for randomly distributed stars bearing a single RGD peptide, even though the average RGD density was lower in the clustered case (Fig. 8.6a).[92] Similar dependencies were obtained when testing cellular adhesion to $(RGD)_n$–bovine serum albumin (BSA) conjugates of different valences n and average densities.[93] These results indicate the existence of a minimum ligand distance for the initiation of FA assembly and the importance of the spatial distribution of epitopes.

Using micellar block copolymer nanolithography, it is possible to control ligand spacing at the nanometer length scale. Hereby, thiol-terminated adhe-sive sequences are covalently linked to gold nanoparticles. Arnold et al could determine the critical ligand distance for FA formation to take place.[63] Each particle served as a chemical anchor for the covalent binding of the adhesion-promoting peptide cRGDfK via a thiol linker. To prevent unspecific protein adsorption, inert PEG was covalently attached to the glass surface between the gold nanoparticles. Cell adhesion was mediated only by the cyclic cRGDfK ligand that specifically addresses $\alpha_v\beta_3$ integrin. Due to steric hindrance, only one integrin can bind to a single functionalized gold dot. Thus, the ligand sepa-ration was associated with the integrin separation in the cell (Fig. 8.6b). It could be shown that a separation distance of cRGDfK ligands of 73 nm pro-vided very limited cell attachment, whereas interligand distances below 58 nm promoted stable cell adhesion.

Furthermore, experiments employing single-cell force microscopy (SCFM) revealed that the lateral spacing of individual integrin receptor–ligand bonds

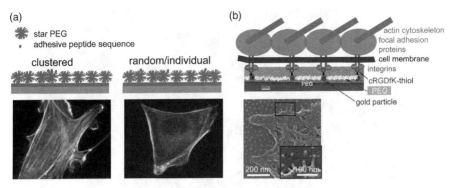

Figure 8.6 Nanoscale patterning affects cell adhesion. (a) RGD peptides are presented on star polymers to vary the total average concentration and the spatial distribution. The actin cytoskeleton of a cell adhering to a 9-RGD star polymer substrate (left) and a 1-RGD star polymer substrate is imaged by fluorescence microscopy. Adapted from Maheshwari et al.[92] by permission of The Company of Biologists Ltd. © 2000. (b) Biofunctionalization of the gold nanopattern and specific cell interactions: scheme of the biofunctionalized substrate on the basis of a high-resolution transmission electron micrograph of gold particles (side view) depicting the interaction of cRGDfK ligands with integrin receptors linked to the actin cytoskeleton via FA proteins. Bottom: Scanning electron micrographs show parts of critical point-dried cells on biofunctionalized nanopatterns with ~60-nm particle separation. The inset shows a close-up of ultrasmall cellular protrusions with a diameter of ~10 to ~20 nm and a length of ~30 to ~50 nm, interacting selectively with the cRGDfK-functionalized gold nanoparticles. Adapted from Arnold et al.[56] (See color insert.)

determines the strength of the cell–substrate bond and, thus, cell ECM interaction forces. When integrin ligand spacing exceeded 90 nm, focal contact formation was impaired and detachment forces were significantly decreased compared to a ligand separation of less than 50 nm.[94] Moreover, a strong dependence on adhesion time during the first 10 minutes of cell–substrate interaction suggests an active, cooperative cell response that is controlled by the spacing between individually activated integrins.[95]

8.5.3 Micro-Nanopatterns to Uncouple Local from Global Density

Nanopatterned surfaces with increasing interligand distances concomitantly exhibit a reduced average ligand density. Therefore, a ligand spacing effect cannot be differentiated from a density effect. Substrates where micrometer-sized nanostructured patches are surrounded by bare substratum overcome this constraint. These micro-nanostructured surfaces can help to differentiate whether a cell response really results from the induced proximity of the ligand-coupled receptor clusters or simply depends on the amount of bound receptor. Arnold et al. approached this question by designing surfaces with 58-nm-spaced nanoparticles in micropatches where the average (global) concentration of particles was lower (90 dots/µm²) than on surfaces with an extended

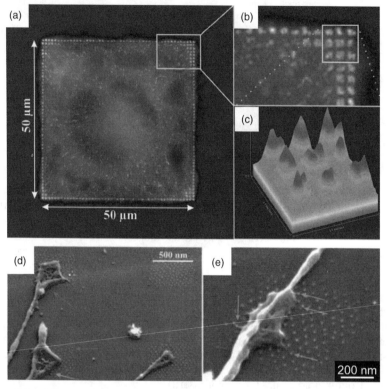

Figure 8.7   Cell adhesion to micro-nanostructured substrates with interligand distances of 58 nm. (a) Live cell fluorescence microscopy image of a REF52-yellow fluorescent protein (YFP)-paxillin cell plated for 2 hours on a 50-μm square divided into 500 × 500 nm squares, separated by 500 nm. (b) Close-up of (a) illustrating the contact site formation on squares. (c) YFP-paxillin fluorescence intensity distribution on cellular adhesion sites. (d,e) Scanning electron micrographs of filopodial structures on biofunctionalized hierarchical nanopatterns (500-nm squares separated by 1000 nm). Red arrows indicate mature contact structures, and blue arrows show ultrasmall cellular protrusions in contact with the adhesive gold nanoparticles. Reproduced from Arnold et al.[98] by permission of The Royal Society of Chemistry, © 2009. http://dx.doi.org/10.1039/B815634D (See color insert.)

nanopattern with a spacing of 73 nm (190 dots/μm^2).[63] As indicated in the fluorescence image in Figure 8.7a–c, cells adhere and form FAs on the micropattern visualized by the FA protein paxillin and are confined to the structured area. Scanning electron micrographs showed cell interaction with biofunctionalized gold particles and no interaction with bare areas where no adhesive ligand was present (Fig. 8.7d,e). Although less binding sites were available on the micro-nanopatterned substrate, cells could adhere and form stable FAs in contrast to the 73-nm-spaced nanopattern. These experiments show that it is not the global ligand number that is critical for inducing cell adhesion and FA assembly, but rather the local dot-to-dot separation, namely, the spatial confinement of integrin receptors.

8.5.4 Nanoscale Gradients to Induce Cell Polarization and Directed Migration

Cell polarization and directed cell migration play a crucial role in many physiological processes such as embryonic development, immune response, and angiogenesis, as well as in pathological processes, like inflammation and cancer metastasis.[96]

All tissue cells depend on external anchorage for survival and thus will switch to a migratory behavior to explore their environment if the substratum beneath them does not provide sufficient binding possibilities. An adhesion gradient presented by spatially organized adhesive peptide sites will therefore guide cell movement toward denser areas, a process called haptotaxis. Such gradients are presented by ECM components in different tissues of the body. Since a separation distance in cRGDfK ligands of 73 nm supported only very limited cell attachment, whereas interligand distances of 58 nm were able to promote stable cell adhesion, it can be hypothesized that nanoscale gradients spanning this interligand distance regime would provoke a kind of biased cellular response.

Figure 8.8a,b shows the adhesion of cells to a nanoscale distance gradient substrate ranging from an interligand spacing of 50–80 nm. With increasing interparticle distances, the numbers of attached cells as well as the projected cell area become significantly smaller. Along the gradient, at interligand distances of 55–75 nm, cells are highly elongated and oriented toward the gradient axis (not shown).[86] It is assumed that the polarization of the cell body and hence the induction of directed cell migration toward smaller RGD spacings can only take place at a distinct range of interparticle distances where the cell is capable of forming FAs. By visualizing actin filaments and FA proteins, the presence of such structures and their distribution were investigated, particularly on larger interligand distances of up to 70 nm, where the cell area was found to be reduced but gradient sensing still took place. On a homogeneously spaced pattern of 50 nm, cells do not orient and feature well-developed major vinculin clusters that are distributed symmetrically over the periphery of the cell and well-established actin fibers (Fig. 8.8c). On a gradient with a local interparticle spacing of 70 nm, cells elongate and polarize toward the gradient (Fig. 8.8c). Vinculin aggregates are rather randomly organized but are asymmetrically distributed between the cell front and rear. The actin fibers are very fine but are still aligned and connect FAs on both ends of the cell.

Furthermore, directed cell migration and cell polarization were investigated with respect to interligand distances. The range of interligand distances where cells are able to transduce the anisotropy from the substrate into a functional response clearly depends on cell adhesion. The importance of cell adhesion and, therefore, optimal integrin clustering for oriented cell polarization is

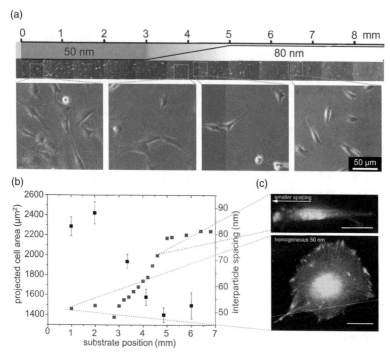

Figure 8.8 Cell adhesion to nanoscale distance gradient substrates. (a) Stitched phase-contrast micrographs showing the adhesion of MC3T3 osteoblasts to different areas of the gradient substrate. Close-up shows images at substrate areas offering 50-, 60-, 70-, and 80-nm interparticle spacing. (b) Projected cell area after 23 hours' cell culture on a substrate including a 2-mm spacing gradient from 50 to 80 nm. (c) Bottom: immuno-fluorescence images of MC3T3 osteoblasts after 23 hours of adhesion on a homogeneously nanopatterned area with 50 nm. Top: along the gradient on a section having a spacing of approximately 70 nm. Smaller spacings are on the left side of the image. Cells are stained for vinculin (green) and actin (red). Scale bars correspond to 20 μm. Adapted from Arnold et al.[56] and Hirschfeld-Warneken et al.[86] (See color insert.)

summarized in an overview graph in Figure 8.9. Only a gradient nanopattern in the intermediate interligand distance regime triggers a directed response. For analysis, the gradient substrates ranged from 45 to 130 nm with a constant gradient strength of 18 ± 4 nm/mm. On very dense nanopatch spacing positions around 55 nm, cells displayed a recognizable asymmetric cell shape in the direction of the gradient axis but did not show any migration. A further increase in interligand distances to larger than 65 nm led to an oriented polarization of the cell capable of pursuing the gradient by active directed migration. Once the ligand spacing exceeded 85 nm, the cell morphology was highly elongated but was no longer oriented toward the gradient axis, and cells migrated randomly in all directions. When approaching ligand distances of

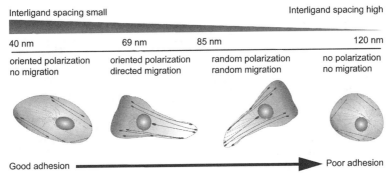

Figure 8.9 Schematic of cell morphologies on different substrates. Depending on the spacing, cells show oriented cell body polarization and directed migration. Cells were analyzed after 24 hours on substrates with a gradient strength of 18 ± 4 nm/mm. Adapted from Aydin et al.[105] by permission of Carl Hanser Verlag, © 2011.

130 nm, cells lost their eccentricity, adhered very poorly, and were not able to migrate anymore.

The most striking finding is that cells can sense small but consistent differences in ligand spacing presented along the front and the back of their body; this difference, which is as little as 1 nm across the cell diameter, seems to affect cell polarization and directed migration. By coupling opposite FAs via actin filaments and myosin-driven contractility, it is very likely that cells test the mechanical stability of spatially distributed FAs and, therefore, migrate toward smaller-spaced peptide arrays. Taken together, these results point out the relevance of nanometer-scale gradients of ECM cues in directing integrin receptor clustering-based responses.

8.5.5   Substrate Elasticity Determines Cell Fate

As introduced earlier, gold nanoparticle arrays can be transferred to PEG-DA hydrogels. These anchor points, embedded in the gel, can then be functionalized with, for example, adhesive peptides or other proteins of interest as described earlier. This transfer lithography approach allows for decoupling the interparticle spacing and, consequently, the spacing of biochemical factors from the rigidity of the underlying substrate, that is, the biophysical cues.[61] In nature, the native ECM or cellular microenvironments are, from a physical point of view, complex, multidimensional parameter spaces. With the help of transfer lithography, the simultaneous influence of different environmental parameters, such as adhesive ligand availability and substrate compliance, on the cellular behavior can be investigated.

Therefore, an artificial substrate system, mimicking the biophysical and biochemical properties of the ECM in connective tissues (Fig. 8.10b), was applied to fibroblasts as a cellular model system. Cell behavior, described as

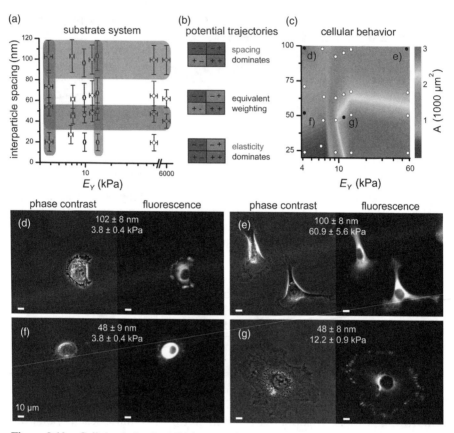

Figure 8.10 Cellular behavior within an artificial, multidimensional parameter space. A two-dimensional space of environmental parameters (substrate elasticity E_Y and nanoparticle spacing L) was spun over several orders of magnitude. (a) Each data point represents a single substrate employed in cell adhesion experiments. Highlighted substrates were selected to quantify cellular sensing thresholds. (b) Possible trajectories of cellular reactions, thus, possible color-coded spreading area on different substrates. (c) Color-coded and interpolated cellular spreading area as trajectories or regions in the two-dimensional space of environmental parameters. White points represent the discrete nature of gained spreading area values. Black marks clarify substrate properties of phase contrast and fluorescence micrographs (d–g) of rat embryonic fibroblasts (REF) stably transfected with paxillin fused to yellow fluorescent protein (REF-YFP-pax) on elastic nanopatterned substrates 24 hours after seeding. Adapted from Aydin et al.[105] by permission of Carl Hanser Verlag, © 2011. (See color insert.)

the trajectories within this two-dimensional space of environmental parameters, was then quantified.[105] Cell spreading areas were determined by analyzing phase contrast and fluorescence microscopy images of cells on different substrates (Fig. 8.10d–g) and were assembled in color-coded plots (Fig. 8.10c). These experiments revealed two tactile set points, that is, thresholds in cellular sensing behavior, at $E_Y \approx 8$ kPa and $L \approx 65$ nm, respectively. According to the hierarchical phase model in cellular behavior[97] and using the obtained threshold values, cellular reaction can theoretically be qualified as positive (+, high spreading area) or negative (–, low spreading area) depending on the substrate properties. Figure 8.10b illustrates possible cellular behavior with regard to the importance or dominance of a particular environmental parameter. Comparison of these theoretical considerations with obtained spreading area values (Fig. 8.10c) clearly identifies the elasticity of the cellular microenvironment as the dominant parameter in cellular sensing processes.

8.6 CONCLUSION

In recent years, nanoscopic control of surface structures and signaling that is related to properties at the nanoscale has increasingly become the focus of biomedical research. Here, we introduce several state-of-the-art patterning and functionalization techniques. In more detail, we describe the concept of the self-assembly-driven process of block copolymer nanolithography for synthesizing hexagonally ordered gold nanoparticle arrays. Advanced patterns such as particle spacing gradients can be obtained by pure self-assembly, while the combination with standard top-down technology allows for generating asymmetric patterns. Moreover, these structures can be transferred to polymeric hydrogels and functionalized with active biomolecules. Nanopatterned surfaces represent a valuable platform for investigating the impact of the spatial distribution of peptides and viscoelastic properties of a surface on cell adhesion.

REFERENCES

1. Torres, A.J., Wu, M., Holowka, D., & Baird, B. Nanobiotechnology and cell biology: micro-and nanofabricated surfaces to investigate receptor-mediated signaling. *Annual Reviews of Biophysics* **37**, 265–288 (2008).

2. Jonkheijm, P., Weinrich, D., Schroder, H., Niemeyer, C.M., & Waldmann, H. Chemical strategies for generating protein biochips. *Angewandte Chemie (International ed. in English)* **47**, 9618–9647 (2008).

3. Holland-Nell, K. & Beck-Sickinger, A.G. Specifically immobilised aldo/keto reductase AKR1A1 shows a dramatic increase in activity relative to the randomly immobilised enzyme. *Chembiochem* **8**, 1071–1076 (2007).

4. Hearn, M.T. & Acosta, D. Applications of novel affinity cassette methods: use of peptide fusion handles for the purification of recombinant proteins. *Journal of Molecular Recognition* **14**, 323–369 (2001).

5. Miller, D.M., 3rd., Olson, J.S., Pflugrath, J.W., & Quiocho, F.A. Rates of ligand binding to periplasmic proteins involved in bacterial transport and chemotaxis. *The Journal of Biological Chemistry* **258**, 13665–13672 (1983).

6. Terpe, K. Overview of tag protein fusions: from molecular and biochemical fundamentals to commercial systems. *Applied Microbiology and Biotechnology* **60**, 523–533 (2003).

7. Waugh, D.S. Making the most of affinity tags. *Trends in Biotechnology* **23**, 316–320 (2005).

8. Lesaicherre, M.L., Lue, R.Y., Chen, G.Y., Zhu, Q., & Yao, S.Q. Intein-mediated biotinylation of proteins and its application in a protein microarray. *Journal of the American Chemical Society* **124**, 8768–8769 (2002).

9. Duckworth, B.P., Xu, J., Taton, T.A., Guo, A., & Distefano, M.D. Site-specific, covalent attachment of proteins to a solid surface. *Bioconjugate Chemistry* **17**, 967–974 (2006).

10. Soellner, M.B., Dickson, K.A., Nilsson, B.L., & Raines, R.T. Site-specific protein immobilization by Staudinger ligation. *Journal of the American Chemical Society* **125**, 11790–11791 (2003).

11. Lata, S., Gavutis, M., Tampe, R., & Piehler, J. Specific and stable fluorescence labeling of histidine-tagged proteins for dissecting multi-protein complex formation. *Journal of the American Chemical Society* **128**, 2365–2372 (2006).

12. Lata, S. & Piehler, J. Stable and functional immobilization of histidine-tagged proteins via multivalent chelator headgroups on a molecular poly(ethylene glycol) brush. *Analytical Chemistry* **77**, 1096–1105 (2005).

13. Johnson, D. & Martin, L. Controlling protein orientation at interfaces using histidine tags: an alternative to Ni/NTA. *Journal of the American Chemical Society* **127**, 2018–2019 (2005).

14. Marin, V.L., Bayburt, T.H., Sligar, S.G., & Mrksich, M. Functional assays of membrane-bound proteins with SAMDI-TOF mass spectrometry. *Angewandte Chemie (International ed. in English)* **46**, 8796–8798 (2007).

15. Zompa, L. Metal complexes of cyclic triamines. 2. Stability and electronic spectra of nickel (II), copper (II), and zinc (II) complexes containing nine-through twelve-membered cyclic triamine ligands. *Inorganic Chemistry* **17**, 2531–2536 (1978).

16. Kumar, A. & Whitesides, G.M. Features of gold having micrometer to centimeter dimensions can be formed through a combination of stamping with an elastomeric stamp and an alkanethiol "ink" followed by chemical etching. *Applied Physics Letters* **63**, 2002–2004 (1993).

17. Whitesides, G.M., Ostuni, E., Takayama, S., Jiang, X., & Ingber, D.E. Soft lithography in biology and biochemistry. *Annual Review of Biomedical Engineering* **3**, 335–373 (2001).

18. Renault, J.P. et al. Fabricating arrays of single protein molecules on glass using microcontact printing. *Journal of Physical Chemistry. B, Condensed Phase* **107**, 703–711 (2003).

19. Coyer, S.R., Garcia, A.J., & Delamarche, E. Facile preparation of complex protein architectures with sub-100-nm resolution on surfaces. *Angewandte Chemie (International ed. in English)* **46**, 6837–6840 (2007).

20. Guo, L.J. Nanoimprint lithography: methods and material requirements. *Advanced Materials* **19**, 495–513 (2007).

21. Truskett, V.N. & Watts, M.P.C. Trends in imprint lithography for biological applications. *Trends in Biotechnology* **24**, 312–317 (2006).

22. Falconnet, D., Koenig, A., Assi, F., & Textor, M. A combined photolithographic and molecular-assembly approach to produce functional micropatterns for applications in the biosciences. *Advanced Functional Materials* **14**, 749–756 (2004).

23. Falconnet, D. et al. A novel approach to produce protein nanopatterns by combining nanoimprint lithography and molecular self-assembly. *Nano Letters* **4**, 1909–1914 (2004).

24. Hoff, J.D., Cheng, L.J., Meyhofer, E., Guo, L.J., & Hunt, A.J. Nanoscale protein patterning by imprint lithography. *Nano Letters* **4**, 853–857 (2004).

25. Maury, P. et al. Creating nanopatterns of his-tagged proteins on surfaces by nanoimprint lithography using specific NiNTA-histidine interactions. *Small* **3**, 1584–1592 (2007).

26. Austin, M.D. et al. Fabrication of 5 nm line width and 14 nm pitch features by nanoimprint lithography. *Applied Physics Letters* **84**, 5299–5301 (2004).

27. Chou, S.Y., Krauss, P.R., Zhang, W., Guo, L., & Zhuang, L. Sub-10 nm imprint lithography and applications. *Journal of Vacuum Science & Technology. B* **15**, 2897–2904 (1997).

28. Hua, F. et al. Polymer imprint lithography with molecular-scale resolution. *Nano Letters* **4**, 2467–2472 (2004).

29. Denis, F.A., Pallandre, A., Nysten, B., Jonas, A.M., & Dupont-Gillain, C.C. Alignment and assembly of adsorbed collagen molecules induced by anisotropic chemical nanopatterns. *Small* **1**, 984–991 (2005).

30. Turchanin, A. et al. Molecular self-assembly, chemical lithography, and biochemical tweezers: a path for the fabrication of functional nanometer-scale protein arrays. *Advanced Materials* **20**, 471–477 (2008).

31. Zhang, G.J. et al. Nanoscale patterning of protein using electron beam lithography of organosilane self-assembled monolayers. *Small* **1**, 833–837 (2005).

32. Christman, K.L. et al. Positioning multiple proteins at the nanoscale with electron beam cross-linked functional polymers. *Journal of the American Chemical Society* **131**, 30–31 (2009).

33. Piner, R.D., Zhu, J., Xu, F., Hong, S., & Mirkin, C.A. "Dip-pen" nanolithography. *Science* **283**, 661–663 (1999).

34. Salaita, K., Wang, Y., & Mirkin, C.A. Applications of dip-pen nanolithography. *Nature Nanotechnology* **2**, 145–155 (2007).

35. Noy, A. et al. Fabrication of luminescent nanostructures and polymer nanowires using dip-pen nanolithography. *Nano Letters* **2**, 109–112 (2002).

36. Gundiah, G. et al. Dip-pen nanolithography with magnetic Fe_2O_3 nanocrystals. *Applied Physics Letters* **84**, 5341–5343 (2004).

37. Demers, L.M. et al. Direct patterning of modified oligonucleotides on metals and insulators by dip-pen nanolithography. *Science* **296**, 1836–1838 (2002).

38. Lee, K.B., Lim, J.H., & Mirkin, C.A. Protein nanostructures formed via direct-write dip-pen nanolithography. *Journal of the American Chemical Society* **125**, 5588–5589 (2003).

39. Lee, S.W. et al. Biologically active protein nanoarrays generated using parallel dip-pen nanolithography. *Advanced Materials* **18**, 1133–1136 (2006).

40. Lim, J.H. et al. Direct-write dip-pen nanolithography of proteins on modified silicon oxide surfaces. *Angewandte Chemie (International ed. in English)* **42**, 2309–2312 (2003).

41. Lee, K.B., Park, S.J., Mirkin, C.A., Smith, J.C., & Mrksich, M. Protein nanoarrays generated by dip-pen nanolithography. *Science* **295**, 1702–1705 (2002).

42. Salaita, K. et al. Sub-100 nm, centimeter-scale, parallel dip-pen nanolithography. *Small* **1**, 940–945 (2005).

43. Salaita, K. et al. Massively parallel dip-pen nanolithography with 55.000-pen two-dimensional arrays. *Angewandte Chemie (International ed. in English)* **45**, 7220–7223 (2006).

44. Huo, F. et al. Polymer pen lithography. *Science* **321**, 1658–1660 (2008).

45. Wang, Y. et al. A self-correcting inking strategy for cantilever arrays addressed by an inkjet printer and used for dip-pen nanolithography. *Small* **4**, 1666–1670 (2008).

46. Xu, S. & Liu, G. Nanometer-scale fabrication by simultaneous nanoshaving and molecular self-assembly. *Langmuir* **13**, 127–129 (1997).

47. Staii, C., Wood, D.W., & Scoles, G. Verification of biochemical activity for proteins nanografted on gold surfaces. *Journal of the American Chemical Society* **130**, 640–646 (2008).

48. Krishnamoorthy, S., Hinderling, C., & Heinzelmann, H. Nanoscale patterning with block copolymers. *Materials Today* **9**, 40–47 (2006).

49. Bates, F.S. & Fredrickson, G.H. Block copolymer thermodynamics: theory and experiment. *Annual Review of Physical Chemistry* **41**, 525–557 (1990).

50. Gao, Z. & Eisenberg, A. A model of micellization for block copolymers in solutions. *Macromolecules* **26**, 7353–7360 (1993).

51. Israelachvili, J.N. *Intermolecular and Surface Forces*, 2nd edn. London; Orlando, FL: Academic Press (1992).

52. Israelachvili, J.N. Self-assembly in two dimensions: surface micelles and domain formation in monolayers. *Langmuir* **10**, 3774–3781 (1994).

53. Izzo, D. & Marques, C.M. Formation of micelles of diblock and triblock copolymers in a selective solvent. *Macromolecules* **26**, 7189–7194 (1993).

54. Spatz, J.P., Röscher, A., Sheiko, S., Krausch, G., & Möller, M. Noble metal loaded block Ionomers: micelle organization, adsorption of free chains and formation of thin films. *Advanced Materials* **7**, 731–735 (1995).

55. Glass, R., Möller, M., & Spatz, J.P. Block copolymer micelle nanolithography. *Nanotechnology* **14**, 1153–1160 (2003). doi:10.1088/0957-4484/14/10/314.

56. Arnold, M. et al. Induction of cell polarization and migration by a gradient of nanoscale variations in adhesive ligand spacing. *Nano Letters* **8**, 2063–2069 (2008). doi:10.1021/nl801483w

57. Möller, M. et al. Ordering and packing periodicity of Au-containing block copolymer micelles. *PMSE Preprints* **90**, 255–256 (2004).

58. Darhuber, A.A., Troian, S.M., Miller, S.M., & Wagner, S. Morphology of liquid microstructures on chemically patterned surfaces. *Journal of Applied Physics* **87**, 7768–7775 (2000).

59. Lohmüller, T., Bock, E., & Spatz, J.P. Synthesis of quasi-hexagonal ordered arrays of metallic nanoparticles with tuneable particle size. *Advanced Materials* **20**, 2297–2302 (2008).

60. Blümmel, J. et al. Protein repellent properties of covalently attached PEG coatings on nanostructured SiO(2)-based interfaces. *Biomaterials* **28**, 4739–4747 (2007).

61. Aydin, D. et al. Polymeric substrates with tunable elasticity and nanoscopically controlled biomolecule presentation. *Langmuir: The ACS Journal of Surfaces and Colloids*, **26**(19), 15472–15480 (2010). doi:10.1021/la103065x

62. Gräter, S.V. et al. Mimicking cellular environments by nanostructured soft interfaces. *Nano Letters* **7**, 1413–1418 (2007).

63. Arnold, M. et al. Activation of integrin function by nanopatterned adhesive interfaces. *ChemPhysChem* **5**, 383–388 (2004).

64. Aydin, D. et al. Micro-nanostructured protein arrays—a tool for geometrically controlled ligand presentation. *Small* **5**, 1014–1018 (2009).

65. Wolfram, T., Belz, F., Schön, T., & Spatz, J.P. Site-specific presentation of single recombinant proteins in defined nanoarrays. *Biointerphases* **2**, 44–48 (2007).

66. Glass, R. et al. Micro-nanostructured interfaces fabricated by the use of inorganic block copolymer micellar monolayers as negative resist for electron-beam lithography. *Advanced Functional Materials* **13**, 569–575 (2003).

67. Glass, R. et al. Block copolymer micelle nanolithography on non-conductive substrates. *New Journal of Physics* **6**, 1–17 (2004).

68. Gorzolnik, B., Mela, P., & Möller, M. Nano-structured micropatterns by combination of block copolymer self-assembly and UV photolithography. *Nanotechnology* **17**, 5027–5032 (2006).

69. Mela, P. et al. Low-ion-dose FIB modification of monomicellar layers for the creation of highly ordered metal nanodot arrays. *Small* **3**, 1368–1373 (2007).

70. Yun, S.H. et al. Micropatterning of a single layer of nanoparticles by lithographical methods with diblock copolymer micelles. *Nanotechnology* **17**, 450–454 (2006).

71. Chen, J., Mela, P., Möller, M., & Lensen, M. Microcontact deprinting: a technique to pattern gold nanoparticles. *ACS Nano* **3**, 1451–1456 (2009).

72. De Gennes, P.G., Brochard-Wyart, F., & Que′re′, D. Capillarity and Wetting Phenomena: Drops, Bubbles, Pearls, Waves. *Springer Science + Business Media* (2004).

73. Darhuber, A.A., Troian, S.M., Davis, J.M., Miller, S.M., & Wagner, S. Selective dip-coating of chemically micropatterned surfaces. *Journal of Applied Physics* **88**, 5119–5126 (2000).

74. Landau, L. & Levich, B. Dragging of a liquid by a moving plate. *Acta Physicochimica USSR* **17**, 42–54 (1942).

75. Wilson, S.D.R. The drag-out problem in film coating theory. *Journal of Engineering Mathematics* **16**, 209–221 (1982).

76. Engler, A.J., Sen, S., Sweeney, H.L., & Discher, D.E. Matrix elasticity directs stem cell lineage specification. *Cell* **126**, 677–689 (2006).

77. Vogel, V. & Sheetz, M. Local force and geometry sensing regulate cell functions. *Nature Reviews. Molecular Cell Biology* **2006**, 265–275 (2004).

78. Gilmore, A.P. Anoikis. *Cell Death and Differentiation* **12**(Suppl 2), 1473–1477 (2005).

79. Discher, D.E., Janmey, P., & Wang, Y.L. Tissue cells feel and respond to the stiffness of their substrate. *Science* **310**, 1139–1143 (2005).

80. Giancotti, F.G. & Ruoslahti, E. Integrin signaling. *Science* **285**, 1028–1032 (1999).

81. Ruoslahti, E. & Pierschbacher, M.D. New perspectives in cell adhesion: RGD and integrins. *Science* **238**, 491–497 (1987).

82. Bershadsky, A., Kozlov, M., & Geiger, B. Adhesion-mediated mechanosensitivity: a time to experiment, and a time to theorize. *Current Opinion in Cell Biology* **18**, 472–481 (2006).

83. Chen, C.S. Mechanotransduction—a field pulling together? *Journal of Cell Science* **121**, 3285–3292 (2008).

84. Biggs, M.J.P., Richards, R.G., Gadegaard, N., Wilkinson, C.D.W., & Dalby, M.J. The effects of nanoscale pits on primary human osteoblast adhesion formation and cellular spreading. *Journal of Materials Science. Materials in Medicine* **18**, 399–404 (2007).

85. Brunetti, V. et al. Neurons sense nanoscale roughness with nanometer sensitivity. *Proceedings of the National Academy of Sciences of the United States of America* **107**, 6264–6269 (2010).

86. Hirschfeld-Warneken, V.C. et al. Cell adhesion and polarisation on molecularly defined spacing gradient surfaces of cyclic RGDfK peptide patches. *European Journal of Cell Biology* **87**, 743–750 (2008).

87. Meller, D., Peters, K., & Meller, K. Human cornea and sclera studied by atomic force microscopy. *Cell and Tissue Research* **288**, 111–118 (1997).

88. Ploetz, C., Zycband, E.I., & Birk, D.E. Collagen fibril assembly and deposition in the developing dermis: segmental deposition in extracellular compartments. *Journal of Structural Biology* **106**, 73–81 (1991).

89. Xiong, J.-P. et al. Crystal structure of the extracellular segment of integrin alphaV beta3 in complex with an Arg-Gly-Asp ligand. *Science* **296**, 151–155 (2002).

90. Xiong, J.P. et al. Crystal structure of the extracellular segment of integrin alphaV beta3. *Science* **294**, 339–345 (2001).

91. Hynes, R.O. Integrins: bidirectional, allosteric signaling machines. *Cell* **110**, 673–687 (2002).

92. Maheshwari, G., Brown, G., Lauffenburger, D.A., Wells, A., & Griffith, L.G. Cell adhesion and motility depend on nanoscale RGD clustering. *Journal of Cell Science* **113**, 1677–1686 (2000).

93. Danilov, Y.N. & Juliano, R.L. (Arg-Gly-Asp)n-Albumin conjugates as a model substratum for integrin-mediated cell adhesion. *Experimental Cell Research* **182**, 186–196 (1989).

94. Selhuber-Unkel, C. et al. Cell adhesion strength is controlled by intermolecular spacing of adhesion receptors. *Biophysical Journal* **98**, 543–551 (2010).

95. Walter, N., Selhuber, C., Kessler, H., & Spatz, J.P. Cellular unbinding forces of initial adhesion processes on nanopatterned surfaces probed with magnetic tweezers. *Nano Letters* **6**, 398–402 (2006).

96. Lauffenburger, D.A. & Horwitz, A.F. Cell migration: a physically integrated molecular process. *Cell* **84**, 359–369 (1996).

97. Döbereiner, H., Dubin-Thaler, B., Giannone, G., & Sheetz, M. Force sensing and generation in cell phases: analyses of complex functions. *Journal of Applied Physiology* **98**, 1542–1546 (2005).

98. Arnold, M. et al. Cell interactions with hierarchically structured nano-patterned adhesive surfaces. *Soft Matter* **5**, 72–77 (2009). http://dx.doi.org/10.1039/B815634D.

99. Guignet, E.G., Hovius, R., & Vogel, H. Reversible site-selective labeling of membrane proteins in live cells. *Nature Biotechnology* **22**, 440–444 (2004).

100. Wegner, G.J., Lee, H.J., & Corn, R.M. Characterization and optimization of peptide arrays for the study of epitope-antibody interactions using surface plasmon resonance imaging. *Analytical Chemistry* **74**, 5161–5168 (2002).

101. Eliasson, M. et al. Chimeric IgG-binding receptors engineered from staphylococcal protein A and streptococcal protein G. *The Journal of Biological Chemistry* **263**, 4323–4327 (1988).

102. Tolbert, T. & Wong, C. Intein-mediated synthesis of proteins containing carbohydrates and other molecular probes. *Journal of the American Chemical Society* **122**, 5421–5428 (2000).

103. Duckworth, B.P., Zhang, Z., Hosokawa, A., & Distefano, M.D. Selective labeling of proteins by using protein farnesyltransferase. *Chembiochem* **8**, 98–105 (2007).

104. Kho, Y. et al. A tagging-via-substrate technology for detection and proteomics of farnesylated proteins. *Proceedings of the National Academy of Sciences of the United States of America* **101**, 12479–12484 (2004).

105. Aydin, D., Hirschfeld-Warneken, V. C., Louban, I., & Spatz, J. P. Intelligent induction of active biosystem responses at interfaces. *International Journal of Materials Research*, **102**(7), 796–808. Carl Hanser Verlag (2011).

CHAPTER 9

Responsive Polymer Coatings for Smart Applications in Chromatography, Drug Delivery Systems, and Cell Sheet Engineering

ROGÉRIO P. PIRRACO, MASAYUKI YAMATO, YOSHIKATSU AKIYAMA, KENICHI NAGASE, MASAMICHI NAKAYAMA, ALEXANDRA P. MARQUES, RUI L. REIS, and TERUO OKANO

9.1 INTRODUCTION

The use of intelligent surfaces as interfaces to control the behavior of biomolecules is an increasingly popular strategy. Intelligent surfaces are surfaces that have one or more properties being controlled by external stimuli. The most common way to obtain an intelligent surface is to introduce a smart polymer onto the surface of a material. Our laboratory focuses on the use of poly(N-isopropylacrylamide) (PIPAAm) as a smart polymer for creating thermoresponsive surfaces.[1] In aqueous solutions, PIPAAm has a reversible phase transition temperature of 32°C.[1] This property allows the hydrophilic/hydrophobic character of the polymer to be controlled by changing the temperature of the surrounding medium. This can be used as an "on–off" switch for modulating the interactions between the polymer and various biomolecules. Therefore, PIPAAm has been used to produce intelligent surfaces for diverse applications. By modulating temperature, the separation of biomolecules can be controlled by using PIPAAm-modified chromatographic matrices.[2–16] The alterations of the hydrophobicity of PIPAAm provoked by temperature changes allow the affinity of PIPAAm-grafted surfaces to be modulated for separating solutes, resulting in a temperature-responsive chromatographic system. Temperature alterations also result in changes of the

Intelligent Surfaces in Biotechnology: Scientific and Engineering Concepts, Enabling Technologies, and Translation to Bio-Oriented Applications, First Edition.
Edited by H. Michelle Grandin and Marcus Textor.

PIPAAm chain conformation. This property is used to produce temperature-responsive polymeric micelles with thermoresponsive cores or coronas for drug delivery purposes.[17-27] The expansion and shrinking of the coronas can be controlled by changing temperature, and thus the capture or release of a drug can be regulated. PIPAAm-grafted cell culture substrates for producing cell sheets are, however, the most addressed subject in our laboratory.[1,28-45] These culture substrate surfaces are cell adhesive when temperature is above the phase transition temperature, also called "lower critical solution temperature (LCST)," but the substrates become nonadhesive for cells when the temperature is lower than LCST. Our concept of "cell sheet engineering" is based on this very property of thermoresponsive culture dishes. Cells can be cultured on the dishes until they are confluent and then harvested as a single contiguous cell sheet composed of cells and their intact extracellular matrix (ECM) capable of being transplanted, just by lowering the temperature below LCST. Our laboratory has successfully applied this concept to the regeneration of a variety of tissues.[46-66] The following sections of this chapter will present in more detail the applications of thermoresponsive surfaces for chromatographic purposes, for the production of drug delivery nanoparticles, and for cell sheet engineering.

9.2 TEMPERATURE-RESPONSIVE CHROMATOGRAPHY

9.2.1 Hydrophobic Chromatography

By taking advantage of the temperature-dependent hydrophilic/hydrophobic conformations of PIPAAm-grafted surfaces as described previously, temperature-responsive chromatography systems having a PIPAAm-grafted stationary phase are now being explored as a new chromatographic method. By controlling temperature, the chromatographic matrices are able to tailor the hydrophobic interaction between PIPPAm-grafted substrates and analytes, thereby leading to the modulation of captured analytes.

Kanazawa et al. prepared PIPAAm-grafted silica beads as a chromatographic stationary phase through an activated ester–amine coupling method and obtained the elution profiles of five mixed steroids using the prepared stationary phase and Milli-Q water as the mobile phase (Fig. 9.1).[6] The order of hydrophobicity of the steroids, as given by their log P values, determined their elution order. They also verified that increasing the column temperature resulted in higher retention times of the steroids. These results were attributed to the thermoresponsive hydrophilic/hydrophobic alteration of PIPAAm-grafted stationary-phase surfaces. At low temperatures, the PIPAAm-grafted silica bead surface becomes hydrophilic because the grafted polymer becomes hydrated, leading to weak hydrophobic interactions with the hydrophobic analytes. With temperatures above LCST, PIPAAm-grafted silica beads become hydrophobic because of the dehydration of grafted PIPAAm,

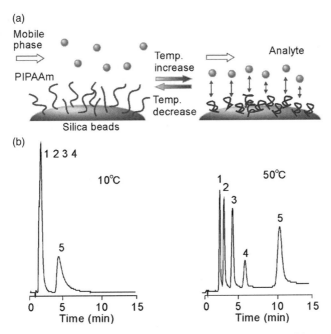

Figure 9.1 Concept of temperature-responsive chromatography: (a) hydration and dehydration of grafted poly(*N*-isopropylacrylamide) (PIPAAm) on silica beads in response to an external temperature change and (b) chromatograms of steroid analytes separated on PIPAAm-grafted silica beads. Peaks: 1, hydrocortisone; 2, prednisolone; 3, dexamethasone; 4, hydrocortisone acetate; 5, testosterone.

resulting in strong hydrophobic interactions with the analytes. This work demonstrated the feasibility of using PIPAAm-grafted surfaces as temperature-controlled stationary phases in a new chromatographic system.

A way to improve separation efficiency in these temperature-responsive chromatographic systems is through the incorporation of hydrophobic monomers into grafted PIPAAm, thereby enhancing the interaction with analytes. Kanazawa et al. grafted hydrophobized thermoresponsive copolymer, poly(IPAAm-*co*-*n*-butylmethacrylate) (BMA) onto (aminopropyl)silica beads.[3,5] The copolymer-grafted beads were then used as a column packing material. Again, the elution profile of five steroids was obtained, and, in this case, the capacity factor of analytes on the copolymer-grafted beads was observed to be larger than those on PIPAAm homopolymer-grafted beads. The amount of incorporated BMA increased the retention times of steroids proportionately. The temperature-responsive elution profiles of the analytes were, therefore, strongly affected by the hydrophobic nature of the grafted polymer chains. In the same works,[3,5] the separation of peptides, specifically insulin chains A and B, as well as β-endorphin (fragments 1–27), using the same hydrophobic copolymer-grafted silica beads, was investigated. For a

BMA content of 3.2% in the grafted copolymer, these three peptides were successfully separated at 30°C with a 0.5 mol/L NaCl aqueous mobile phase (pH 2.1). Moreover, the number of hydrophobic amino acid residues in the peptides was found to correlate with the retention times, indicating that the hydrophobic interactions between the copolymers and the analytes determined the separation efficacy. In a later work from the same authors,[4] phenylthiohydantoin (PTH)-derivatized amino acid analyses were performed using poly(IPAAm-co-BMA) hydrogel-modified silica beads as chromatographic matrices. The authors observed that the separation of amino acids was controlled by manipulating the column temperature in spite of using an isocratic aqueous mobile phase. Retention times of PTH amino acids increased beyond the copolymer transition temperature, thus reflecting their greater partitioning on the grafted copolymer due to the increased dehydration and hydrophobic aggregation of the copolymer chains.

Polymer graft conformation on bead surfaces is also important in separation efficiency. Yakushiji et al. prepared cross-linked PIPAAm hydrogel-modified silica beads as thermoresponsive chromatography matrices and observed the elution behavior of hydrophobic steroids from the prepared PIPAAm-grafted silica beads.[67] Using the prepared silica beads, the separation of hydrophobic steroids was accomplished even at low temperatures. This is a consequence of the penetration of the analytes into the PIPAAm hydrogel layer. At low temperature, the modified PIPAAm highly hydrates and expands its network, allowing steroid molecules to penetrate into the hydrogel layer.

Nagase et al. also prepared PIPAAm brush-grafted silica beads using a surface-initiated atom transfer radical polymerization (ATRP).[13] The amount of PIPAAm grafted onto the silica bead surfaces exceeded, by nearly one order of magnitude, that previously reported with polymer hydrogel-modified silica beads prepared by conventional radical polymerization. This is attributed to the densely grafted structure of PIPAAm brushes on the silica bead surface. Relatively longer retention times of steroids were observed on PIPAAm brush-grafted columns, compared with those previously reported for other PIPAAm-grafted silica beads, indicating that the densely grafted PIPAAm chains result in even stronger hydrophobic interactions with steroids by simply changing the column temperature.

9.2.2 Ion-Exchange Chromatography

Many biological substances such as peptides, nucleic acids, and proteins have both hydrophobic and ionic sites in their molecular structures. Therefore, ion-exchange chromatography is considered to be a useful separation technique for these biomolecules. However, conventional ion-exchange chromatography uses excessive amounts of salt in the mobile phase for modulating electrostatic interactions, leading to the denaturation and deactivation of biomolecules. Thus, thermoresponsive ion-exchange chromatography, of which electrostatic properties are modulated by changing temperatures, was

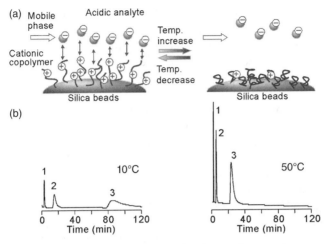

Figure 9.2   Concept of temperature-responsive ion-exchange chromatography: (a) electrostatic property alteration of grafted thermoresponsive cationic copolymer on silica beads in response to an external temperature change and (b) chromatograms of adenosine nucleotide analytes separated on thermoresponsive cationic copolymer-grafted silica beads. Peaks: 1, AMP; 2, ADP; 3, ATP.

developed using isopropylacrylamide (IPAAm) copolymers having charged groups (Fig. 9.2).

The first attempt for thermoresponsive ion-exchange chromatography was performed by using poly(IPAAm-*co*-acrylic acid) (AAc) hydrogel-modified silica beads as chromatographic matrices.[9] The elution behavior of catecholamine derivatives from poly(IPAAm-*co*-AAc)-grafted silica beads was studied as a function of changing the temperature and pH of the mobile phase. Optimal separation of these analytes was achieved at a rather high temperature of 50°C and at pH 7. This was attributed to (i) the increased hydrophobicity of the grafted copolymer and (ii) the enhanced electrostatic interaction between the copolymer and the analytes at that pH. Also, the charged copolymers exhibited a thermally modulated charge density change.[10,68] Thus, the copolymer-grafted silica beads exhibited simultaneous hydrophilic/hydrophobic and charge density alterations under thermal stimuli, leading to the modulated retention of charged biological analytes.

In other work, *N-tert*-butylacrylamide (tBAAm) was added to poly(IPAAm-*co*-AAc) copolymer for increasing the hydrophobic interactions with analytes.[11] A cross-linked poly(IPAAm-*co*-AAc-*co*-tBAAm) hydrogel was grafted to the surface of silica beads and then used as column matrices. These columns were used for the chromatographic separation of angiotensin subtypes I–III. The combined electrostatic and hydrophobic interactions had a greater effect in the retention times of these analytes. At temperatures below the copolymer transition temperature, there were both hydrophobic and electrostatic interactions between the analytes and the grafted copolymer on the silica beads. When the temperature was increased above the transition temperature, the charge densities of the copolymer were greatly diminished, resulting in decreased electrostatic interaction with the angiotensin subtypes and, consequently, reduced retention times.

The use of temperature-responsive chromatography can also be applied to the separation of acidic biological substances. A cationic copolymer, poly(IPAAm-co-N,N-dimethylaminopropylacrylamide (DMAPAAm)-co-BMA), was grafted onto silica beads as a chromatographic stationary phase.[2,7] Using this system, the regulation of the retention time of adenosine nucleotides with an aqueous mobile phase was investigated. At lower temperatures, the retention times for adenosine nucleotides were found to be larger due to the electrostatic interactions between the analyte and the positively charged grafted copolymer. With increasing temperature, the retention times of adenosine nucleotides decreased because the charge density of the grafted copolymer decreased with increasing the hydrophobicity of the vicinity of cationic amino group.[7,8,68] The same type of stationary phase was used to separate oligonucleotides and oligodeoxythymidines using mobile phases at different pH values. Using a pH-4.5 mobile phase, the retention times of oligodeoxythymidines decreased with increasing temperature. This was explained by a decrease in the electrostatic interaction between the grafted copolymer and the dissociated oligodeoxythymidines with increasing temperature. In contrast, using a pH-3.0 mobile phase, the retention times of the analytes increased with increasing temperature because oligodeoxythymidines are unable to dissociate at this pH value, and only hydrophobic interaction retained them.

As mentioned earlier, PIPAAm brush-grafted silica beads prepared by surface-initiated ATRP exhibit strong interactions with analytes.[13] Thus, thermoresponsive ionic copolymer brush silica beads were prepared by surface-initiated ATRP and were utilized as a thermoresponsive ion-exchange chromatography stationary phase. P(IPAAm-co-(dimethylamino) ethylmethacrylate) (DMAEMA) brush-grafted silica beads were prepared by using surface-initiated ATRP as thermoresponsive cationic chromatography matrices.[14] The prepared chromatography matrices exhibited longer retention times of adenosine nucleotides and oligonucleotides compared with those on thermoresponsive cationic hydrogel-modified beads. Also, poly(IPAAm-co-AAc-co-tBAAm) brush-grafted silica beads were prepared as thermoresponsive anionic chromatography matrices.[12] The prepared bead-packed column showed the chromatograms of catecholamine derivatives and angiotensin subtypes with high resolution peaks. These results were attributed to the strong electrostatic interactions between the copolymer brush surfaces and the analytes because the copolymers with ionic groups were densely grafted on silica beads surfaces. Thus, thermoresponsive ionic copolymer brush-grafted silica beads are applicable to ion-exchange chromatography and demonstrate strong, thermally modulated, and electrostatic interactions.[12,14]

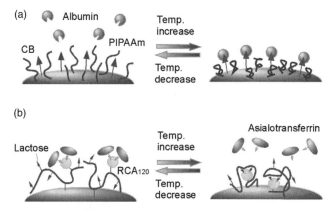

Figure 9.3 Concept of temperature-responsive affinity chromatography: (a) thermally modulated affinity between albumin and Cibacron Blue (CB) and (b) thermally modulated affinity between asialotransferrin, lactose, and RCA_{120}.

9.2.3 Affinity Chromatography

Besides hydrophilic/hydrophobic changes, PIPAAm also exhibits conformational changes with temperature. This particular characteristic was used to develop an innovative affinity chromatography system where the affinity of a target molecule was controlled by modulating temperature (Fig. 9.3).[15,16] In the first attempt of this work,[15] Cibacron Blue (CB), a molecule known to have a high affinity to albumin, was covalently immobilized onto amino-functionalized polymethacrylate bead matrices with an appropriate spacer length. The matrix surfaces were coimmobilized with end-carboxyl PIPAAm, synthesized through radical telomerization using 3-mercapto-propionic acid (MPA) as a chain transfer agent (Fig. 9.3a). At high temperature, the grafted PIPAAm was dehydrated and collapsed, and albumin tended to interact with CB, resulting in the adsorption of albumin to the stationary surface. With decreasing temperature, the grafted PIPAAm became hydrated, adopting a chain length extending beyond the immobilized CB and resulting in desorption of the adsorbed albumin. Thus, this chromatographic system allowed us to modulate the affinity between CB and albumin, demonstrating the feasibility of the thermally modulated separation of targeted biomolecules.

The temperature-induced conformational change in grafted PIPAAm was further used in another type of affinity chromatography where a ligand was able to be moved in response to external stimuli (Fig. 9.3b).[16] *Ricinus communis* agglutinin (RCA_{120}), a galactose-specific lectin, and lactose were introduced into the PIPAAm chain by sequential substitution reactions onto poly[N-(acryloyloxy)succinimide], first with isopropylamine and then with a mixture of RCA_{120} and β-lactosylamine The resulting copolymer was then attached to Sepharose beads. A glycoprotein target, asialotransferrin, was loaded onto a column packed with the copolymer immobilized beads. At 5°C, the column retained the glycoprotein target. By increasing the column temperature to 30°C, most of the asialotransferrins could be eluted. This temperature-induced elution was explained by the sugar-induced recognition of RCA_{120}. With an increase in column temperature, the grafted copolymer was dehydrated and collapsed. Coimmobilized RCA_{120} ligand and lactose hapten were brought into closer proximity to each other, resulting in the immobilized lactose displacing the affinity-bound asialotransferrin from the immobilized RCA_{120} lectin.

9.3 TEMPERATURE-RESPONSIVE POLYMER MICELLES

The use of polymeric micelles for hydrophobic drug solubilization in water and drug targeting purposes has increased since the 1990s. Polymeric micelles are nanosized entities made of amphiphilic block or graft copolymers that assemble into a core–shell architecture in aqueous media,[69,70] and the structure provides them with high structural stability.[24,27,71] Hydrophobic inner cores can incorporate a large amount of hydrophobic drug while maintaining their total water solubility due to the presence of hydrophilic outer shells.[72] The nanometric size (10–200 nm) of the polymeric micelles precludes their detection by the reticuloendothelial system, a part of the body's defense system, and assures long circulation in the bloodstream[73,74]. All these factors contribute to their successful use as drug delivery systems for solid tumors through passive targeting, taking advantage of a specific tumor feature, that is, the enhanced permeability and retention (EPR) effect. The latter effect is based on the vascular hyperpermeability and poor lymphatic drainage at solid tumor sites,[75,76] resulting in a large accumulation of macromolecules in tumor interstitium. For applied or clinically tested targeted drug carrier systems, neither target-selective drug delivery nor release has been completely controlled. Great improvements in the selectivity of these systems could be obtained if an additional targeting methodology could be added. For instance, an increased drug release rate, after accumulation at target sites, would be one way to improve the selectivity of the systems. Therefore, drug carrier systems that can efficiently deliver and release anticancer drugs at cancer sites in response to external or internal stimuli have been extensively studied.[77–85] These stimuli can be of a physiological nature, specific to the target site,[77–79,86,87] or induced artificially from the exterior, such as temperature variation, light, or ultrasound.[80–85] The use of temperature variation as stimulus presents many advantages. It is relatively noninvasive, easy to use, and already employed in medical applications. As a result, temperature-responsive micelles can present as an extremely valid option for drug carrier systems. These micelles comprise a block of a thermoresponsive polymer as one part of the core–shell structure. The most studied thermoresponsive polymer is PIPAAm since its LCST is very close to human physiological temperature. Depending on the nature of the other polymer block, two types of temperature-responsive micelles can

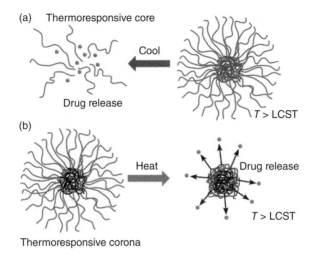

Figure 9.4   Schematic of temperature-responsive polymeric micelles either with a thermoresponsive core (a) or thermoresponsive corona (b). (See color insert.)

be designed: Either they have a temperature-responsive outer corona or a temperature-responsive inner core (Fig. 9.4).

9.3.1   Temperature-Responsive Corona

Polymeric micelles possessing a temperature-responsive corona are composed of block copolymers with a hydrophobic chain and a temperature-responsive chain. Below LCST, the micelles are formed with a hydrophobic inner core and a temperature-responsive corona. When the temperature is raised above LCST, the corona becomes hydrophobic and shrinks. With this type of behavior, it is possible to promote drug release at the desired site by local hyperthermia or focused ultrasound application.

End-functionalized PIPAAm was used to prepare block copolymers with hydrophobic polymer segments. Hydroxyl-semitelechelic PIPAAm and carboxylic-semitelechelic hydrophobic polymers were synthesized by telomerization with 2-mercaptoethanol and 3-mercapropropionic acid as telogens, respectively.[19,21] The copolymers were obtained by a coupling reaction of the hydrophobic groups of PIPAAm with the activated terminal carboxylic groups of the hydrophobic polymers. As expected, temperature modulation across LCST induced the hydration/dehydration state of the thermoresponsive coronas. When temperature was above LCST, the coronas became hydrophobic and shrunk. Turbidity measurements showed that the phase transition temperature for micelles made of poly(N-isopropylacrylamide)-b-poly(n-butyl methacrylate) (PIPAAm-b-PBMA) diblock copolymers was similar to that of an IPAAm homopolymer,[21] indicating that the cointroduction of hydrophobic poly(n-butyl methacrylate) (PBMA) was unable to influence micellar phase transition temperature in contrast to other reports.[20,25,88] In the latter works, hydrophobic groups located on freely mobile PIPAAm chain termini promoted the dehydration of proximal IPAAm units while also disturbing polymer hydration, which resulted in lowering the LCST values. No change, however, was observed in LCST, when PIPAAm was connected to the inner core-forming hydrophobic polymer segment due to a clearly defined phase separation between the micellar hydrophilic corona and the hydrophobic core.[22]

Two aspects that significantly influence the thermoresponsive behavior of polymeric micelles are the hydrophobicity and polarity of the outermost surface functionality. Well-defined diblock copolymers of thermoresponsive poly(N-isopropylacrylamide-co-N,N-dimethylacrylamide) (PID) and hydrophobic polymer segments, poly(benzyl methacrylate) (PID-b-PBzMA), possessing different temperature-responsive PID chain lengths, were synthesized by a reversible addition–fragmentation chain transfer radical (RAFT) polymerization.[25] The introduction of a comonomer, N,N-dimethylacrylamide, adjusted LCST to be around 40°C,[23] conveniently above the physiological temperature. Using these copolymers, temperature-responsive polymeric micelles were produced with coronas functionalized with phenyl or hydroxyl groups. These functional groups had a great influence on the thermoresponse of the polymeric micelles without affecting critical micelle concentration (CMC) or particle size.[25] The LCST of hydroxylated PID/PBzMA micelles (40 mol % dimethylacrylamide (DMAAm) in the PID chain) was around 40°C, unaffected by the thermoresponsive polymer molecular weight. Although the molecular weight and composition of the PID chains were equivalent in hydroxylated micelles and in micelles with coronas functionalized with phenyl groups, a shift of the phase transition temperature to lower values was verified to occur. This shows that the hydrophobic phenyl groups placed in the outermost part of the micellar corona promoted the dehydration of the temperature-responsive segments, which in turn affected the micellar solubility and aggregation state. Therefore, these data indicate that the temperature-responsive behavior of polymeric micelles can be controlled by the modulation of surface hydrophobicity.[25] Accordingly, in another work, micelles comprising mixtures of phenyl- and hydroxyl block copolymers were found to demonstrate only one sharp transition temperature at 34.4°C. This temperature lies between the LCSTs of pure phenyl-modified micelles and hydroxyl-modified micelles.[26] This means that temperature-responsive polymers under close-packed conditions produced in micelle corona are likely to be influenced significantly by the surrounding polymer chains and/or end-functional groups, inducing phase transitions cooperatively.[26] Thus, monodispersed micelles' thermoresponse can be regulated by blending well-defined diblock copolymers with temperature-responsive segments having hydrophobic and/or hydrophilic termini without any variations in CMC value or micelle size.[26]

There is no doubt that thermoresponsive micelles have a substantial potential for the development of smart drug release systems. PIPAAm micelles were

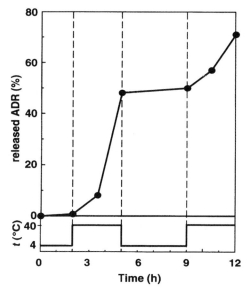

Figure 9.5   On–off switched drug release measured by UV absorbance (485 nm) from PIPAAm-*b*-PBMA micelles containing Adriamycin (ADR) responding to temperature changes.

made with two different types of hydrophobic segments, PBMA and polystyrene (PS), and were tested for the release of an anticancer drug, doxorubicin (Dox).[19,21] Micelle formation was associated with the loading of the drug by dialysis. For PIPAAm-*b*-PS micelles, there was no drug release above and below LCST. In the case of PIPAAm-*b*-PBMA micelles, the drug release was inhibited below LCST but accelerated above LCST. In fact, by applying a 4–40°C cycle to the loaded micelles, an on–off drug release response was observed by UV absorbance at 485 nm (Fig. 9.5).[19,21] This can be explained by the rigidity of the PS inner core, inhibiting a structural change of the micelles due to the thermoresponse of the corona, because their glassy transition temperature (60°C) is quite high compared to their LCST. The physicochemical properties of hydrophobic polymer segments are therefore a key aspect of the thermally modulated drug release profile.

In another work, temperature-responsive micelles comprising poly(*N*-isopropylacrylamide-*co*-*N*,*N*-dimethylacrylamide)-*b*-poly(D,L-lactide) (PID-*b*-PLA), which possess biodegradable cores and exhibit their LCST at 40°C, were designed to be used with clinical hyperthermia treatment. Dox-loaded PID-*b*-PLA micelles were put in contact with cultured endothelial cells for investigating the temperature-controlled cytotoxic activity.[23] At a physiological temperature of 37°C, which is below LCST, almost no cytotoxic effect was observed. Above LCST, at 42.5°C, the cytotoxic activity of the micelles over cultured endothelial cells was quite high, indicating that the drug release rate increased six times in comparison with micelles at 37°C.[23] Micelles (without

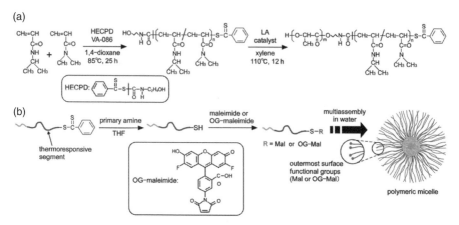

Figure 9.6 (a) Synthesis of poly(IPAAm-*co*-DMAAm)-*b*-PLA diblock copolymers. (b) Conversion of thermoresponsive polymer termini and formation of polymeric micelles. HECPD: 2-[N-(2-hydroxyethyl)-carbamoyl]prop-2-yl dithiobenzoate; THF: tetrahydrofuran; OG: Oregon Green 488; SH: sulfhydryl group. (See color insert.)

drug) are found to have no cytotoxic effect to the cells. These results show that polymeric micelles possessing temperature-responsive coronas are greatly attractive for a multitargeting tumor therapeutic system by combination with local hyperthermia.

Cellular internalization and intracellular distribution of thermoresponsive micelles were studied using fluorescently labeled PID-*b*-PLA micelles.[18] Well-defined diblock copolymers of PID blocks and PLA blocks were formed using a combination of RAFT and ring-opening polymerization. Chain terminal fluorescent probe introduction onto the PID segments was achieved by the reaction of maleimide derivatives with polymer thiol groups produced from aminolyzed terminal dithiobenzoate (Fig. 9.6). Intracellular uptake was significantly increased only at a temperature above the micelle LCST due to the enhancement of interactions between cells and micelles mediated through the thermoresponsive phase transition of micelle coronas. Moreover, the studied thermoresponsive micelles were found to have no significant cytotoxic effect.[18] Thermally induced cellular uptake systems using temperature-responsive polymeric micelles can be useful as intracellular delivery tools for anticancer drugs, genes, and peptides.

9.3.2 Temperature-Responsive Core

This type of polymeric micelle is composed of block copolymers with both temperature-responsive segments and hydrophilic segments. Below LCST, these copolymers disperse independently in water. When temperature is increased above LCST; the temperature-responsive segment becomes hydrophobic and aggregates. This leads to the formation of core–shell-type micelles possessing temperature-responsive cores. Hydrophobic drugs can be incorporated into the micellar cores above LCST and quickly released below LCST.

Poly(ethylene glycol)-*b*-PIPAAm (PEG-*b*-PIPAAm) is a commonly used block copolymer for forming polymeric micelles with thermosensitive cores. Highly hydrated poly(ethylene glycol) (PEG) chains, as hydrophilic outer corona-forming segments, stabilize the dispersions. The properties of micelles made with PEG-*b*-PIPAAm copolymers and their derivatives have been extensively studied.[80,89–93] One possible advantage of these micellar systems with a temperature-responsive core is a rapid drug release after temperature stimulus. Since below LCST the core–shell structure disappears, drug release appears without any delay by a simple diffusion process. However, if a temperature reduction is needed for drug release in clinical applications, hypothermia will be a method to be applied. This method, based on lowering the temperature, limits its application to a specific location in the human body, possibly, the surface of our body or near surface areas. One promising strategy to overcome this was presented by Neradovic and colleagues.[94,95] In their work, functionalized nanoparticles composed of PEG-*b*-poly(IPAAm-*co*-*N*-(2-hydroxypropyl) methacrylamide-dilactate) (poly(IPAAm-*co*-HPMAm-dilactate)-b-PEG) copolymers were developed. The introduction of hydrolytically sensitive poly(lactide) chains elevated LCST to 45°C after hydrolysis, resulting in a collapsed core–shell structure at normal body temperature.[95] However, the nanoparticles presented a large size of approximately 200 nm, which is a downfall for EPR-mediated drug delivery to tumor tissues. To overcome this issue, the same group developed a way to downsize the particles.[96] By a "heat shock" treatment, where a small volume of poly(IPAAm-*co*-HPMAm-dilactate)-*b*-PEG kept below its LCST was added to a large volume of heated water, polymeric micelles with the narrow size distribution of 50–70 nm were formed. The resulting micelles presented an adequate size to be applied in drug delivery applications.

Another possible advantage of micelles with a temperature-responsive core is that drugs can be incorporated just by heating aqueous copolymer solution above the temperature-responsive segment LCST. Therefore, unlike micelles with temperature-responsive coronas where dialysis is a conventional method for loading drugs, no organic solvent is needed to incorporate drugs into the micelles. On the other hand, due to the inherent temperature-responsive nature of the inner core, there is a restriction on the type and strength of possible interactions for drug incorporation. The nature of these interactions is of paramount importance since it will determine the efficiency of drug incorporation, drug release rate, and temperature response.

9.4 TEMPERATURE-RESPONSIVE CULTURE SURFACES

9.4.1 Temperature-Responsive Culture Dishes

Our laboratory first proposed the use of temperature-responsive surfaces for cell culture more than 20 years ago.[1] These dishes allow cells to be cultured and then, after reaching confluency, to harvest all the cells retaining an ECM deposited during culture as a single contiguous cell sheet by simply lowering temperature. For the original fabrication of these dishes, IPAAm monomers are dissolved in 2-propanol and then are uniformly spread over tissue culture polystyrene (TCPS) dishes.[1,18] For polymerizing and covalent grafting onto TCPS dishes, these are irradiated with an electron beam (EB). Although requiring the use of expensive equipment, EB methodology offers many advantages over other techniques for graft polymerization. The technique is able to provide a uniform covalent polymer grafting over the entire TCPS surface in only a few steps and is suitable for large-scale production. Other groups reported plasma polymerization to produce PIPAAm-grafted surfaces; however, plasma polymerization was successful for only small areas.[97] Furthermore, x-ray photoelectron spectroscopy (XPS) analysis showed that, upon cell sheet recovery, there was a greater quantity of residual proteins left on PIPAAm-TCPS dishes polymerized with plasma than that on dishes polymerized with EB irradiation.[29]

Using EB methodology, the thickness of the grafted PIPAAm layer is controlled by the concentration of the monomers and radiation energy. In fact, the thickness of the grafted polymer is critical for the adhesion behavior of cells. It was determined that for obtaining optimal cell adhesion and detachment, PIPAAm layer on a TCPS surface should have a thickness of 20 nm and a density range of 0.8–2.2 $\mu g/cm^2$ (Fig. 9.7).[28,45] It was also shown that by increasing the thickness and density of grafted PIPAAm layers, the contact angle of the surface both above and below LCST decreased, indicating that the surfaces became more hydrophobic.[28] This is related to the mobility of PIPAAm chains. For the thicker layers of grafted PIPAAm, there is a greater mobility of PIPAAm chains and, even above LCST, the hydrophobic environment in the vicinity of basal PS surface is insufficient to promote the dehydration and aggregation of the outermost chains. However, for thin or ultrathin PIPAAm layers, the mobility of the PIPAAm chains is more restricted, and the chains at the interface with the substrate, which have decreased hydration due to the hydrophobicity of PS, manage to drive the dehydration of the outermost chains.[28] This results in a slightly hydrophobic and cell-adherent surface. It thus becomes clear that controlling the thickness of grafted PIPAAm is a

(a)   (b)

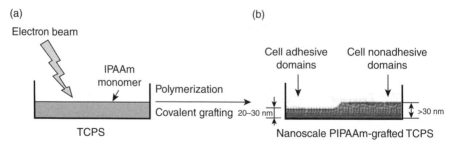

Figure 9.7 Principle of nanoscale-thick thermoresponsive surfaces for cell adhesion/deadhesion.

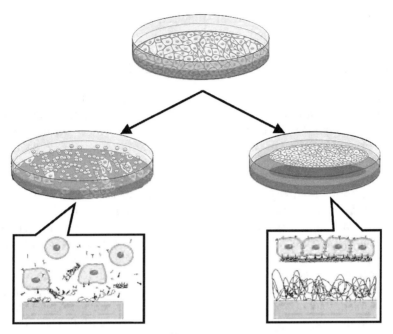

Figure 9.8 Confluent cells are subjected to two types of cell harvesting methods. The first is conventional trypsinization, in which nearly all membrane proteins, as well as deposited ECM, are digested (left). Therefore, all the cells are harvested as single cells. On the contrary, cell sheet harvesting by temperature reduction does not need proteolytic enzymes, such that all the cultured cells are harvested as a single contiguous cell sheet together with deposited ECM (right). Green materials depict deposited ECM. (See color insert.)

critical issue for obtaining the desired temperature-switchable attachment/detachment behavior of the cultured cells.

Our PIPAAm-TCPS dishes are hydrophilic below the PIPAAm LCST of 32°C resulting in cell repellency. When temperature rises above 32°C, PIPAAm chains dehydrate and collapse; cells are then able to adhere and proliferate.[28,45] Furthermore, after cell culture in these dishes, when temperature falls below LCST, attached cells detach themselves spontaneously without the use of proteolytic enzymes (Fig. 9.8). This spontaneous detachment is in fact an active detachment process since it involves ATP consumption as demonstrated using the inhibitors of ATP synthesis and tyrosine kinases.[45] Other works have focused on understanding the detachment mechanisms at the cytoskeletal and intracellular signaling levels.[98–100] From all of these works, we can conclude that intracellular signal transduction is necessary for cells to detach from temperature-responsive TCPS dishes. Moreover, cell detachment behavior from temperature-responsive TCPS dishes is profoundly cell type dependent. The nature and amount of ECM produced by cells is a critical factor for cell detachment from temperature-responsive dishes. Since different cell types produce different types of ECM, the time required for detachment varies and, in some cases, no detachment is observed.[36]

9.4.2 Temperature-Responsive Surfaces on Porous Substrates

As discussed in the previous sections, the hydration of PIPAAm-grafted surfaces is essential for cell detachment from those surfaces. It is then obvious that water supply to the temperature-responsive polymer will be a limiting factor for cell detachment speed. In conventional PIPAAm-TCPS dishes with confluent cell sheets, water only accesses grafted PIPAAm through the periphery of the dish, resulting in the limited speed of detachment. The speed of cell sheet detachment is a key factor because of its direct influence on the manipulation of the cell sheets. Quick cell sheet detachment can reduce processing time necessary to stratify multiple cell sheets. Furthermore, in a surgical setting, rapid cell sheet recovery from a dish can decrease transplantation time and increase the opportunity of a good clinical outcome. To address the issue of cell sheet detachment speed, PIPAAm-grafted porous poly(ethylene terephthalate) membranes were developed.[37] The rationale was to decrease cell sheet detachment time by allowing water to access the PIPAAm layer, not only from the periphery of the sheet but also from beneath through the pores of the membrane. Successful grafting of PIPAAm to porous membranes was verified by an electron spectroscopy and attenuated total reflection–Fourier transform infrared (FTIR). In terms of surface roughness, PIPAAm-grafted membranes were found by AFM to be smoother than ungrafted surfaces. However, the microporous structure was intact. The cell sheet detachment time on the porous membranes was found to decrease to half of that on PIPAAm-grafted TCPS dishes.[37]

This concept was further expanded in a more recent work where PEG was cografted with PIPAAm in porous membranes.[34] By introducing PEG (0.5 wt%) in grafted porous membranes, the detachment time was found to be almost half of that of the first porous membranes because PEG is a hydrophilic polymer, accelerates the hydration of PIPAAm layer, and therefore reduces the detachment time.

Temperature-responsive porous membranes were then applied to the culture of canine[38] and human[39] epithelial cells without the use of feeder layers or FBS. For allowing medium to supply the basal side of cells, the pores of the temperature-responsive membrane were found to be useful.

9.4.3 Functionalization of Temperature-Responsive Surfaces

Functionalization of temperature-responsive surfaces enables certain surface properties to be tailored in order to respond to the demands of a specific application. AAc was previously incorporated into PIPAAm, producing PIPAAm/AAc copolymers, in order to add reactive carboxylic groups to the polymer chain.[101–103] It was verified, however, that adding increased amounts of AAc to PIPAAm resulted in a shift of the LCST to values higher than 37°C,[104] and the surface was too strongly hydrated to allow cells to attach. Therefore, 2-carboxyisopropylacrylamide (CIPAAm) having both a side chain similar to IPAAm and a carboxylic group was synthesized.[105] Surfaces grafted with poly(IPAAm-*co*-CIPAAm) were found to be weakly hydrophobic, similar to PIPAAm-grafted surfaces and TCPS, and the surface allowed cells to attach.[32] When the temperature was decreased below LCST, cells cultured on poly(IPAAm-*co*-CIPAAm)-grafted surfaces detached themselves spontaneously. Furthermore, the detachment was faster than PIPAAm-only grafted surfaces. This is due to the hydrophilic nature of the carboxylic group of CIPAAm, which accelerates the hydration of the copolymer below LCST, resulting in quicker cell detachment.

Taking advantage of the carboxylic groups in the previously described copolymer, a cell adhesion peptide, Arg-Gly-Asp-Ser (RGDS), was immobilized onto poly(IPAAm-*co*-CIPAAm)-grafted TCPS dishes.[30,31] The surface allowed cells to adhere in the absence of serum when temperature was above LCST and dehydrated copolymer chains exposed the RGDS ligands (Fig. 9.9). Below LCST, cells detached themselves spontaneously. In addition to allowing the culture of cells in the absence of serum, this system further gave an on–off control for the interaction between determined cell surface proteins and their immobilized ligands, which may prove to be a very powerful tool for the study of cell–protein interactions.

This concept was further extended by combining streptavidin immobilized on temperature-responsive culture dishes with biotinylated RGDS peptides.[40] RGDS was spaced to biotin by fusion with repetitive glycine motifs with variable lengths. In fact, the length of the glycine spacers influenced cell adhesion, and 12 motifs of glycine were proven to be the preferred value for optimal

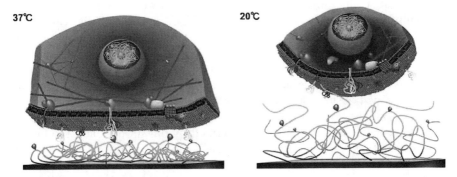

37°C   20°C

Figure 9.9   Schematic illustration of temperature-responsive affinity control between integrin receptors and RGDS ligands. At 37°C, the temperature-responsive polymer shrinks to expose RGD ligands (red beads) to the integrin receptors of cell membranes (yellow). Upon temperature reduction, the polymer swells to push cells out from the surface. (See color insert.)

cell adhesion. In these conditions, cell detachment at 20°C was improved in comparison to regular temperature-responsive dishes.

All of the described methods may become critical tools for regenerative medicine since they allow cells not only to be recovered as cell sheets without the use of trypsin but also to be cultured without the use of serum, an undesired xenogeneic factor in clinical settings.

9.4.4   Temperature-Responsive Surface Patterning

Heterotypic cell interactions are critical for the normal function of most tissues in the human body. *In vitro*, those heterotypic interactions can be recreated by the use of cocultures. Our laboratory aimed at producing patterned temperature-responsive culture surfaces for allowing heterotypic cells to coculture and to recover them as patterned cocultured cell sheets for regenerative medical applications. Surfaces patterned with grafts of both PIPAAm and cografted poly(IPAAm-*n*-butyl methacrylate) (P(IPAAm-BMA)) were prepared. The latter copolymer was previously studied as a grafting material to produce temperature-responsive dishes.[106] With this copolymer, LCST was found to be reduced. In fact, by regulating the amount of BMA added to PIPAAm, it was possible to regulate the transition temperature of the dishes. Cells adhered normally to the dishes at 37°C, and the detachment was found to be strongly dependent on the BMA content of the copolymer. Increasing amounts of BMA in the copolymer resulted in decreasing LCST. This adjustment provided strict control of the transition temperature and cell detachment through a controlled BMA amount added to the copolymer.[106] Combined grafting of BMA and PIPAAm on the same surface resulted in areas with different transition temperatures across the pattern. Metal masks were used to graft and polymerize the desired patterns by EB radiation.[43,44] Hepatocytes were seeded at 27°C and were allowed to adhere only in P(IPAAm-BMA) cografted areas since this copolymer has an LCST lower than that of PIPAAm. The culture temperature was increased to 37°C, and endothelial cells were then seeded. The cells adhered to PIPAAm-grafted areas for creating the patterned coculture of hepatocytes and endothelial cells. When the temperature was lowered to 20°C, below both polymers' LCST, a cell monolayer was harvested as a patterned cell sheet with intact heterotypic cellular interactions. Resembled work using microcontact patterning was also recently completed.[33] In this work, elastomeric polydimethylsiloxane (PDMS) stamps were prepared with a maskless technique already described by our group,[35] and the microcontact printing of fibronectin was made on temperature-responsive TCPS dishes. First, rat hepatocytes were seeded on TCPS dishes printed with fibronectin under serum-free conditions. These cells attached only on the fibronectin domains. Sequentially, endothelial cells were seeded in the presence of serum. Double fluorescent staining showed that endothelial cells successfully adhered between hepatocyte domains. Upon temperature reduction, cells were successfully recovered as a coculture cell sheet.

The techniques described earlier paved the way to produce novel tissue-engineered constructs by layering patterned coculture cell sheets in an organ-like fashion.

9.5 CELL SHEET ENGINEERING

9.5.1 Characterization of Harvested Cell Sheets

As referred in other sections, upon decreasing the temperature, depending on the type of cell, cell sheets released from PIPAAm-TCPS dishes tend to shrink or wrinkle. This impairs both their efficient therapeutic application and their correct characterization. Usually, polyvinylidene difluoride (PVDF) membranes are used as carriers to avoid shrinkage, but not all types of cell sheets adhere correctly to the membrane due to decreased cell membrane interaction. Therefore, the use of fibrin or gelatin hydrogels as carriers for stacked myoblast/endothelial cell sheet constructs was proposed.[41] Fibrin hydrogels attached very strongly to myoblast cell sheets and allowed cell sheets to be manipulated easily. However, the fibrin–cell sheet complex interferes with the microscopic evaluation of the cell sheet. Gelatin, on the other hand, can be removed after cell sheet manipulation by melting at 37°C[41]. The impact of such strategies on cell sheets' viability was tested using a LIVE/DEAD assay with 3',6'-di(O-acetyl)-4',5'-bis[N,N-bis(carboxymethyl)amino-methyl]fluorescein, tetraacetoxymethyl ester (calcein AM) and ethidium homodimer-1. No damage to the cells was found. Furthermore, the size and shape of cell sheets remained virtually unchanged before and after the manipulation, proving the feasibility of the hydrogels to serve as cell sheet construct carriers and, thus, increasing the potential analytical approaches for their characterization.

Another type of cell sheet hydrogel carrier, based on polyelectrolytes, has been proposed.[42] Polyelectrolytes are polymers that have an electrolyte group that becomes dissociated in solution and gives a charge to the polymer. We prepared a polyion complex (PIC) hydrogel by mixing poly(N,N-dimethylacrylamide-co-2-acrylamido-2-methylpropane sulfonic acid) (poly(DMAAm-co-AMPS)), an anionic water-soluble polymer, and poly(N,N-dimethylacrylamide-co-2-acryloxyethyltrimethylammonium chloride) (poly(DMAAm-co-AETA-Cl)), a cationic water-soluble polymer. By varying the composition of the two electrolytes, several PICs were prepared. EB irradiation and a set of Teflon rings were used to immobilize the PIC on porous membranes (Fig. 9.10). The resulting hydrogels were successfully used as carriers to transfer cell sheets. After cell sheet transplantation, the PIC hydrogel easily released the cell sheet by adding a warm medium. LIVE/DEAD assays showed that no significant damage was made to the cell sheets.[42] It was therefore shown that these PIC hydrogels are promising candidates to serve as cell sheet carriers.

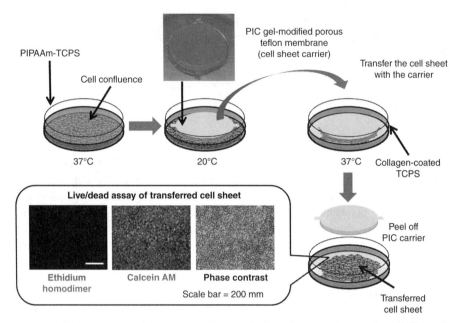

Figure 9.10 Schematic illustration of the transfer of a cell sheet using a PIC gel-modified porous Teflon membrane (cell sheet carrier). Inset shows microscopy images of a LIVE/DEAD assay of the transferred cell sheet. (See color insert.)

9.5.2 Applications in Regenerative Medicine

Many hopes have been placed in the fields of tissue engineering and regenerative medicine for solving many problems in tissue and organ regeneration. Many obstacles, however, still subsist due to current technique limitations. Promising results have been achieved by the injection of cell suspensions in damaged sites[107–114] or by the transplantation with biodegradable scaffolds.[115,116] Nevertheless, individual techniques have their own critical drawbacks. Migration of injected cells and consequent low efficiency in delivering the cells to the desired anatomic site are recurrent.[117,118] Biodegradable scaffolds with cultured cells have the limitation of oxygen and nutrient supply to the cells in the core of construct. This results in cell necrosis at the bulk of the construct.[119–121] Furthermore, foreign body response to an implanted biomaterial is a frequent reaction in the host and causes, as a consequence, the formation of fibrotic tissues surrounding the implant.[122]

The use of cell sheets in these fields, termed cell sheet engineering, avoids most of the problems previously described. Cells are recovered from temperature-sensitive dishes as a cohesive sheet where all cell–cell and cell–ECM connections are preserved.[53,54] The ECM beneath the cell sheets acts as a natural glue that enables cell sheets to be applied in virtually all anatomic sites. Furthermore, since cell sheets comprise only cells and their ECM, using autologous cells avoids an immune rejection of implanted cell sheets. Following all these advantages, our group has applied cell sheet engineering to the regeneration of various tissues as discussed next.

In the field of opthalmology, clinical trials to treat unilateral or bilateral total corneal stem cell deficiencies due to alkali burns or Stevens–Johnson syndrome were made. Using autologous limbal stem cells (for the unilateral cases)[56] or autologous oral mucosa epithelial cells (for the bilateral case),[57] patients with such diseases were successfully treated. In the bilateral cases, a 3 × 3 mm specimen of oral mucosa was taken form each patient. Epithelial cells were isolated from the specimen, seeded in temperature-responsive culture inserts, and cultured in the presence of 3T3 feeder layer on the bottom of culture wells (Fig. 9.11). After 14 days, epithelial cell sheets were recovered by decreasing the temperature to 20°C. The conjunctival and subconjunctival scar tissue from the cornea was removed up to 3 mm outside the limbus to reexpose the corneal stroma. The harvested cell sheet was placed over the corneal stroma, and no sutures were applied since the sheet strongly adhered to the tissue. Within 1 week, the complete reepithelialization of the corneal surfaces appeared in all four treated eyes. All the patients' corneal transparencies were restored and the postoperative visual acuities remarkably improved. During a mean follow-up period of 14 months, all corneal surfaces remained transparent without any complications.

For the treatment of esophageal ulcerations, we developed a method where the ESD was combined with the endoscopic transplantation of autologous oral mucosal epithelial cell sheets.[58,59] These types of ulcerations are a major postoperative burden for many patients that can result in stenosis.[58] Using our method (Fig. 9.12), we were able to treat patients who underwent esophageal endoscopic mucosal resection (EMR) or endoscopic submucosal dissection (ESD) due to esophageal carcinoma by endoscopic transplantation of autologous oral mucosal epithelial cell sheets.[59] Cells, isolated from the patient's own oral mucosa, were seeded on temperature-responsive culture inserts and were cultured with autologous serum for 2 weeks. Cell sheets were harvested by reducing the culture temperature to 20°C and were transplanted with endoscopic forceps onto the esophageal ulceration after EMR or ESD. It was verified that after cell sheet transplantation, the EMR or ESD area did not contract significantly and retained its original shape and size and that 3 weeks after the procedure, the wound was healed completely.

The application of cell sheet engineering in periodontology has also been tested using animal models.[46,47,49,51] In a recent work using beagle dogs as an animal model, periodontal ligament cell sheets were layered and, using a woven polyglycolic acid support, were transplanted to dental root surfaces having three-wall periodontal defects in an autologous manner, and bone defects were filled with porous β-tricalcium phosphate.[51] Both new bone and cementum, connecting with well-oriented collagen fibers, was found only after the cell sheet transplantation, thereby suggesting that cell sheet engineering may be very useful for periodontal regeneration in clinical settings.

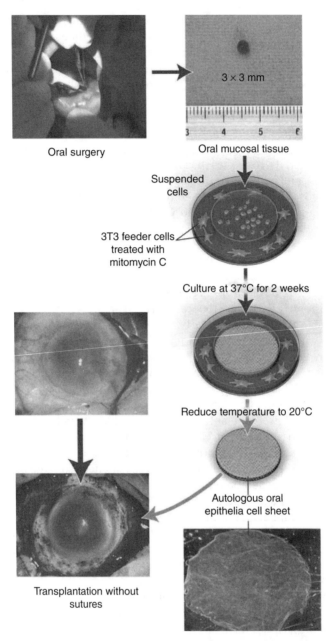

Figure 9.11 The removal of oral mucosal tissue (3 by 3 mm) from a patient's cheek. Isolated epithelial cells are seeded onto temperature-responsive cell-culture inserts. After 2 weeks at 37°C, these cells grow to form multilayered sheets of epithelial cells. The viable cell sheet is harvested, with intact cell-to-cell junctions along with the extracellular matrix, in a transplantable form simply by reducing the temperature of the culture to 20°C for 30 minutes. The cell sheet is then transplanted directly to the diseased eye without sutures. (See color insert.)

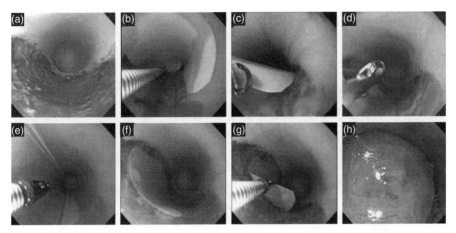

Figure 9.12 Endoscopic transplantation of autologous oral mucosal epithelial cell sheets. After endoscopic submucosal dissection, a flat esophageal ulcer is created (a). The cultured oral mucosal epithelial cell sheet, attached to a white polyvinylidene difluoride (PVDF) support membrane, is then grasped by endoscopic forceps and transferred to the dissection site (b) and gently placed on the ulcer wound bed (c). After carefully withdrawing the endoscopic forceps (d), the endoscopic mucosal resection tube is used to apply gentle pressure to the PVDF support membrane and the underlying cell sheet (e). The cell sheet along with the support membrane is then left undisturbed for 10 minutes to allow for direct attachment to the host tissues (f). The support membrane is then easily removed (g), leaving the autologous cell sheet on the ulcer wound bed (h).

Recently, our group proposed cell sheet engineering to supply a potential therapy for diabetes type I.[61] In this work, rat pancreatic islet cells were cultured on laminin 5-coated temperature-responsive culture dishes. Cell sheets were recovered and implanted subcutaneously in rats. Pancreatic cell sheets were found to remain biofunctional, producing insulin and glucagon 7 days after the transplantation. This opens a new perspective for the treatment of type I diabetes and other islet-dependent diseases.

Myocardial tissue regeneration was also vastly studied by our group using cell sheet engineering.[48,50,52,55,60,62–66,123] This is addressed in the next subsection of this chapter.

9.5.3 Thick Tissue Reconstruction

As discussed earlier in this chapter, the unique properties of temperature-responsive dishes enable the harvesting of confluent cells as sheets with their ECM. The ECM contains adhesive proteins and serves as a natural glue; in addition to facilitating cell sheet adhesion to anatomic sites, it also allows the cell sheets to adhere to other sheets upon layering. Using this principle, we

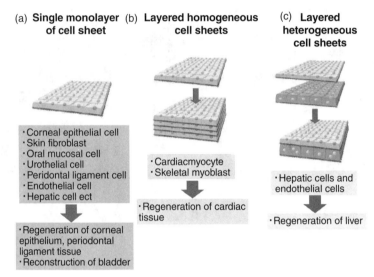

Figure 9.13 Schematic drawing of regeneration or reconstruction of tissue and organ by various cell sheet methods including (a) single-monolayer cell sheet and (b) layering of homogeneous 3-D tissue or (c) layering of heterogeneous 3-D tissue. (See color insert.)

materialized the production of three-dimensional tissues by sequentially layering cell sheets (Fig. 9.13).[63,64,66] Cell types such as mesenchymal stem cells,[123] cardiac myocytes,[60,62–65] and skeletal myoblasts[50,52,55] have been used to produce cell sheets that were tested in animal models. Layered cardiomyocyte sheets showed spontaneous beating that was synchronized between two sheets for a specific time period.[48,64] Thus, by layering these cell sheets, it was possible to fabricate a cardiac patch that could be transplanted to a defective heart. Skeletal myoblast sheet transplantation was tested in various animal models.[50,52,55] In a rat ischemic model, cardiac function and hematopoietic cell numbers were increased, while fibrosis was decreased.[55] Similarly, in a dilated cardiomyopathy hamster model, the transplantation of myoblast sheets improved cardiac function and decreased fibrosis with a consequent increase in life span.[52] Also, in a pacing-induced canine heart failure model, skeletal myoblast sheets decreased myocardial remodeling.[50] This body of results led us to commence clinical trials, which are currently ongoing, using these sheets. We hypothesized that adding endothelial cells to our established cell sheets in a coculture model could increase the efficiency of cell sheet transplantation. In this sense, we produced fibroblast cell sheets and cardiomyocyte cell sheets cocultured with endothelial progenitor cells (EPCs) and applied them in rat infarction models.[124,125] In both cases, EPC contributed to the neovascularization of the constructs that presented an increased capability to improve cardiac function. Furthermore, we proved that diffusion limitations related with engineered tissue thickness could be circumvented by polysurgery.[63] In this work, the

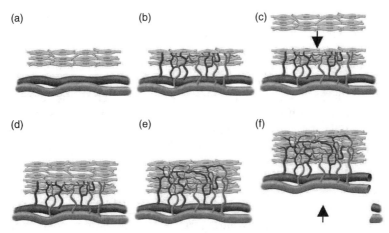

Figure 9.14 Schematic illustration of the concept used for bioengineering multilayer grafts with surgically connectable vessels. (a) First, a graft is transplanted over a surgically accessible artery and vein. (b) In this case, the graft is supplied with both new vasculature and blood directly from these existing vessels. (c,d) After sufficient vascularization has occurred, a second graft is transplanted onto the first graft. (e,f) Finally, the microvascularized construct, accompanied by graftable vessels harvested from the host, is fully perfused by host vessels and surgically resected. Ectopic transplantation of such a graft is then possible. (See color insert.)

multistep transplantation of three-layer-thick myocardial cell sheets at a rat ectopic site originated vascularized, cell-dense myocardial tissues. We were able to produce 1-mm-thick tissues, synchronously beating after the transplantation of a total of 30 cell sheets in 10 steps. These tissues were also fabricated over a surgically connectable artery and vein, which made possible their transplantation to other ectopic sites with direct vessel anastomosis (Fig. 9.14). This strategy can be applied to a variety of tissues and allows one of the biggest challenges in tissue engineering, vascularization in a construct to be materialized.

In summary, the entire body of work developed by our group regarding thick tissue reconstruction, and cardiac tissue in particular, strongly suggests that cell sheet engineering is an extremely promising, ever-evolving technology for the fields of tissue engineering and regenerative medicine.

9.6 CONCLUSIONS

We have taken advantage of the temperature-responsive properties of PIPAAm for creating innovative technologies in the fields of chromatography and drug delivery. Moreover, we recognized the specific requirements of those different applications and combined PIPAAm with specific monomers to obtain copolymers with different characteristics. With this strategy, we were able to manipulate the final polymer attributes such as hydrophobicity/hydrophilicity, conformation, polarity, and electrostatic properties, significantly boosting the range of applications of PIPAAm-based temperature-responsive polymers.

Furthermore, cell sheet engineering has been applied to the regeneration of various tissues with a high degree of success. We have proposed our technique for application in periodontology and in the treatment of esophagic ulcerations, and we are currently pursuing the transition to the clinical settings in those cases. More importantly, we have carried or are carrying phase I clinical trials for the use of cell sheets in corneal defects and in myocardial tissue regeneration.

We believe that the future advancements in this technology will transform cell sheet engineering in a revolutionary tool in the various fields described here. Further refinement of temperature-responsive chromatographic matrices will allow the establishment of this "green" technique as standard due to its reduced use of dangerous solvents. The use of temperature-responsive micelles for drug delivery is one of the most promising techniques for targeted cancer therapy, and its success will depend greatly on how efficiently hyperthermia or ultrasounds can be applied at the cancer site. Meanwhile, cell sheet engineering will be proposed for the regeneration of an increasing number of tissues, and the great challenges ahead relate to the ability to engineer complex tissue architectures as well as vascular networks for thick tissues.

REFERENCES

1. Yamada, N. et al. Thermo-responsive polymeric surfaces; control of attachment and detachment of cultured cells. *Macromolecular Chemistry Rapid Communications* **11**, 571–576 (1990).

2. Ayano, E., Sakamoto, C., Kanazawa, H., Kikuchi, A., & Okano, T. Separation of nucleotides with an aqueous mobile phase using pH- and temperature-responsive polymer modified packing materials. *Analytical Sciences* **22**, 539–543 (2006).

3. Kanazawa, H. et al. Temperature-responsive liquid chromatography. 2. Effects of hydrophobic groups in N-isopropylacrylamide copolymer-modified silica. *Analytical Chemistry* **69**, 823–830 (1997).

4. Kanazawa, H., Sunamoto, T., Matsushima, Y., Kikuchi, A., & Okano, T. Temperature-responsive chromatographic separation of amino acid phenylthiohydantoins using aqueous media as the mobile phase. *Analytical Chemistry* **72**, 5961–5966 (2000).

5. Kanazawa, H. et al. Analysis of peptides and proteins by temperature-responsive chromatographic system using N-isopropylacrylamide polymer-modified columns. *Journal of Pharmaceutical and Biomedical Analysis* **15**, 1545–1550 (1997).

6. Kanazawa, H. et al. Temperature-responsive chromatography using poly(N-isopropylacrylamide)-modified silica. *Analytical Chemistry* **68**, 100–105 (1996).

7. Kikuchi, A., Kobayashi, J., Okano, T., Iwasa, T., & Sakai, K. Temperature-modulated interaction changes with adenosine nucleotides on intelligent cationic, thermoresponsive surfaces1. *Journal of Bioactive and Compatible Polymers* **22**, 575 (2007).

8. Kikuchi, A. & Okano, T. Temperature-responsive, polymer-modified surfaces for green chromatography. *Macromolecular Symposia* **207**, 217–228 (2004).

9. Kobayashi, J., Kikuchi, A., Sakai, K., & Okano, T. Aqueous chromatography utilizing pH-/temperature-responsive polymer stationary phases to separate ionic bioactive compounds. *Analytical Chemistry* **73**, 2027–2033 (2001).

10. Kobayashi, J., Kikuchi, A., Sakai, K., & Okano, T. Aqueous chromatography utilizing hydrophobicity-modified anionic temperature-responsive hydrogel for stationary phases. *Journal of Chromatography A* **958**, 109–119 (2002).

11. Kobayashi, J., Kikuchi, A., Sakai, K., & Okano, T. Cross-linked thermoresponsive anionic polymer-grafted surfaces to separate bioactive basic peptides. *Analytical Chemistry* **75**, 3244–3249 (2003).

12. Nagase, K. et al. Preparation of thermoresponsive anionic copolymer brush surfaces for separating basic biomolecules. *Biomacromolecules* **11**, 215–223 (2010).

13. Nagase, K. et al. Interfacial property modulation of thermoresponsive polymer brush surfaces and their interaction with biomolecules. *Langmuir* **23**, 9409–9415 (2007).

14. Nagase, K. et al. Preparation of thermoresponsive cationic copolymer brush surfaces and application of the surface to separation of biomolecules. *Biomacromolecules* **9**, 1340–1347 (2008).

15. Yoshizako, K. et al. Regulation of protein binding toward a ligand on chromatographic matrixes by masking and forced-releasing effects using thermoresponsive polymer. *Analytical Chemistry* **74**, 4160–4166 (2002).

16. Yamanaka, H. et al. Affinity chromatography with collapsibly tethered ligands. *Analytical Chemistry* **75**, 1658–1663 (2003).

17. Akimoto, J., Nakayama, M., Sakai, K., & Okano, T. Molecular design of outermost surface functionalized thermoresponsive polymeric micelles with biodegradable cores. *Journal of Polymer Science, Part A, Polymer Chemistry* **46**, 7127–7137 (2008).

18. Akimoto, J., Nakayama, M., Sakai, K., & Okano, T. Temperature-induced intracellular uptake of thermoresponsive polymeric micelles. *Biomacromolecules* **10**(6), 1331–1336 (2009).

19. Chung, J.E., Yokoyama, M., & Okano, T. Inner core segment design for drug delivery control of thermo-responsive polymeric micelles. *Journal of Controlled Release* **65**, 93–103 (2000).

20. Chung, J.E. et al. Reversibly thermo-responsive alkyl-terminated poly(N-isopropylacrylamide) core-shell micellar structures. *Colloids and Surfaces. B, Biointerfaces* **9**, 37–48 (1997).

21. Chung, J.E. et al. Thermo-responsive drug delivery from polymeric micelles constructed using block copolymers of poly(N-isopropylacrylamide) and poly(butylmethacrylate). *Journal of Controlled Release* **62**, 115–127 (1999).

22. Hamaguchi, T. et al. NK105, a paclitaxel-incorporating micellar nanoparticle formulation, can extend in vivo antitumour activity and reduce the neurotoxicity of paclitaxel. *British Journal of Cancer* **92**, 1240 (2005).

23. Kohori, F. et al. Control of adriamycin cytotoxic activity using thermally responsive polymeric micelles composed of poly(N-isopropylacrylamide-co-N, N-dimethylacrylamide)-b-poly(d, l-lactide). *Colloids and Surfaces. B, Biointerfaces* **16**, 195–205 (1999).

24. Mizumura, Y. et al. Incorporation of the anticancer agent KRN5500 into polymeric micelles diminishes the pulmonary toxicity. *Cancer Science* **93**, 1237–1243 (2002).

25. Nakayama, M. & Okano, T. Polymer terminal group effects on properties of thermoresponsive polymeric micelles with controlled outer-shell chain lengths. *Biomacromolecules* **6**, 2320–2327 (2005).

26. Nakayama, M. & Okano, T. Unique thermoresponsive polymeric micelle behavior via cooperative polymer corona phase transitions. *Macromolecules* **41**, 504–507 (2008).

27. Yokoyama, M. et al. Selective delivery of adiramycin to a solid tumor using a polymeric micelle carrier system. *Journal of Drug Targeting* **7**, 171–186 (1999).

28. Akiyama, Y., Kikuchi, A., Yamato, M., & Okano, T. Ultrathin poly(N-isopropylacrylamide) grafted layer on polystyrene surfaces for cell adhesion/detachment control. *Langmuir* **20**, 5506–5511 (2004).

29. Akiyama, Y., Kushida, A., Yamato, M., Kikuchi, A., & Okano, T. Surface characterization of poly(N-isopropylacrylamide) grafted tissue culture polystyrene by electron beam irradiation, using atomic force microscopy, and X-ray photoelectron spectroscopy. *Journal of Nanoscience and Nanotechnology* **7**, 796–802 (2007).

30. Ebara, M. et al. Temperature-responsive cell culture surfaces enable "on-off" affinity control between cell integrins and RGDS ligands. *Biomacromolecules* **5**, 505–510 (2004).

31. Ebara, M. et al. Immobilization of cell-adhesive peptides to temperature-responsive surfaces facilitates both serum-free cell adhesion and noninvasive cell harvest. *Tissue Engineering* **10**, 1125–1135 (2004).

32. Ebara, M. et al. Copolymerization of 2-carboxyisopropylacrylamide with N-isopropylacrylamide accelerates cell detachment from grafted surfaces by reducing temperature. *Biomacromolecules* **4**, 344–349 (2003).

33. Elloumi Hannachi, I. et al. Fabrication of transferable micropatterned-co-cultured cell sheets with microcontact printing. *Biomaterials* **30**, 5427–5432 (2009).

34. Hyeong Kwon, O., Kikuchi, A., Yamato, M., & Okano, T. Accelerated cell sheet recovery by co-grafting of PEG with PIPAAm onto porous cell culture membranes. *Biomaterials* **24**, 1223–1232 (2003).

35. Itoga, K., Yamato, M., Kobayashi, J., Kikuchi, A., & Okano, T. Cell micropatterning using photopolymerization with a liquid crystal device commercial projector. *Biomaterials* **25**, 2047–2053 (2004).

36. Kushida, A. et al. Temperature-responsive culture dishes allow nonenzymatic harvest of differentiated Madin-Darby canine kidney (MDCK) cell sheets. *Journal of Biomedical Materials Research* **51**, 216–223 (2000).

37. Kwon, O.H., Kikuchi, A., Yamato, M., Sakurai, Y., & Okano, T. Rapid cell sheet detachment from poly(N-isopropylacrylamide)-grafted porous cell culture membranes. *Journal of Biomedical Materials Research* **50**, 82–89 (2000).

38. Murakami, D. et al. The effect of micropores in the surface of temperature-responsive culture inserts on the fabrication of transplantable canine oral mucosal epithelial cell sheets. *Biomaterials* **27**, 5518–5523 (2006).

39. Murakami, D. et al. Fabrication of transplantable human oral mucosal epithelial cell sheets using temperature-responsive culture inserts without feeder layer cells. *Journal of Artificial Organs* **9**, 185–191 (2006).

40. Nishi, M. et al. The use of biotin–avidin binding to facilitate biomodification of thermoresponsive culture surfaces. *Biomaterials* **28**, 5471–5476 (2007).

41. Sasagawa, T. et al. Design of prevascularized three-dimensional cell-dense tissues using a cell sheet stacking manipulation technology. *Biomaterials* **31**(7), 1646–1654 (2009).

42. Tang, Z., Kikuchi, A., Akiyama, Y., & Okano, T. Novel cell sheet carriers using polyion complex gel modified membranes for tissue engineering technology for cell sheet manipulation and transplantation. *Reactive and Functional Polymers* **67**, 1388–1397 (2007).

43. Tsuda, Y., Kikuchi, A., Yamato, M., Chen, G., & Okano, T. Heterotypic cell interactions on a dually patterned surface. *Biochemical and Biophysical Research Communications* **348**, 937–944 (2006).

44. Tsuda, Y. et al. The use of patterned dual thermoresponsive surfaces for the collective recovery as co-cultured cell sheets. *Biomaterials* **26**, 1885–1893 (2005).

45. Yamato, M. et al. Signal transduction and cytoskeletal reorganization are required for cell detachment from cell culture surfaces grafted with a temperature-responsive polymer. *Journal of Biomedical Materials Research* **44**, 44–52 (1999).

46. Akizuki, T. et al. Application of periodontal ligament cell sheet for periodontal regeneration: a pilot study in beagle dogs. *Journal of Periodontal Research* **40**, 245–251 (2005).

47. Flores, M.G. et al. Cementum-periodontal ligament complex regeneration using the cell sheet technique. *Journal of Periodontal Research* **43**, 364–371 (2008).

48. Haraguchi, Y., Shimizu, T., Yamato, M., Kikuchi, A., & Okano, T. Electrical coupling of cardiomyocyte sheets occurs rapidly via functional gap junction formation. *Biomaterials* **27**, 4765–4774 (2006).

49. Hasegawa, M., Yamato, M., Kikuchi, A., Okano, T., & Ishikawa, I. Human periodontal ligament cell sheets can regenerate periodontal ligament tissue in an athymic rat model. *Tissue Engineering* **11**, 469–478 (2005).

50. Hata, H. et al. Grafted skeletal myoblast sheets attenuate myocardial remodeling in pacing-induced canine heart failure model. *The Journal of Thoracic and Cardiovascular Surgery* **132**, 918–924 (2006).

51. Iwata, T. et al. Periodontal regeneration with multi-layered periodontal ligament-derived cell sheets in a canine model. *Biomaterials* **30**, 2716–2723 (2009).

52. Kondoh, H. et al. Longer preservation of cardiac performance by sheet-shaped myoblast implantation in dilated cardiomyopathic hamsters. *Cardiovascular Research* **69**, 466 (2006).

53. Kushida, A., Yamato, M., Isoi, Y., Kikuchi, A., & Okano, T. A noninvasive transfer system for polarized renal tubule epithelial cell sheets using temperature-responsive culture dishes. *European Cells & Materials* **10**, 23–30 (2005).

54. Kushida, A. et al. Decrease in culture temperature releases monolayer endothelial cell sheets together with deposited fibronectin matrix from temperature-responsive culture surfaces. *Journal of Biomedical Materials Research* **45**, 355–362 (1999).

55. Memon, I.A. et al. Repair of impaired myocardium by means of implantation of engineered autologous myoblast sheets. *The Journal of Thoracic and Cardiovascular Surgery* **130**, 1333–1341 (2005).

56. Nishida, K. et al. Functional bioengineered corneal epithelial sheet grafts from corneal stem cells expanded ex vivo on a temperature-responsive cell culture surface. *Transplantation* **77**, 379 (2004).

57. Nishida, K. et al. Corneal reconstruction with tissue-engineered cell sheets composed of autologous oral mucosal epithelium. *New England Journal of Medicine* **351**, 1187 (2004).

58. Ohki, T. et al. Treatment of oesophageal ulcerations using endoscopic transplantation of tissue-engineered autologous oral mucosal epithelial cell sheets in a canine model. *British Medical Journal* **55**, 1704 (2006).

59. Ohki, T. et al. Endoscopic transplantation of human oral mucosal epithelial cell sheets-world's first case of regenerative medicine applied to endoscopic treatment. *Gastrointestinal Endoscopy* **69**, AB253–AB254 (2009).

60. Sekine, H., Shimizu, T., Kosaka, S., Kobayashi, E., & Okano, T. Cardiomyocyte bridging between hearts and bioengineered myocardial tissues with mesenchymal transition of mesothelial cells. *Journal of Heart and Lung Transplantation* **25**, 324–332 (2006).

61. Shimizu, H. et al. Bioengineering of a functional sheet of islet cells for the treatment of diabetes mellitus. *Biomaterials* **30**, 5943–5949 (2009).

62. Shimizu, T. et al. Long-term survival and growth of pulsatile myocardial tissue grafts engineered by the layering of cardiomyocyte sheets. *Tissue Engineering* **12**, 499–507 (2006).

63. Shimizu, T. et al. Polysurgery of cell sheet grafts overcomes diffusion limits to produce thick, vascularized myocardial tissues. *The FASEB Journal* **20**, 708–710 (2006).

64. Shimizu, T. et al. Fabrication of pulsatile cardiac tissue grafts using a novel 3-dimensional cell sheet manipulation technique and temperature-responsive cell culture surfaces. *Circulation Research* **90**, e40 (2002).

65. Shimizu, T., Yamato, M., Kikuchi, A., & Okano, T. Two-dimensional manipulation of cardiac myocyte sheets utilizing temperature-responsive culture dishes augments the pulsatile amplitude. *Tissue Engineering* **7**, 141–151 (2001).

66. Shimizu, T., Yamato, M., Kikuchi, A., & Okano, T. Cell sheet engineering for myocardial tissue reconstruction. *Biomaterials* **24**, 2309–2316 (2003).

67. Yakushiji, T. et al. Effects of cross-linked structure on temperature-responsive hydrophobic interaction of Poly(N-isopropylacrylamide) hydrogel-modified surfaces with steroids. *Analytical Chemistry* **71**, 1125–1130 (1999).

68. Feil, H., Bae, Y.H., Feijen, J., & Kim, S.W. Mutual influence of pH and temperature on the swelling of ionizable and thermosensitive hydrogels. *Macromolecules* **25**, 5528–5530 (1992).

69. Tuzar, Z. & Kratochvil, P. Block and graft copolymer micelles in solution. *Advances in Colloid and Interface Science* **6**, 201–232 (1976).

70. Wilhelm, M. et al. Poly(styrene-ethylene oxide) block copolymer micelle formation in water: a fluorescence probe study. *Macromolecules* **24**, 1033–1040 (1991).

71. Cheon Lee, S., Kim, C., Chan Kwon, I., Chung, H., & Young Jeong, S. Polymeric micelles of poly(2-ethyl-2-oxazoline)-block-poly(-caprolactone) copolymer as a carrier for paclitaxel. *Journal of Controlled Release* **89**, 437–446 (2003).

72. Lavasanifar, A., Samuel, J., & Kwon, G.S. Poly(ethylene oxide)-block-poly(L-amino acid) micelles for drug delivery. *Advanced Drug Delivery Reviews* **54**, 169–190 (2002).

73. Gref, R. et al. Biodegradable long-circulating polymeric nanospheres. *Science* **263**, 1600 (1994).

74. Peracchia, M.T. et al. PEG-coated nanospheres from amphiphilic diblock and multiblock copolymers: investigation of their drug encapsulation and release characteristics. *Journal of Controlled Release* **46**, 223–231 (1997).

75. Matsumura, Y. & Maeda, H. A new concept for macromolecular therapeutics in cancer chemotherapy: mechanism of tumoritropic accumulation of proteins and the antitumor agent smancs. *Cancer Research* **46**, 6387–6392 (1986).

76. Maeda, H., Seymour, L.W., & Miyamoto, Y. Conjugates of anticancer agents and polymers: advantages of macromolecular therapeutics in vivo. *Bioconjugate Chemistry* **3**, 351–362 (1992).

77. Na, K., Seong Lee, E., & Bae, Y.H. Adriamycin loaded pullulan acetate/sulfonamide conjugate nanoparticles responding to tumor pH: pH-dependent cell interaction, internalization and cytotoxicity in vitro. *Journal of Controlled Release* **87**, 3–13 (2003).

78. Lee, E.S., Na, K., & Bae, Y.H. Super pH-sensitive multifunctional polymeric micelle. *Nano Letters* **5**, 325–329 (2005).

79. Rae, Y. et al. Preparation and biological characterization of polymeric micelle drug carriers with intracellular pH-triggered drug release property: tumor permeability, controlled subcellular drug distribution, and enhanced in vivo antitumor efficacy. *Bioconjugate Chemistry* **16**, 122–130 (2005).

80. Topp, M.D.C., Dijkstra, P.J., Talsma, H., & Feijen, J. Thermosensitive micelle-forming block copolymers of poly(ethylene glycol) and poly(N-isopropylacrylamide). *Macromolecules* **30**, 8518–8520 (1997).

81. Cammas, S. et al. Thermo-responsive polymer nanoparticles with a core-shell micelle structure as site-specific drug carriers. *Journal of Controlled Release* **48**, 157–164 (1997).

82. Chilkoti, A., Dreher, M.R., Meyer, D.E., & Raucher, D. Targeted drug delivery by thermally responsive polymers. *Advanced Drug Delivery Reviews* **54**, 613–630 (2002).

83. Jiang, J., Tong, X., & Zhao, Y. A new design for light-breakable polymer micelles. *Journal of the American Chemical Society* **127**, 8290–8291 (2005).

84. Gao, Z.G., Fain, H.D., & Rapoport, N. Controlled and targeted tumor chemotherapy by micellar-encapsulated drug and ultrasound. *Journal of Controlled Release* **102**, 203–222 (2005).

85. Marin, A. et al. Drug delivery in pluronic micelles: effect of high-frequency ultrasound on drug release from micelles and intracellular uptake. *Journal of Controlled Release* **84**, 39–47 (2002).

86. Putnam, D. & Kopecek, J. Polymer conjugates with anticancer activity. *Advances in Polymer Science* **122**, 55–124 (1995).

87. Duncan, R., Dimitrijevic, S., & Evagorou, E.G. The role of polymer conjugates in the diagnosis and treatment of cancer. *STP Pharma Sciences* **6**, 237–263 (1996).

88. Chung, J.E., Yokoyama, M., Aoyagi, T., Sakurai, Y., & Okano, T. Effect of molecular architecture of hydrophobically modified poly(N-isopropylacrylamide) on the formation of thermoresponsive core-shell micellar drug carriers. *Journal of Controlled Release* **53**, 119–130 (1998).

89. Rao, J., Xu, J., Luo, S., & Liu, S. Cononsolvency-induced micellization of pyrene end-labeled diblock copolymers of N-isopropylacrylamide and oligo (ethylene glycol) methyl ether methacrylate. *Langmuir* **23**, 11857–11865 (2007).

90. Zhang, W. et al. Micellization of thermo-and pH-responsive triblock copolymer of poly(ethylene glycol)-b-poly(4-vinylpyridine)-b-poly(N-isopropylacrylamide). *Macromolecules* **38**, 8850–8852 (2005).

91. Maeda, Y., Taniguchi, N., & Ikeda, I. Changes in the hydration state of a block copolymer of poly(N-isopropylacrylamide) and poly(ethylene oxide) on thermo-sensitive micellization in water. *Macromolecular Rapid Communications* **22**, 1390–1393 (2001).

92. Chiang, Y., Chern, C., & Chiu, H.C. Thermally responsive interactions between the PEG and PNIPAAm grafts attached to the PAAc backbone and the corresponding structural changes of polymeric micelles in water. *Macromolecules* **38**, 23 (2005).

93. Nedelcheva, A.N., Vladimirov, N.G., Novakov, C.P., & Berlinova, I.V. Associative block copolymers comprising poly(N-isopropylacrylamide) and poly(ethylene oxide) end-functionalized with a fluorophilic or hydrophilic group. Synthesis and aqueous solution properties. *Journal of Polymer Science. Part A, Polymer Chemistry* **42**, 5736–5744 (2004).

94. Neradovic, D., Hinrichs, W.L.J., Kettenes-van den Bosch, J.J., & Hennink, W.E. Poly(N-isopropylacrylamide) with hydrolyzable lactic acid ester side groups: a new type of thermosensitive polymer. *Macromolecular Rapid Communications* **20**, 577–581 (1999).

95. Neradovic, D., Van Nostrum, C.F., & Hennink, W.E. Thermoresponsive polymeric micelles with controlled instability based on hydrolytically sensitive N-isopropylacrylamide copolymers. *Macromolecules* **34**, 7589–7591 (2001).

96. Neradovic, D., Soga, O., Van Nostrum, C.F., & Hennink, W.E. The effect of the processing and formulation parameters on the size of nanoparticles based on block copolymers of poly(ethylene glycol) and poly(N-isopropylacrylamide) with and without hydrolytically sensitive groups. *Biomaterials* **25**, 2409–2418 (2004).

97. Pan, Y.V., Wesley, R.A., Luginbuhl, R., Denton, D.D., & Ratner, B.D. Plasma polymerized N-isopropylacrylamide: synthesis and characterization of a smart thermally responsive coating. *Biomacromolecules* **2**, 32–36 (2001).

98. Harris, A.K., Wild, P., & Stopak, D. Silicone rubber substrata: a new wrinkle in the study of cell locomotion. *Science* **208**, 177 (1980).

99. Yamato, M., Adachi, E., Yamamoto, K., & Hayashi, T. Condensation of collagen fibrils to the direct vicinity of fibroblasts as a cause of gel contraction. *Journal of Biochemistry* **117**, 940 (1995).

100. Ingber, D.E., Dike, L., Sims, J., & Hansen, L. Cellular tensegrity: exploring how mechanical changes in the cytoskeleton regulate cell growth, migration and tissue pattern during morphogenesis. *Mechanical Engineering of the Cytoskeleton in Developmental Biology* **173**, 173–224 (1994).

101. Houseman, B.T. & Mrksich, M. The microenvironment of immobilized Arg-Gly-Asp peptides is an important determinant of cell adhesion. *Biomaterials* **22**, 943–955 (2001).

102. Stile, R.A., Chung, E., Burghardt, W.R., & Healy, K.E. Poly(N-isopropylacrylamide)-based semi-interpenetrating polymer networks for tissue engineering applications. Effects of linear poly(acrylic acid) chains on rheology. *Journal of Biomaterials Science, Polymer Edition* **15**, 865–878 (2004).

103. Stile, R.A. & Healy, K.E. Thermo-responsive peptide-modified hydrogels for tissue regeneration. *Biomacromolecules* **2**, 185–194 (2001).

104. Chen, G. & Hoffman, A.S. Graft copolymers that exhibit temperature-induced phase transitions over a wide range of pH. *Nature* **373**, 49–52 (1995).

105. Aoyagi, T., Ebara, M., Sakai, K., Sakurai, Y., & Okano, T. Novel bifunctional polymer with reactivity and temperature sensitivity. *Journal of Biomaterials Science, Polymer Edition* **11**, 101–110 (2000).

106. Tsuda, Y. et al. Control of cell adhesion and detachment using temperature and thermoresponsive copolymer grafted culture surfaces. *Journal of Biomedical Materials Research* **69**, 70–78 (2004).

107. Hagege, A.A. et al. Skeletal myoblast transplantation in ischemic heart failure: long-term follow-up of the first phase I cohort of patients. *Circulation* **114**, I–108–I–113 (2006).

108. Bjorklund, A. & Lindvall, O. Cell replacement therapies for central nervous system disorders. *Nature Neuroscience* **3**, 537–544 (2000).

109. Drucker-Colin, R. & Verdugo-Diaz, L. Cell transplantation for Parkinson's disease: present status. *Cellular and Molecular Neurobiology* **24**, 301–316 (2004).

110. Horslen, S.P. et al. Isolated hepatocyte transplantation in an infant with a severe urea cycle disorder. *Pediatrics* **111**, 1262 (2003).

111. Durdu, S. et al. Autologous bone-marrow mononuclear cell implantation for patients with Rutherford grade II-III thromboangiitis obliterans. *Journal of Vascular Surgery* **44**, 732–739 (2006).

112. Nanjundappa, A., Raza, J.A., Dieter, R.S., Mandapaka, S., & Cascio, W.E. Cell transplantation for treatment of left-ventricular dysfunction due to ischemic heart failure: from bench to bedside. *Expert Review of Cardiovascular Therapy* **5**, 125–131 (2007).

113. Gao, L.R. et al. Effect of intracoronary transplantation of autologous bone marrow-derived mononuclear cells on outcomes of patients with refractory chronic heart failure secondary to ischemic cardiomyopathy. *The American Journal of Cardiology* **98**, 597–602 (2006).

114. Menasché, P. et al. Autologous skeletal myoblast transplantation for severe postinfarction left ventricular dysfunction. *Journal of the American College of Cardiology* **41**, 1078–1083 (2003).

115. Atala, A., Bauer, S.B., Soker, S., Yoo, J.J., & Retik, A.B. Tissue-engineered autologous bladders for patients needing cystoplasty. *The Lancet* **367**, 1241–1246 (2006).

116. Quarto, R. et al. Repair of large bone defects with the use of autologous bone marrow stromal cells. *The New England Journal of Medicine* **344**, 385 (2001).

117. Del Priore, L.V. et al. Retinal pigment epithelial cell transplantation after subfoveal membranectomy in age-related macular degeneration clinicopathologic correlation. *American Journal of Ophthalmology* **131**, 472–480 (2001).

118. Yang, J. et al. Cell sheet engineering: recreating tissues without biodegradable scaffolds. *Biomaterials* **26**, 6415–6422 (2005).

119. Kneser, U. et al. Long-term differentiated function of heterotopically transplanted hepatocytes on three-dimensional polymer matrices. *Journal of Biomedical Materials Research* **47**, 494–503 (1999).

120. Holy, C.E., Shoichet, M.S., & Davies, J.E. Engineering three-dimensional bone tissue in vitro using biodegradable scaffolds: investigating initial cell-seeding density and culture period. *Journal of Biomedical Materials Research* **51**, 376–382 (2000).

121. Ishaug-Riley, S.L., Crane-Kruger, G.M., Yaszemski, M.J., & Mikos, A.G. Three-dimensional culture of rat calvarial osteoblasts in porous biodegradable polymers. *Biomaterials* **19**, 1405–1412 (1998).

122. Badylak, S.F. & Gilbert, T.W. Immune response to biologic scaffold materials. *Seminars in Immunology* **20**, 109–116 (2008).

123. Miyahara, Y. et al. Monolayered mesenchymal stem cells repair scarred myocardium after myocardial infarction. *Nature Medicine* **12**, 459–465 (2006).

124. Kobayashi, H. et al. Fibroblast sheets co-cultured with endothelial progenitor cells improve cardiac function of infarcted hearts. *Journal of Artificial Organs* **11**, 141–147 (2008).

125. Sekine, H. et al. Endothelial cell coculture within tissue-engineered cardiomyocyte sheets enhances neovascularization and improves cardiac function of ischemic hearts. *Circulation* **118**, S145 (2008).

Page numbers appearing in bold refer to figures and methods boxes and page numbers appearing in italic refer to tables.

Intelligent Surfaces in Biotechnology: Scientific and Engineering Concepts, Enabling Technologies, and Translation to Bio-Oriented Applications, First Edition.
Edited by H. Michelle Grandin and Marcus Textor.
© 2012 John Wiley & Sons, Inc. Published 2012 by John Wiley & Sons, Inc.

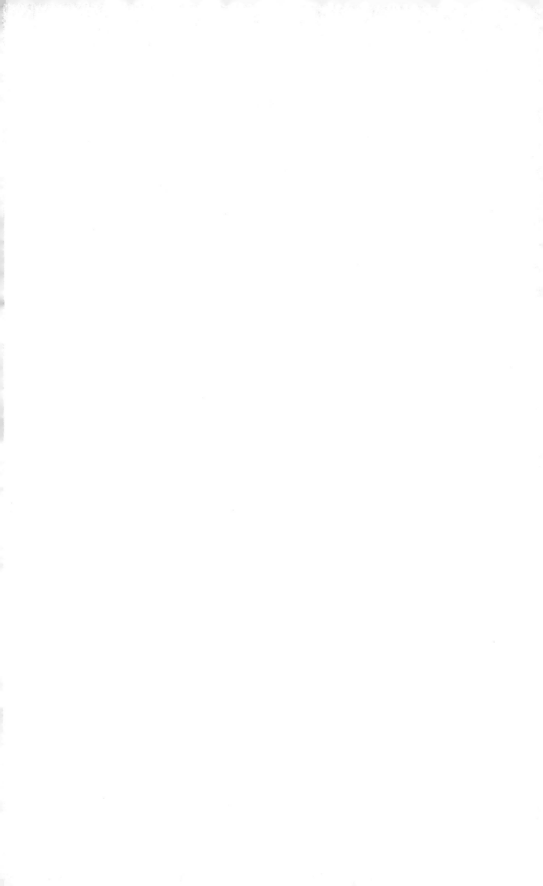